SCHWARTZ'S
PRINCIPLES OF SURGERY
ABSITE and Board Review

NOTICE

SCHWARTZ'S
PRINCIPLES OF SURGERY
ABSITE and Board Review
10th Edition

Edited by

F. Charles Brunicardi, MD, FACS
Moss Foundation Chair in Gastrointestinal and Personalized Surgery
Professor and Vice Chair Surgical Services
Chief of General Surgery, UCLA Santa Monica Medical Center
Department of Surgery
David Geffen School of Medicine at UCLA
Los Angeles, California

Associate Editors

Dana K. Andersen, MD, FACS
Program Director
Division of Digestive Diseases and Nutrition
National Institute of Diabetes and Digestive and
Kidney Diseases
National Institutes of Health
Bethesda, Maryland

Timothy R. Billiar, MD, FACS
George Vance Foster Professor and Chairman
Department of Surgery
University of Pittsburgh School of Medicine
Pittsburgh, Pennsylvania

David L. Dunn, MD, PhD, FACS
Executive Vice President for Health Affairs
Professor of Surgery, Microbiology and Immunology
University of Louisville
Louisville, Kentucky

John G. Hunter, MD, FACS
Mackenzie Professor and Chair
Department of Surgery
Oregon Health & Science University
Portland, Oregon

Jeffrey B. Matthews, MD, FACS
Surgeon-in-Chief and Chairman
Department of Surgery
Dallas B. Phemister Professor of Surgery
Chicago, Illinois

Raphael E. Pollock, MD, PhD, FACS
Professor and Director
Division of Surgical Oncology Chief of Surgical Services
The James Comprehensive Cancer Center
The Ohio State University Wexner Medical Center
Columbus, Ohio

James X. Wu, MD
General Surgery Resident
Department of Surgery
UCLA David Geffen School of Medicine
Los Angeles, California

New York   Chicago   San Francisco   Athens   London   Madrid   Mexico City
Milan   New Delhi   Singapore   Sydney   Toronto

Schwartz's Principles of Surgery: ABSITE and Board Review, 10th Edition

Previous editions copyright 2011, 2007 by The McGraw-Hill Companies, Inc.

1 2 3 4 5 6 7 8 9 0   ROV/ROV   20 19 18 17 16

ISBN 978-0-07-183891-7
MHID 0-07-183891-0

This book was set in Minion Pro by Cenveo® Publisher Services.
The editors were Brian Belval and Christie Naglieri
The production supervisor was Catherine Saggese
Project management was provided by Tanya Punj, Cenveo Publisher Services.
RR Donnelley was the printer and binder.

This book is printed on acid-free paper.

Library of Congress Cataloging-in-Publication Data

Schwartz's principles of surgery. ABSITE and board review / edited by
F. Charles Brunicardi ; associate editors, Dana K. Andersen, Timothy R. Billiar,
David L. Dunn, John G. Hunter, Raphael E. Pollock, Jeffrey B. Matthews.—Tenth edition.
        p. ; cm.
    Principles of surgery. ABSITE and board review
    Should be used in conjunction with the tenth edition of Schwartz's principles
of surgery.
    Includes index.
    ISBN 978-0-07-183891-7 (pbk., alk. paper)—ISBN 0-07-183891-0
    I. Brunicardi, F. Charles, editor.   II. Schwartz's principles of surgery. Tenth edition.
Complemented by (expression):   III. Title: Principles of surgery. ABSITE and board
review.
    [DNLM: 1. Surgical Procedures, Operative—Examination Questions.   WO 18.2]
    RD31
    617.0076—dc23
                                                                                    2015020914

International Edition. ISBN 978-1-259-25124-5; MHID 1-259-25124-1. Copyright 2016 by McGraw-Hill Education. Exclusive rights by McGraw-Hill Education for manufacture and export. This book cannot be re-exported from the country to which it is consigned by McGraw-Hill Education. The International Edition is not available in North America.

McGraw-Hill Education books are available at special quantity discounts to use as premiums and sales promotions or for use in corporate training programs. To contact a representative, please visit the Contact Us pages at www.mhprofessional.com

CONTENTS

Dana K. Andersen, MD, FACS
Program Director
Division of Digestive Diseases and Nutrition
National Institute of Diabetes and Digestive and
    Kidney Diseases
National Institutes of Health
Bethesda, Maryland

Timothy R. Billiar, MD, FACS
George Vance Foster Professor and Chairman
Department of Surgery
University of Pittsburgh School of Medicine
Pittsburgh, Pennsylvania

F. Charles Brunicardi, MD, FACS
Moss Foundation Chair in Gastrointestinal
    and Personalized Surgery
Professor and Vice Chair Surgical Services
Chief of General Surgery, UCLA Santa Monica
    Medical Center
Department of Surgery
David Geffen School of Medicine at UCLA
Los Angeles, California

Mary Condron, MD
Resident
Department of Surgery
Oregon Health & Science University
Portland, Oregon

Christopher Connelly, MD
Resident
Department of Surgery
Oregon Health & Science University
Portland, Oregon

Mackenzie Cook, MD
General Surgery Resident
Department of Surgery
Oregon Health & Science University
Portland, Oregon

David L. Dunn, MD, PhD, FACS
Executive Vice President for Health Affairs
Professor of Surgery, Microbiology and Immunology
University of Louisville
Louisville, Kentucky

John G. Hunter, MD, FACS
Mackenzie Professor and Chair
Department of Surgery
Oregon Health & Science University
Portland, Oregon

Scott Louis, MD
Surgery Resident
Oregon Health & Science University
Portland, Oregon

Jeffrey B. Matthews, MD, FACS
Surgeon-in-Chief and Chairman
Department of Surgery
Dallas B. Phemister Professor of Surgery
Chicago, Illinois

Fernando Mier, MD
Advanced GI and Bariatric Surgery Fellow
Department of General and Gastrointestinal Surgery
Oregon Health and Science University
Portland, Oregon

Alexis Moren, MD
General Surgery Resident
Oregon Health & Science University
Portland, Oregon

Raphael E. Pollock, MD, PhD, FACS
Professor and Director
Division of Surgical Oncology Chief of Surgical Services
The James Comprehensive Cancer Center
The Ohio State University Wexner Medical Center
Columbus, Ohio

Tana Lynn Repella, MD, PhD
General Surgery Resident
Department of Surgery
Oregon Health & Science University
Portland, Oregon

Julia C. Swanson, MD
Congenital Cardiac Surgery Fellow
Department of Surgery
Texas Children's Hospital
Houston, Texas

Erica Swenson, DO
General Surgery Resident
Department of Surgery
Oregon Health & Science University
Portland, Oregon

Patrick R. Varley, MD
Resident
Department of General Surgery
University of Pittsburgh Medical Center
Pittsburgh, Pennsylvania

James X. Wu, MD
General Surgery Resident
Department of Surgery
UCLA David Geffen School of Medicine
Los Angeles, California

Estin Yang, MD, MPH
Resident Physician
Department of Surgery
Oregon Health & Science University
Portland, Oregon

CONTRIBUTORS

This 10th edition of *Schwartz's Principles of Surgery: ABSITE and Board Review* marks a milestone of excellence in surgical education for the betterment of craft, quality of care, and the edification of surgical students and colleagues alike. With 842 questions spanning the 49 updated chapters of this edition, including two new chapters, Fundamental Principles of Leadership Training in Surgery and Global Surgery, this is the comprehensive companion text for reviewing and assessing the information compiled in the main book and for preparation for the American Board of Surgery In-Training Examination (ABSITE).

Contributors of the primary book have updated the questions for each chapter since the last edition in an effort to continue to provide a high level of review on the most up-to-date information and techniques currently taught and employed in the operating theater. We have maintained the proven format of providing the answer-bearing portion of the text immediately following the question and answer as an efficient method for reinforcement and recall. The user may read the question followed by the answer as a form of review, or by covering the right-hand column of the page, the user can complete the questions in a more authentic test format and uncover the answers for review/scoring.

To Brian Belval, Christie Naglieri, and all at McGraw-Hill, we are thankful for the continued belief in and support of this book. We wish to thank Katie Elsbury for her dedication to the organization and editing of this book.

F. Charles Brunicardi, MD, FACS

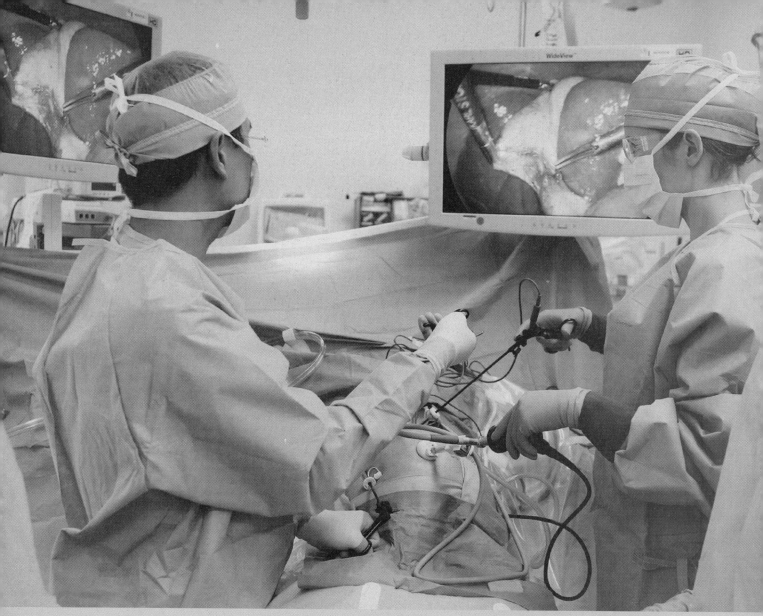

PART I

Basic Considerations

CHAPTER 1

Leadership

1. The fundamental principles of leadership are
   A. Vision and willingness
   B. Command and control
   C. Time management and mentoring
   D. Coaching, pacesetting, and democratic

   Answer: A
   Vision and willingness are the two fundamental principles of leadership. Command and control is a colloquial term for the previously predominant style of leadership in surgery based on fear and intimidation. Time management and mentorship are key leadership skills. Coaching, pacesetting, and democratic are leadership styles. (See Schwartz 10th ed., p. 3.)

2. Effective communication is a key component of leadership, given that miscommunication is a leading cause of medical errors. Which of the following statements is FALSE regarding communication?
   A. *To Err Is Human,* a publication by the US Institute of Medicine, identified medical errors as the eighth leading cause of death in the United States, causing 100,000 deaths annually.
   B. Effective communication that ensures all team members understand daily goals of care for an ICU patient can significantly decrease patient's length of stay in the ICU.
   C. Communication errors are often simply due to negligence and failure to transmit information.
   D. Information transfer and communication errors cause delays in patient care and can cause serious adverse events.
   E. Improved communication in OR among the cardiac surgery patients is associated with decreased adverse outcomes.

   Answer: C
   Communication errors are often caused by miscommunication due to hierarchical differences, concerns with upward influence, conflicting roles and role ambiguity, and interpersonal conflict. (See Schwartz 10th ed., p. 6.)

3. Daniel Goleman of the *Harvard Business Review* described six key leadership styles. Which of the following statements is FALSE regarding leadership styles?
   A. The coercive style of leadership is antiquated and is no longer effective in surgery.
   B. Democratic leadership is useful for building team consensus and minimizing conflict, but may frustrate team members if there is no clear, unifying vision.
   C. The pacesetter leads by example and sets high standards for his team, but typically takes over the tasks of something falling behind instead of building them up.
   D. The authoritative leader is often the most effective, and focuses on directing the team toward a common vision, allowing team members to give room for innovation and experimentation, and supporting their efforts.

   Answer: A
   Though it is no longer appropriate as the predominant leadership style, during times of duress when a clear, single leader is needed, a coercive leadership style may be prudent. This is most appropriate in emergency trauma settings. Excessive coercive leadership can erode team members' sense of responsibility, motivation, sense of participation in a shared vision, and ultimately, performance. (See Schwartz 10th ed., p. 9.)

4. Which is FALSE regarding modern conflict resolution techniques?
   A. Based upon objectivity and willingness to listen.
   B. Should seek a solution that benefits all involved and which is based upon core values of the organization.
   C. Traditional command-and-control technique based on fear and intimidation can lead to sanctions and lawsuits.
   D. Conflict resolution is more successful when both sides can admit they share some fault.

Answer: D

Modern conflict resolution techniques are based upon objectivity, willingness to listen, and pursuit of principle-based solutions. For example, an effective style of conflict resolution is the utilization of the "abundance mentality" model, which attempts to achieve a solution that benefits all involved and is based upon core values of the organization, as opposed to the utilization of the traditional fault-finding model, which identifies sides as right or wrong. Application of the abundance mentality in surgery elevates the conflict above the affected parties and focuses on the higher unifying goal of improved patient care. Morbidity and mortality (M&M) conferences are managed in this style and have the purpose of practice improvement and improving overall quality of care within the system, as opposed to placing guilt or blame on the surgeon or surgical trainees for the complication being reviewed. The traditional style of command-and-control technique based on fear and intimidation is no longer welcome in any health care system and can lead to sanctions, lawsuits, and removal of hospital privileges or position of leadership. (See Schwartz 10th ed., p. 7.)

Systemic Response to Injury and Metabolic Support

1. C-reactive protein (CRP)
   A. Is secreted in a circadian rhythm with higher levels in the morning
   B. Increases after eating a large meal
   C. Does not increase in response to stress in patients with liver failure
   D. Is less sensitive than erythrocyte sedimentation rate as a marker of inflammation

Answer: C
The acute phase proteins are nonspecific biochemical markers produced by hepatocytes in response to tissue injury, infection, or inflammation. Interleukin (IL)-6 is a potent inducer of acute phase proteins that can include proteinase inhibitors, coagulation and complement proteins, and transport proteins. Clinically, only C-reactive protein (CRP) has been consistently used as a marker of injury response due to its dynamic reflection of inflammation. Importantly, CRP levels do not show diurnal variations and are not affected by feeding. Only pre-existing liver failure will impair CRP production. Therefore, it has become a useful biomarker of inflammation as well as response to treatment. Its accuracy surpasses that of the erythrocyte sedimentation rate. (See Schwartz 10th ed., p.17.)

2. Which of the following is true regarding the inflammatory response following traumatic injury?
   A. There is an acute proinflammatory response caused by stimulation of the adaptive immune system.
   B. There is an anti-inflammatory response that leads to a return to homeostasis accompanied suppression of the innate immune system.
   C. The degree of inflammation is proportional to injury severity.
   D. Systemic inflammation following trauma is related to the immune response to microbes.

Answer: C
The degree of the systemic inflammatory response following trauma is proportional to injury severity and is an independent predictor of subsequent organ dysfunction and resultant mortality. Recent work has provided insight into the mechanisms by which immune activation in this setting is triggered. The clinical features of the injury-mediated systemic inflammatory response, characterized by increased body temperature, heart rate, respirations, and white blood cell count, are similar to those observed with infection. While significant efforts have been devoted to establishing a microbial etiology for this response, it is now widely accepted that systemic inflammation following trauma is sterile. (See Schwartz 10th ed., p.14.)

3. High-mobility group protein B1 (HMGB1)
   A. Is associated with the best-characterized damage-associated molecular pattern (DAMP), detectable in the circulation within 30 minutes of trauma
   B. Is a protein secreted by immune-competent cells stimulated by pathogen-associated molecular patterns (PAMPs) or inflammatory cytokines
   C. Is also secreted by endothelial cells, platelets, and also as a part of cell death
   D. All of the above

4. The most abundant amino acid in the human body is
   A. Carnitine
   B. Arginine
   C. Glutamine
   D. Methionine

5. What is the role of mitochondrial DAMPs in the injury-mediated inflammatory response?
   A. Mitochondrial DNA induces production of HMGB1.
   B. Mitochondrial DNA and peptides from damaged mitochondria activate the macrophage inflammasome.
   C. Mitochondrial DNA and peptides modulate the anti-inflammatory response that suppresses the adaptive immune system.
   D. Mitochondrial DNA is directly toxic to the liver and lung in high amounts.

6. Which is FALSE regarding the hypothalamic-pituitary-adrenal (HPA) axis and injury-associated stress?
   A. The HPA is initiated by the hypothalamus producing corticotropin-releasing hormone (CRH) in response to inflammatory cytokines.
   B. CRH acts on the anterior pituitary to stimulate adrenocorticotropin hormone (ACTH) secretion.
   C. CRH simulates the zona fasciculata of the adrenal gland to synthesize and secrete glucocorticoids.
   D. Insufficient cortisol in response to critical illness can lead to tachycardia, hypotension, weakness, hypoglycemia, hyponatremia, and hyperkalemia.

Answer: D

The best-characterized DAMP in the context of the injury-associated inflammatory response is high-mobility group protein B1 (HMGB1), which is rapidly released into the circulation within 30 minutes following trauma. Subsequent studies have proven, however, that HMGB1 is actively secreted from immune-competent cells stimulated by PAMPs (eg, endotoxin) or by inflammatory cytokines (eg, tumor necrosis factor and interleukin-1). Stressed nonimmune cells, such as endothelial cells, and platelet also actively secrete HMGB1. Finally, passive release of HMGB1 can occur following cell death, whether it is programmed or uncontrolled (necrosis). The diverse proinflammatory biological responses that result from HMGB1 signaling include: (1) the release of cytokines and chemokines from macrophage/monocytes and dendritic cells; (2) neutrophil activation and chemotaxis; (3) alterations in epithelial barrier function, including increased permeability; and (4) increased procoagulant activity on platelet surfaces; among others. (See Schwartz 10th ed., p.15.)

Answer: C

Glutamine is the most abundant amino acid in the human body, comprising nearly two-thirds of the free intracellular amino acid pool. (See Schwartz 10th ed., p. 53.)

Answer: B

Mitochondrial proteins and/or DNA can act as DAMPs by triggering an inflammatory response to necrosis and cellular stress. Specifically, the release of mitochondrial DNA (mtDNA) and formyl peptides from damaged or dysfunctional mitochondria has been implicated in activation of the macrophage inflammasome, a cytosolic signaling complex that responds to cellular stress. With stress or tissue injury, mtDNA and peptides are released from damaged mitochondria where they can contribute to a sterile inflammatory response. From an evolutionary perspective, given that eukaryotic mitochondria derive from bacterial origin, it would make sense that they retain bacterial features capable of eliciting a strong response that is typically associated with a pathogen trigger. (See Schwartz 10th ed., p. 16.)

Answer: C

CRH acts on the anterior pituitary to stimulate the secretion of adrenocorticotropin hormone (ACTH) into the systemic circulation. ACTH acts on the zona fasciculata of the adrenal glands to synthesize and secrete glucocorticoids. Cortisol is the major glucocorticoid in humans and is essential for survival during significant physiologic stress. The resulting increase in cortisol levels following trauma has several important anti-inflammatory actions. Adrenal insufficiency represents a clinical syndrome highlighted largely by inadequate amounts of circulating cortisol and aldosterone. Classically, adrenal insufficiency is described in patients with atrophic adrenal glands caused by exogenous steroid administration who undergo a stressor such as surgery. These patients subsequently manifest signs and symptoms such as tachycardia, hypotension, weakness, nausea, vomiting, and fever. (See Schwartz 10th ed., p. 20.)

7. Nutritional formulas used to treat pulmonary failure typically increase the fat intake of a patient's total caloric intake to
   A. 50%
   B. 20%
   C. 80%
   D. 10%

Answer: A

In pulmonary failure formulas, fat content is usually increased to 50% of the total calories, with a corresponding reduction in carbohydrate content. The goal is to reduce carbon dioxide production and alleviate ventilation burden for failing lungs. (See Schwartz 10th ed., p. 54.)

CHAPTER 3

Fluid and Electrolyte Management of the Surgical Patient

1. Metabolic acidosis with a normal anion gap (AG) occurs with
   A. Diabetic acidosis
   B. Renal failure
   C. Severe diarrhea
   D. Starvation

   Answer: C
   Metabolic acidosis with a normal anion gap (AG) results from either acid administration (HCl or NH_4^+) or a loss of bicarbonate from gastrointestinal (GI) losses, such as diarrhea, fistulas (enteric, pancreatic, or biliary), ureterosigmoidostomy, or from renal loss. The bicarbonate loss is accompanied by a gain of chloride, thus the AG remains unchanged. (See Schwartz 10th ed., p. 74.)

2. All are possible causes of postoperative hyponatremia EXCEPT
   A. Excess infusion of normal saline intraoperatively.
   B. Administration of antipsychotic medication.
   C. Transient decrease in antidiuretic hormone (ADH) secretion.
   D. Excess oral water intake.

   Answer: C
   Hyponatremia is caused by excess free water (dilution) or decreased sodium (depletion). Thus, excessive intake of free water (oral or IV) can lead to hyponatremia. Also, medications can cause water retention and subsequent hyponatremia, especially in older patients. Primary renal disease, diuretic use, and secretion of antidiuretic hormone (ADH) are common causes of sodium depletion. ADH can be released transiently postoperatively, or less frequently, in syndrome of inappropriate ADH secretion. Lastly, pseudohyponatremia can be seen on laboratory testing when high serum glucose, lipid, or protein levels compromise sodium measurements. (See Schwartz 10th ed., p. 69.)

3. Which of the following is an early sign of hyperkalemia?
   A. Peaked T waves
   B. Peaked P waves
   C. Peaked (shortened) QRS complex
   D. Peaked U waves

   Answer: A
   Symptoms of hyperkalemia are primarily GI, neuromuscular, and cardiovascular. GI symptoms include nausea, vomiting, intestinal colic, and diarrhea; neuromuscular symptoms range from weakness to ascending paralysis to respiratory failure; while cardiovascular manifestations range from electrocardiogram (ECG) changes to cardiac arrhythmias and arrest. ECG changes that may be seen with hyperkalemia include

   Peaked T waves (early change)
   Flattened P wave
   Prolonged PR interval (first-degree block)
   Widened QRS complex
   Sine wave formation
   Ventricular fibrillation

   (See Schwartz 10th ed., p. 71.)

4. Hypocalcemia may cause which of the following?
   A. Congestive heart failure
   B. Atrial fibrillation
   C. Pancreatitis
   D. Hypoparathyroidism

Answer: A

Mild hypocalcemia can present with muscle cramping or digital/perioral paresthesias. Severe hypocalcemia leads to decreased cardiac contractility and heart failure. ECG changes of hypocalcemia include prolonged QT interval, T-wave inversion, heart block, and ventricular fibrillation. Hypoparathyroidism and severe pancreatitis are potential causes of hypocalcemia. (See Schwartz 10th ed., p. 72.)

5. The next most appropriate test to order in a patient with a pH of 7.1, P_{CO_2} of 40, sodium of 132, potassium of 4.2, and chloride of 105 is
   A. Serum bicarbonate
   B. Serum magnesium
   C. Serum ethanol
   D. Serum salicylate

Answer: A

Metabolic acidosis results from an increased intake of acids, an increased generation of acids, or an increased loss of bicarbonate. In evaluating a patient with a low serum bicarbonate level and metabolic acidosis, first measure the AG, an index of unmeasured anions.

$$AG = [Na] - [Cl + HCO_3]$$

Metabolic acidosis with an increased AG occurs from either exogenous acid ingestion (ethylene glycol, salicylate, or methanol) or endogenous acid production of β-hydroxybutyrate and acetoacetate in ketoacidosis, lactate in lactic acidosis, or organic acids in renal insufficiency. (See Schwartz 10th ed., p. 74.)

6. Which of the following is FALSE regarding hypertonic saline?
   A. Is an arteriolar vasodilator and may increase bleeding
   B. Should be avoided in closed head injury
   C. Should not be used for initial resuscitation
   D. Increases cerebral perfusion

Answer: B

Hypertonic saline (7.5%) has been used as a treatment modality in patients with closed head injuries. It has been shown to increase cerebral perfusion and decrease intracranial pressure, thus decreasing brain edema. However, there also have been concerns of increased bleeding because hypertonic saline is an arteriolar vasodilator. (See Schwartz 10th ed., p. 76.)

7. Normal saline is
   A. 135 mEq NaCl/L
   B. 145 mEq NaCl/L
   C. 148 mEq NaCl/L
   D. 154 mEq NaCl/L

Answer: D

Sodium chloride is mildly hypertonic, containing 154 mEq of sodium that is balanced by 154 mEq of chloride. The high chloride concentration imposes a significant chloride load upon the kidneys and may lead to a hyperchloremic metabolic acidosis. It is an ideal solution, however, for correcting volume deficits associated with hyponatremia, hypochloremia, and metabolic alkalosis. (See Schwartz 10th ed., p. 76.)

8. Fluid resuscitation using albumin
   A. Is associated with coagulopathy
   B. Is available as 1% or 5% solutions
   C. Can lead to pulmonary edema
   D. Decreased factor XIII

Answer: C

Albumin is available as 5% (osmolality of 300 mOsm/L) or 25% (osmolality of 1500 mOsm/L). Due to increased intravascular oncotic pressure, fluid is drawn into the intravascular space, leading to pulmonary edema when albumin is used for resuscitation for hypovolemic shock. Hydroxyethyl starch solutions are associated with postoperative bleeding in cardiac and neurosurgery patients. (See Schwartz 10th ed., p. 77.)

9. Water constitutes what percentage of total body weight?
   A. 30–40%
   B. 40–50%
   C. 50–60%
   D. 60–70%

Answer: C

Water constitutes approximately 50 to 60% of total body weight. The relationship between total body weight and total body water (TBW) is relatively constant for an individual and is primarily a reflection of body fat. Lean tissues, such as muscle and solid organs, have higher water content than fat and bone. As a result, young, lean men have a higher proportion of body weight as water than elderly or obese individuals. An average young adult male will have 60% of his total body weight as TBW, while an average young adult female's will be 50%. The lower percentage of TBW in women correlates with a higher percentage of adipose tissue and lower percentage of muscle mass in most. Estimates of TBW should be adjusted down approximately 10 to 20% in obese individuals and up by 10% in malnourished individuals. The highest percentage of TBW is found in newborns, with approximately 80% of their total body weight composed of water. This decreases to about 65% by 1 year and thereafter remains fairly constant. (See Schwartz 10th ed., p. 65.)

10. If a patient's serum glucose increases by 180 mg/dL, what is the increase in serum osmolality, assuming all other laboratory values remain constant?
   A. Does not change
   B. 8
   C. 10
   D. 12

Answer: C

Osmotic pressure is measured in units of osmoles (osm) or milliosmoles (mOsm) that refer to the actual number of osmotically active particles. For example, 1 millimole (mmol) of sodium chloride contributes to 2 mOsm (one from sodium and one from chloride). The principal determinants of osmolality are the concentrations of sodium, glucose, and urea (blood urea nitrogen [BUN]):

Calculated serum osmolality = 2 sodium + glucose/18 + BUN/2.8

(See Schwartz 10th ed., p. 67.)

11. What is the actual potassium of a patient with pH of 7.8 and serum potassium of 2.2?
   A. 2.2
   B. 2.8
   C. 3.2
   D. 3.4

Answer: D

The change in potassium associated with alkalosis can be calculated by the following formula:

Potassium decreases by 0.3 mEq/L for every 0.1 increase in pH above normal

(See Schwartz 10th ed., p. 71.)

12. The free water deficit of a 70 kg man with serum sodium of 154 is
   A. 0.1 L
   B. 0.7 L
   C. 1 L
   D. 7 L

Answer: D

This is the formula used to estimate the amount of water required to correct hypernatremia

$$\text{Water deficit L} = \frac{\text{serum sodium} - 140}{140} \times \text{TBW}$$

Estimate TBW (total body water) as 50% of lean body mass in men and 40% in women. (See Schwartz 10th ed., p. 69.)

13. A patient with serum calcium of 6.8 and albumin of 1.2 has a corrected calcium of
   A. 7.7
   B. 8.0
   C. 8.6
   D. 9.2

Answer: D

When measuring total serum calcium levels, the albumin concentration must be taken into consideration.

Adjust total serum calcium down by 0.8 mg/dL for every 1 g/dL decrease in albumin. (See Schwartz 10th ed., p. 72.)

14. All the following treatments for hyperkalemia reduce serum potassium EXCEPT
   A. Bicarbonate
   B. Kayexalate
   C. Glucose infusion with insulin
   D. Calcium

Answer: D

When ECG changes are present, calcium chloride or calcium gluconate (5–10 mL of 10% solution) should be administered immediately to counteract the myocardial effects of hyperkalemia. Calcium infusion should be used cautiously in patients receiving digitalis, because digitalis toxicity may be precipitated. Glucose and bicarbonate shift potassium intracellularly. Kayexalate is a cation exchange resin that binds potassium, either given enterally or as an enema. (See Schwarz 10th ed., p. 77.)

15. An alcoholic patient with serum albumin of 3.9, K of 3.1, Mg of 2.4, Ca of 7.8, and PO_4 of 3.2 receives three boluses of IV potassium and has serum potassium of 3.3. You should
    A. Continue to bolus potassium until the serum level is >3.6.
    B. Give $MgSO_4$ IV.
    C. Check the ionized calcium.
    D. Check the BUN and creatinine.

Answer: B

Magnesium depletion is a common problem in hospitalized patients, particularly in the ICU. The kidney is primarily responsible for magnesium homeostasis through regulation by calcium/magnesium receptors on renal tubular cells that sense serum magnesium levels. Hypomagnesemia results from a variety of etiologies ranging from poor intake (starvation, alcoholism, prolonged use of IV fluids, and total parenteral nutrition with inadequate supplementation of magnesium), increased renal excretion (alcohol, most diuretics, and amphotericin B), GI losses (diarrhea), malabsorption, acute pancreatitis, diabetic ketoacidosis, and primary aldosteronism. Hypomagnesemia is important not only for its direct effects on the nervous system but also because it can produce hypocalcemia and lead to persistent hypokalemia. When hypokalemia or hypocalcemia coexist with hypomagnesemia, magnesium should be aggressively replaced to assist in restoring potassium or calcium homeostasis. (See Schwartz 10th ed., p. 73.)

16. Calculate the daily maintenance fluids needed for a 60-kg female
    A. 2060
    B. 2100
    C. 2160
    D. 2400

Answer: B

A 60-kg female would receive a total of 2100 mL of fluid daily: 1000 mL for the first 10 kg of body weight (10 kg × 100 mL/kg/day), 500 mL for the next 20 kg (10 kg × 50 mL/kg/day), and 80 mL for the last 40 kg (40 kg × 20 mL/kg/day). (See Schwartz 10th ed., p. 78.)

17. A patient who has spasms in the hand when a blood pressure cuff is blown up most likely has
    A. Hypercalcemia
    B. Hypocalcemia
    C. Hypermagnesemia
    D. Hypomagnesemia

Answer: B

Asymptomatic hypocalcemia may occur with hypoproteinemia (normal ionized calcium), but symptoms can develop with alkalosis (decreased ionized calcium). In general, symptoms do not occur until the ionized fraction falls below 2.5 mg/dL, and are neuromuscular and cardiac in origin, including paresthesias of the face and extremities, muscle cramps, carpopedal spasm, stridor, tetany, and seizures. Patients will demonstrate hyperreflexia and positive Chvostek sign (spasm resulting from tapping over the facial nerve) and Trousseau sign (spasm resulting from pressure applied to the nerves and vessels of the upper extremity, as when obtaining a blood pressure). Decreased cardiac contractility and heart failure can also accompany hypocalcemia. (See Schwartz 10th ed., p. 72.)

18. The actual AG of a chronic alcoholic with Na 133, K 4, Cl⁻ 101, HCO_3^- 22, albumin of 2.5 mg/dL is
    A. 6
    B. 10
    C. 14
    D. 15

Answer: D

The normal AG is <12 mmol/L and is due primarily to the albumin effect, so that the estimated AG must be adjusted for albumin (hypoalbuminemia reduces the AG).

$$\text{Corrected AG} = \text{actual AG} + [2.5(4.5 - \text{albumin})]$$

(See Schwartz 10th ed., p. 74.)

19. The effective osmotic pressure between the plasma and interstitial fluid compartments is primarily controlled by
    A. Bicarbonate
    B. Chloride ion
    C. Potassium ion
    D. Protein

Answer: D

The dissolved protein in plasma does not pass through the semipermeable cell membrane, and this fact is responsible for the effective or colloid osmotic pressure. (See Schwartz 10th ed., p. 66.)

20. The metabolic derangement most commonly seen in patients with profuse vomiting
    A. Hypochloremic, hypokalemic metabolic alkalosis
    B. Hypochloremic, hypokalemic metabolic acidosis
    C. Hypochloremic, hyperkalemic metabolic alkalosis
    D. Hypochloremic, hyperkalemic metabolic acidosis

Answer: B
Hypochloremic, hypokalemic metabolic alkalosis can occur from isolated loss of gastric contents in infants with pyloric stenosis or in adults with duodenal ulcer disease. Unlike vomiting associated with an open pylorus, which involves a loss of gastric as well as pancreatic, biliary, and intestinal secretions, vomiting with an obstructed pylorus results only in the loss of gastric fluid, which is high in chloride and hydrogen, and therefore results in a hypochloremic alkalosis. Initially the urinary bicarbonate level is high in compensation for the alkalosis. Hydrogen ion reabsorption also ensues, with an accompanied potassium ion excretion. In response to the associated volume deficit, aldosterone-mediated sodium reabsorption increases potassium excretion. The resulting hypokalemia leads to the excretion of hydrogen ions in the face of alkalosis, a paradoxic aciduria. Treatment includes replacement of the volume deficit with isotonic saline and then potassium replacement once adequate urine output is achieved. (See Schwartz 10th ed., p. 74.)

21. Symptoms and signs of extracellular fluid volume deficit include all of the following EXCEPT
    A. Anorexia
    B. Apathy
    C. Decreased body temperature
    D. High pulse pressure

Answer: D
High pulse pressure occurs with extracellular fluid volume excess, but the other symptoms and signs are characteristic of moderate extracellular volume deficit. (See Schwartz 10th ed., p. 68.)

22. A low urinary $[NH_4^+]$ with a hyperchloremic acidosis indicates what cause?
    A. Excessive vomiting
    B. Enterocutaneous fistula
    C. Chronic diarrhea
    D. Renal tubular acidosis

Answer: D
Metabolic acidosis with a normal AG results either from exogenous acid administration (HCl or NH_4^+), from loss of bicarbonate due to GI disorders such as diarrhea and fistulas or ureterosigmoidostomy, or from renal losses. In these settings, the bicarbonate loss is accompanied by a gain of chloride; thus, the AG remains unchanged. To determine if the loss of bicarbonate has a renal cause, the urinary $[NH_4^+]$ can be measured. A low urinary $[NH_4^+]$ in the face of hyperchloremic acidosis would indicate that the kidney is the site of loss, and evaluation for renal tubular acidosis should be undertaken. Proximal renal tubular acidosis results from decreased tubular reabsorption of HCO_3^-, whereas distal renal tubular acidosis results from decreased acid excretion. The carbonic anhydrase inhibitor acetazolamide also causes bicarbonate loss from the kidneys. (See Schwartz 10th ed., p. 74.)

23. When lactic acid is produced in response to injury, the body minimizes pH change by
    A. Decreasing production of sodium bicarbonate in tissues
    B. Excreting carbon dioxide through the lungs
    C. Excreting lactic acid through the kidneys
    D. Metabolizing the lactic acid in the liver

Answer: B
Lactic acid reacts with base bicarbonate to produce carbonic acid. The carbonic acid is broken down into water and carbon dioxide that is excreted by the lungs. Any diminution in pulmonary function jeopardizes this reaction. (See Schwartz 10th ed., p. 73.)

24. What is the best determinant of whether a patient has a metabolic acidosis versus alkalosis?
    A. Arterial pH
    B. Serum bicarbonate
    C. P_{CO_2}
    D. Serum CO_2 level

Answer: A
While bicarbonate, P_{CO_2}, and patient history often can suggest the most likely metabolic derangement, only the measurement of arterial pH confirms acidosis versus alkalosis. (See Schwartz 10th ed., p. 74.)

25. If a patient's arterial P_{CO_2} is found to be 25 mm Hg, the arterial pH will be approximately
    A. 7.52
    B. 7.40
    C. 7.32
    D. 7.28

Answer: D

A low Pa_{CO_2} indicates excess elimination of carbon dioxide by the lungs, and the body pH will fall. Within reasonable physiologic ranges a 15 mm Hg fall in Pa_{CO_2} should produce a 0.12 change from the normal body pH of 7.4. (See Schwartz 10th ed., p. 74.)

26. Which of the following are NOT characteristic findings of acute renal failure?
    A. BUN >100 mg/dL
    B. Hypokalemia
    C. Severe acidosis
    D. Uremic pericarditis
    E. Uremic encephalopathy

Answer: A

Hyperkalemia, severe acidosis, uremic encephalopathy, and uremic pericarditis are all indications of life-threatening problems, and urgent correction is mandatory. Elevation of BUN is commonly seen as well, but is not itself an indication for dialysis. (See Schwartz 10th ed., p. 81.)

27. An elderly diabetic patient who has acute cholecystitis is found to have a serum sodium level of 122 mEq/L and a blood glucose of 600 mg/dL. After correcting the glucose concentration to 100 mg/dL with insulin, the serum sodium concentration would
    A. Decrease significantly unless the patient also received 3% saline
    B. Decrease transiently but return to approximately 122 mEq/L without specific therapy
    C. Remain essentially unchanged
    D. Increase to the normal range without specific therapy

Answer: D

A rise in the extracellular fluid concentration of a substance that does not diffuse passively across cell membranes (eg, glucose or urea) causes an increase in effective osmotic pressure, a transfer of water from cells, and dilutional hyponatremia. For each 100 mg/dL rise in blood glucose above normal, the serum sodium level falls approximately to 3 mEq/L. Alternatively, the serum sodium level would increase by about 15 mEq/L if the blood glucose level fell from 600 to 100 mg/dL. (See Schwartz 10th ed., p. 69.)

28. Excessive administration of normal saline for fluid resuscitation can lead to what metabolic derangement?
    A. Metabolic alkalosis
    B. Metabolic acidosis
    C. Respiratory alkalosis
    D. Respiratory acidosis

Answer: B

Sodium chloride is mildly hypertonic, containing 154 mEq of sodium that is balanced by 154 mEq of chloride. The high chloride concentration imposes a significant chloride load on the kidneys and may lead to a hyperchloremic metabolic acidosis. Sodium chloride is an ideal solution, however, for correcting volume deficits associated with hyponatremia, hypochloremia, and metabolic alkalosis. (See Schwartz 10th ed., p. 74.)

29. The first step in the management of acute hypercalcemia should be
    A. Correction of deficit of extracellular fluid volume
    B. Hemodialysis.
    C. Administration of furosemide.
    D. Administration of mithramycin.

Answer: A

Patients with acute hypercalcemia usually have either acute hyperparathyroidism or metastatic breast carcinoma with multiple bony metastases. These patients develop severe headaches, bone pain, thirst, emesis, and polyuria. Unless treatment is instituted promptly, the symptoms may be rapidly fatal. Immediate correction of the associated deficit of extracellular fluid volume is the most important step in treatment. When effective, this results in the lowering of the serum calcium level by dilution. Once extracellular fluid volume has been replaced, furosemide is effective treatment. Hemodialysis may also be employed, but its effect is less rapid. Mithramycin is very useful in controlling metastatic bone disease, but its effect is slow, and it cannot be depended upon when the patient has acute hypercalcemia. (See Schwartz 10th ed., p. 72.)

30. A victim of a motor vehicle accident arrives in hemorrhagic shock. His arterial blood gases are pH, 7.25; P_{O_2}, 95 mm Hg; P_{CO_2}, 25 mm Hg; HCO_3^-, 15 mEq/L. The patient's metabolic acidosis would be treated best with
    A. Ampule of sodium bicarbonate
    B. Sodium bicarbonate infusion
    C. Lactated Ringer solution
    D. Hyperventilation

Answer: C

In patients suffering from hemorrhagic shock, the presence of a metabolic acidosis early in the postresuscitative period is indicative of tissue hypoxia due to persistent inadequate tissue perfusion. Attempts to correct this problem by administering an alkalizing agent will not solve the basic problem.

However, proper volume replacement by means of a balanced salt solution such as lactated Ringer solution will restore perfusion and correct the metabolic acidosis by ending anaerobic metabolism. (See Schwartz 10th ed., p. 79.)

31. Three days after surgery for gastric carcinoma, a 50-year-old alcoholic male exhibits delirium, muscle tremors, and hyperactive tendon reflexes. Magnesium deficiency is suspected. All of the following statements regarding this situation are true EXCEPT
    A. A decision to administer magnesium should be based on the serum magnesium level.
    B. Adequate cellular replacement of magnesium will require 1 to 3 weeks.
    C. A concomitant calcium deficiency should be suspected.
    D. Calcium is a specific antagonist of the myocardial effects of magnesium.

Answer: A
Magnesium deficiency should be suspected in any malnourished patient who exhibits disturbed neuromuscular or cerebral activity in the postoperative period. Laboratory confirmation often is not reliable, and the syndrome may exist in the presence of a normal serum magnesium level. Hypocalcemia often coexists, particularly in patients who have clinical signs of tetany. Intravenous magnesium can be administered safely to a well-hydrated patient for initial treatment of a severe deficit, but concomitant electrocardiographic monitoring is essential. The electrocardiographic changes associated with acute hypermagnesemia resemble those of hyperkalemia, and calcium chloride or gluconate should be readily available to counteract any adverse myocardial effects of excess magnesium ions. Partial or complete relief of symptoms may follow the initial infusion of magnesium, although continued replacement for a period of 1 to 3 weeks is necessary to replenish cellular stores. (See Schwartz 10th ed., p. 78.)

32. Refeeding syndrome can be associated with all of the following EXCEPT
    A. Respiratory failure
    B. Hyperkalemia
    C. Confusion
    D. Cardiac arrhythmias

Answer: B
With refeeding, a shift in metabolism from fat to carbohydrate substrate stimulates insulin release, which results in the cellular uptake of electrolytes, particularly phosphate, magnesium, potassium, and calcium. However, severe hyperglycemia may result from blunted basal insulin secretion. (See Schwartz 10th ed., p. 81.)

CHAPTER 4

Hemostasis, Surgical Bleeding, and Transfusion

1. Which of the following is NOT one of the four major physiologic events of hemostasis?
   A. Fibrinolysis
   B. Vasodilatation
   C. Platelet plug formation
   D. Fibrin production

Answer: B

Hemostasis is a complex process and its function is to limit blood loss from an injured vessel. Four major physiologic events participate in the hemostatic process: vascular constriction, platelet plug formation, fibrin formation, and fibrinolysis. Though each tend to be activated in order, the four processes are interrelated so that there is a continuum and multiple reinforcements. (See Schwartz 10th ed., p. 85.)

2. Which is required for platelet adherence to injured endothelium?
   A. Thromboxane A$_2$
   B. Glycoprotein (GP) IIb/IIIa
   C. Adenosine diphosphate (ADP)
   D. Von Willebrand factor (vWF)

Answer: D

Platelets do not normally adhere to each other or to the vessel wall but can form a plug that aids in cessation of bleeding when vascular disruption occurs. Injury to the intimal layer in the vascular wall exposes subendothelial collagen to which platelets adhere. This process requires von Willebrand factor (vWF), a protein in the subendothelium that is lacking in patients with von Willebrand disease. vWF binds to glycoprotein (GP) I/IX/V on the platelet membrane. Following adhesion, platelets initiate a release reaction that recruits other platelets from the circulating blood to seal the disrupted vessel. Up to this point, this process is known as *primary hemostasis*. Platelet aggregation is reversible and is not associated with secretion. Additionally, heparin does not interfere with this reaction and thus hemostasis can occur in the heparinized patient. Adenosine diphosphate (ADP) and serotonin are the principal mediators in platelet aggregation. (See Schwartz 10th ed., p. 85.)

3. Which of the following clotting factors is the first factor common to both intrinsic and extrinsic pathways?
   A. Factor I (fibrinogen)
   B. Factor IX (Christmas factor)
   C. Factor X (Stuart-Prower factor)
   D. Factor XI (plasma thromboplasma antecedent)

Answer: C

The intrinsic pathway begins with the activation of factor XII that subsequently activates factors XI, IX, and VII. In this pathway, each of the primary factors is "intrinsic" to the circulating plasma, whereby no surface is required to initiate the process. In the extrinsic pathway, tissue factor (TF) is released or exposed on the surface of the endothelium, binding to circulating factor VII, facilitating its activation to VIIa. Each of these pathways continues on to a common sequence that begins with the activation of factor X to Xa (in the presence of VIIIa). Subsequently, Xa (with the help of factor Va) converts factor II (prothrombin) to thrombin and then factor I (fibrinogen) to fibrin. Clot formation occurs after fibrin monomers are cross-linked to polymers with the assistance of factor XIII. (See Schwartz 10th ed., p. 87.)

4. Which congenital factor deficiency is associated with delayed bleeding after initial hemostasis?
   A. Factor VII
   B. Factor IX
   C. Factor XI
   D. Factor XIII

Answer: D

Congenital factor XIII (FXIII) deficiency, originally recognized by Duckert in 1960, is a rare autosomal recessive disease usually associated with a severe bleeding diathesis. The male-to-female ratio is 1:1. Although acquired FXIII deficiency has been described in association with hepatic failure, inflammatory bowel disease, and myeloid leukemia, the only significant association with bleeding in children is the inherited deficiency. Bleeding is typically delayed because clots form normally but are susceptible to fibrinolysis. Umbilical stump bleeding is characteristic, and there is a high risk of intracranial bleeding. Spontaneous abortion is usual in women with FXIII deficiency unless they receive replacement therapy. Replacement can be accomplished with fresh frozen plasma(FFP), cryoprecipitate, or a FXIII concentrate. Levels of 1 to 2% are usually adequate for hemostasis. (See Schwartz 10th ed., p. 89.)

5. In a previously unexposed patient, when does the platelet count fall in heparin-induced thrombocytopenia (HIT)?
   A. <24 hours
   B. 24–28 hours
   C. 3–4 days
   D. 5–7 days

Answer: D

Heparin-induced thrombocytopenia (HIT) is a form of drug-induced immune thrombocytopenia (ITP). It is an immunological event in which antibodies against platelet factor-4 (PF4) formed during exposure to heparin, affecting platelet activation and endothelial function with resultant thrombocytopenia and intravascular thrombosis. The platelet count typically begins to fall 5 to 7 days after heparin has been started, but if it is a re-exposure, the decrease in count may occur within 1 to 2 days. (See Schwartz 10th ed., p. 90.)

6. Which is NOT an acquired platelet hemostatic defect?
   A. Massive blood transfusion following trauma
   B. Acute renal failure
   C. Disseminated intravascular coagulation (DIC)
   D. Polycythemia vera

Answer: C

Impaired platelet function often accompanies thrombocytopenia but may also occur in the presence of a normal platelet count. The importance of this is obvious when one considers that 80% of overall strength is related to platelet function. The life span of platelets ranges from 7 to 10 days, placing them at increased risk for impairment by medical disorders, prescription, and over-the-counter medications. Impairment of ADP-stimulated aggregation occurs with massive transfusion of blood products. Uremia may be associated with increased bleeding time and impaired aggregation. Defective aggregation and platelet dysfunction is also seen in patients with thrombocythemia, polycythemia vera, and myelofibrosis. DIC is an acquired syndrome characterized by systemic activation of coagulation pathways that result in excessive thrombin generation and the diffuse formation of microthrombi. (See Schwartz 10th ed., p. 92.)

7. What is true about coagulopathy related to trauma?
   A. Acute coagulopathy of trauma is mechanistically similar to DIC.
   B. Coagulopathy can develop in trauma patients following acidosis, hypothermia, and dilution of coagulation factors, though coagulation is normal upon admission.
   C. Acute coagulopathy of trauma is caused by shock and tissue injury.
   D. Acute coagulopathy of trauma is mainly a dilutional coagulopathy.

Answer: C

Traditional teaching regarding trauma-related coagulopathy attributed its development to acidosis, hypothermia, and dilution of coagulation factors. Recent data, however, have shown that over one-third of injured patients has evidence of coagulopathy at the time of admission. More importantly, patients arriving with coagulopathy are at a significantly higher risk of mortality, especially in the first 24 hours after injury. Acute Coagulopathy of trauma is not a simple dilutional coagulopathy but a complex problem with multiple mechanisms. Whereas multiple contributing factors exist, the key initiators to the process of ACoT are shock and tissue injury. ACoT is a separate and distinct process from DIC with its own specific components of hemostatic failure. (See Schwartz 10th ed., p. 93.)

8. What is the best laboratory test for determine degree of anticoagulation with dabigatran and rivaroxaban?
   A. Prothrombin time/international normalized ratio (PT/INR)
   B. partial thromboplastin time (PTT)
   C. Bleeding time
   D. None of the above

Answer: D

Newer anticoagulants, such as dabigatran and rivaroxaban, have no readily available method of detection of the degree of anticoagulation. More concerning is the absence of any available reversal agent. Unlike warfarin, the nonreversible coagulopathy associated with dabigatran and rivaroxaban is of great concern to those providing emergent care to these patients. (See Schwartz 10th ed., p. 94.)

9. A fully heparinized patient develops a condition requiring emergency surgery. After stopping the heparin, what else should be done to prepare the patient?
   A. Nothing, if the surgery can be delayed for 2 to 3 hours.
   B. Immediate administration of protamine 5 mg for every 100 units of heparin most recently administered.
   C. Immediate administration of FFP.
   D. Transfusion of 10 units of platelets.

Answer: A

Certain surgical procedures should not be performed in concert with anticoagulation. In particular, cases where even minor bleeding can cause great morbidity such as the central nervous system and the eye. Emergency operations are occasionally necessary in patients who have been heparinized. The first step in these patients is to discontinue heparin. For more rapid reversal, protamine sulfate is effective. However, significant adverse reactions, especially in patients with severe fish allergies, may be encountered when administering protamine. Symptoms include hypotension, flushing, bradycardia, nausea, and vomiting. Prolongation of the activated partial thromboplastin time (aPTT) after heparin neutralization with protamine may also be a result of the anticoagulant effect of protamine. In the elective surgical patient who is receiving coumarin-derivative therapy sufficient to effect anticoagulation, the drug can be discontinued several days before operation and the prothrombin concentration then checked (level greater than 50% is considered safe). (See Schwartz 10th ed., p. 94.)

10. Primary ITP
    A. Occurs more often in children than adults, but has a similar clinical course.
    B. Includes HIT as a subtype of drug-induced ITP.
    C. Is also known as thrombotic thrombocytopenic purpura (TTP).
    D. Is a disease of impaired platelet production, unknown cause.

Answer: B

Primary immune thrombocytopenia is also known as idiopathic thrombocytopenic purpura (ITP). In children it is usually acute in onset, short-lived, and typically follows a viral illness. In contrast, ITP in adults is gradual in onset, chronic in nature, and has no identifiable cause. Because the circulating platelets in ITP are young and functional, bleeding is less for a given platelet count than when there is failure of platelet production. The pathophysiology of ITP is believed to involve both impaired platelet production and T cell-mediated platelet destruction.

Treatment of drug-induced ITP may simply entail withdrawal of the offending drug, but corticosteroids, gamma globulin, and anti-D immunoglobulin may hasten recovery of the count. HIT is a form of drug-induced ITP. It is an immunological event during which antibodies against platelet factor-4 (PF4) formed during exposure to heparin affect platelet activation and endothelial function with resultant thrombocytopenia and intravascular thrombosis. (See Schwartz 10th ed., p. 90.)

11. Which of the following is the most common intrinsic platelet defect?
    A. Thrombasthenia
    B. Bernard-Soulier syndrome
    C. Cyclooxygenase deficiency
    D. Storage pool disease

Answer: D
The most common intrinsic platelet defect is known as *storage pool disease*. It may involve loss of dense granules (storage sites for adenosine 5′-diphosphate [ADP], adenosine triphosphate [ATP], Ca^{2+}, and inorganic phosphate) and α-granules (storage sites for a large number of proteins, some of which are specific to platelets [eg, PF4 and β-thromboglobulin], while others are present in both platelet α-granules and plasma [eg, fibrinogen, vWF, and albumin]). Dense granule deficiency is the most prevalent of these. It may be an isolated defect or occur with partial albinism in the Hermansky-Pudlak syndrome. Bleeding is variable; depending on how severe the granule defect is. Bleeding is primarily caused by the decreased release of ADP from these platelets. An isolated defect of the α-granules is known as *gray platelet syndrome* because of the appearance of the platelets on Wright's stain. Bleeding is usually mild with this syndrome. A few patients have been reported who have decreased numbers of both dense and α-granules. These patients have a more severe bleeding disorder. Patients with mild bleeding as a consequence of a form of storage pool disease may have decreased bleeding if given DDAVP. It is likely that the high levels of vWF in the plasma after DDAVP somehow compensate for the intrinsic platelet defect. With more severe bleeding, platelet transfusion is required. (See Schwartz 10th ed., p. 89.)

12. Which finding is not consistent with TTP?
    A. Microangiopathic hemolytic anemia
    B. Schistocytes on peripheral blood smear
    C. Fever
    D. Splenomegaly

Answer: D
In TTP, large vWF molecules interact with platelets, leading to activation. These large molecules result from inhibition of a metalloproteinase enzyme, ADAMtS13, which cleaves the large von Willebrand factor molecules. TTP is classically characterized by thrombocytopenia, microangiopathic hemolytic anemia, fever, and renal and neurologic signs or symptoms. The finding of schistocytes on a peripheral blood smear aids in the diagnosis. Plasma exchange with replacement of FFP is the treatment for acute TTP. Additionally, rituximab, a monoclonal antibody against the CD20 protein on B lymphocytes has shown promise as an immunomodulatory therapy directed against patients with acquired TTP, of which the majority are autoimmune-mediated. (See Schwartz 10th ed., p. 91.)

13. What is FALSE regarding coagulation during cardiopulmonary bypass (CPB)?
    A. Contact with circuit tubing and membranes activates inflammatory cascades, and causes abnormal platelet and clotting factor function.
    B. Coagulopathy is compounded by sheer stress.
    C. Following bypass, platelets' morphology and ability to aggregate are irreversibly altered.
    D. Coagulopathy is compounded by hypothermia and hemodilution.

Answer: C
Under normal conditions, homeostasis of the coagulation system is maintained by complex interactions between the endothelium, platelets, and coagulation factors. In patients undergoing cardiopulmonary bypass (CPB), contact with circuit tubing and membranes results in abnormal platelet and clotting factor activation, as well as activation of inflammatory cascades, that ultimately result in excessive fibrinolysis and a combination of both quantitative and qualitative platelet defects. Platelets undergo reversible alterations in morphology and their ability to aggregate, which causes sequestration in the filter, partially degranulated platelets, and platelet fragments. This multifactorial coagulopathy is compounded by the effects of shear stress in the system, induced hypothermia, hemodilution, and anticoagulation. (See Schwartz 10th ed., p. 95.)

14. Following a recent abdominal surgery, your patient is in the ICU with septic shock. Below what level of hemoglobin would a blood transfusion be indicated?
    A. <12 g/dL
    B. <10 g/dL
    C. <8 g/dL
    D. <7 g/dL

Answer: D

A 1988 National Institutes of Health Consensus Report challenged the dictum that a hemoglobin value of less than 10 g/dL or a hematocrit level less than 30% indicates a need for preoperative red blood cell (RBC) transfusion. This was verified in a prospective randomized controlled trial in critically ill patients that compared a restrictive transfusion threshold to a more liberal strategy and demonstrated that maintaining hemoglobin levels between 7 and 9 g/dL had no adverse effect on mortality. In fact, patients with APACHE II scores of ≤20 or patients <55 years actually had a lower mortality.

Despite these results, change in daily clinical practice has been slow. Critically ill patients still frequently receive transfusions, with the pretransfusion hemoglobin approaching 9 g/dL in a recent large observational study. This outdated approach unnecessarily exposes patients to increased risk and little benefit. (See Schwartz 10th ed., p. 98.)

15. Less than 0.5% of transfusions result in a serious transfusion-related complication. What is the leading cause of transfusion-related deaths?
    A. Transfusion-related acute lung injury
    B. ABO hemolytic transfusion reactions
    C. Bacterial contamination of platelets
    D. Iatrogenic hepatitis C infection

Answer: A

Transfusion-related complications are primarily related to blood-induced proinflammatory responses. Transfusion-related events are estimated to occur in approximately 10% of all transfusions, but only less than 0.5% are serious in nature. Transfusion-related deaths, though rare, do occur and are related primarily to transfusion-related acute lung injury (TRALI) (16–22%), ABO hemolytic transfusion reactions (12–15%), and bacterial contamination of platelets (11–18%). (See Schwartz 10th ed., p. 100.)

16. Allergic reactions do not occur with
    A. Packed RBCs
    B. FFP
    C. Cryoprecipitate
    D. None of the above

Answer: D

Allergic reactions are relatively frequent, occurring in about 1% of all transfusions. Reactions are usually mild and consist of rash, urticaria, and flushing. In rare instances, anaphylactic shock develops. Allergic reactions are caused by the transfusion of antibodies from hypersensitive donors or the transfusion of antigens to which the recipient is hypersensitive. Allergic reactions can occur after the administration of any blood product but are commonly associated with FFP and platelets. Treatment and prophylaxis consists of the administration of antihistamines. In more serious cases, epinephrine or steroids may be indicated. (See Schwartz 10th ed., p. 100.)

17. What is the risk of Hepatitis C and HIV-1 transmission with blood transfusion?
    A. 1:10,000,000
    B. 1:1,000,000
    C. 1:500,000
    D. 1:100,000

Answer: B

Transmission of hepatitis C and HIV-1 has been dramatically minimized by the introduction of better antibody and nucleic acid screening for these pathogens. The residual risk among allogeneic donations is now estimated to be less than 1 per 1,000,000 donations and hepatitis B approximately 1 per 300,000 donations. (See Schwartz 10th ed., p. 102.)

18. What is NOT a cause of bleeding due to massive transfusion?
    A. Dilutional coagulopathy
    B. Hypofibrinogenemia
    C. Hypothermia
    D. 2,3-DPG toxicity

Answer: D

Massive blood transfusion is a well-known cause of thrombocytopenia. Bleeding following massive transfusion can occur due to hypothermia, dilutional coagulopathy, platelet dysfunction, fibrinolysis, or hypofibrinogenemia. Another cause of hemostatic failure related to the administration of blood is a hemolytic transfusion reaction. The first sign of a transfusion reaction may be diffuse bleeding. The pathogenesis of this bleeding is thought to be related to the release of ADP from hemolyzed RBCs, resulting in diffuse platelet aggregation, after which the platelet clumps are removed out of the circulation. (See Schwartz 10th ed., p. 104.)

19. The most common cause for a transfusion reaction is
    A. Air embolism
    B. Contaminated blood
    C. Human error
    D. Unusual circulating antibodies

Answer: C

Although contaminated or outdated blood may cause a reaction, the most common cause is human error—blood drawn for typing from the wrong patient, blood incorrectly cross-matched in the laboratory, blood units mislabeled in the laboratory, blood administered to the wrong patient. Most blood banking programs have instituted elaborate checks and balances to minimize these errors. (See Schwartz 10th ed., p. 101.)

20. Frozen plasma prepared from freshly donated blood is necessary when a patient requires
    A. Fibrinogen
    B. Prothrombin
    C. Antihemophilic factor
    D. Christmas factor
    E. Hageman factor

Answer: C

Frozen plasma is required for the transfusion of antihemophilic factor (factor VIII) or proaccelerin (factor V). The other factors are present in banked preparations. (See Schwartz 10th ed., p. 99.)

21. The most common clinical manifestation of a hemolytic transfusion reaction is
    A. Flank pain
    B. Jaundice
    C. Oliguria
    D. A shaking chill

Answer: C

All of the manifestations listed can occur with a hemolytic transfusion reaction. In a large series, oliguria (58%) and hemoglobinuria (56%) were the most common findings. (See Schwartz 10th ed., p. 101.)

22. What type of bacterial sepsis can lead to thrombocytopenia and hemorrhagic disorder?
    A. Gram-negative
    B. Gram-positive
    C. A & B
    D. Encapsulated bacteria

Answer: A

Lastly, severe hemorrhagic disorders due to thrombocytopenia have occurred as a result of gram-negative sepsis. The pathogenesis of endotoxin-induced thrombocytopenia has been suggested that a labile factor V is necessary for this interaction. (See Schwartz 10th ed., p. 104.)

23. After tissue injury, the first step in coagulation is
    A. Binding of factor XII to subendothelial collagen
    B. Cleavage of factor XI to active factor IX
    C. Complexing of factor IX with factor VIII in the presence of ionized calcium conversion of prothrombin to thrombin
    D. Formation of fibrin from fibrinogen

Answer: A

All the listed steps are part of the cascade involved in establishing a firm clot. The process begins with binding of Hageman factor (factor XII) to subendothelial collagen and ends with the conversion of fibrinogen to fibrin. The fibrin forms an insoluble addition that stabilizes the platelet plug. (See Schwartz 10th ed., p. 87.)

24. What are the uses of thromboelastography (TEG)?
    A. Predicting need for lifesaving interventions after arrival for trauma
    B. Predicting 24-hour and 30-day mortality following trauma
    C. Predicting early transfusion of RBC, plasma, platelets, and cryoprecipitate
    D. All of the above

Answer: D

Thromboelastography (TEG) is the only test measuring all dynamic steps of clot formation until eventual clot lysis or retraction. TEG has also been shown to identify, patients who are likely to develop thromboembolic complications postinjury and postoperatively.

Recent trauma data have shown TEG to be useful in predicting early transfusion of RBCs, plasma, platelets, and cryoprecipitate. TEG can also predict the need for lifesaving interventions shortly after arrival and to predict 24-hour and 30-day mortality. Lastly, TEG can be useful to guide administration of tranexamic acid to injured patients with hyperfibrinolysis. (See Schwartz 10th ed., p. 103.)

25. Bank blood is appropriate for replacing each of the following EXCEPT
    A. Factor I (fibrinogen)
    B. Factor II (prothrombin)
    C. Factor VII (proconvertin)
    D. Factor VIII (antihemophilic factor)

Answer: D
Factor VIII is labile, and 60 to 80% of activity is gone 1 week after collection. The other factors listed are stable in banked blood. (See Schwartz 10th ed., p. 99.)

CHAPTER 5

Shock

1. Shock caused by a large tension pneumothorax is categorized as
   A. Trauma shock
   B. Vasodilatory shock
   C. Cardiogenic shock
   D. Obstructive shock

Answer: D

In 1934, Blalock proposed four categories of shock: hypovolemic, vasogenic, cardiogenic, and neurogenic. *Hypovolemic shock,* the most common type, results from loss of circulating blood volume. This may result from loss of whole blood (hemorrhagic shock), plasma, interstitial fluid (bowel obstruction), or a combination. *Vasogenic shock* results from decreased resistance within capacitance vessels, usually seen in sepsis. *Neurogenic shock* is a form of vasogenic shock in which spinal cord injury or spinal anesthesia causes vasodilation due to acute loss of sympathetic vascular tone. *Cardiogenic shock* results from failure of the heart as a pump, as in arrhythmias or acute myocardial infarction (MI).

In recent clinical practice, further classification has described six types of shock: hypovolemic, septic (vasodilatory), neurogenic, cardiogenic, obstructive, and traumatic shock. *Obstructive shock* is a form of cardiogenic shock that results from mechanical impediment to circulation leading to depressed cardiac output rather than primary cardiac failure. This includes etiologies such as pulmonary embolism or tension pneumothorax. In *traumatic shock*, soft tissue and bony injury lead to the activation of inflammatory cells and the release of circulating factors, such as cytokines and intracellular molecules that modulate the immune response. Recent investigations have revealed that the inflammatory mediators released in response to tissue injury (damage-associated molecular patterns [DAMPs]) are recognized by many of the same cellular receptors (pattern recognition receptors [PRRs]) and activate similar signaling pathways as do bacterial products elaborated in sepsis (pathogen-associated molecular patterns [PAMPs]), such as lipopolysaccharide. These effects of tissue injury are combined with the effects of hemorrhage, creating a more complex and amplified deviation from homeostasis. (See Schwartz 10th ed., p. 109.)

2. What is true about baroreceptors?
   A. Volume receptors can be activated in hemorrhage with reduction in left atrial pressure.
   B. Receptors in the aortic arch and carotid bodies inhibit the autonomic nervous system (ANS) when stretched.
   C. When baroreceptors are stretched, they induced increased ANS output and produce constriction of peripheral vessels.
   D. None of the above.

Answer: B

Baroreceptors also are an important afferent pathway in initiation of adaptive responses to shock. Volume receptors, sensitive to changes in both chamber pressure and wall stretch, are present within the atria of the heart. They become activated with low volume hemorrhage or mild reductions in right atrial pressure. Receptors in the aortic arch and carotid bodies respond to alterations in pressure or stretch of the arterial wall, responding to larger reductions in intravascular volume or pressure. These receptors normally inhibit induction of the autonomic nervous system (ANS). When activated, these baroreceptors diminish their output, thus disinhibiting the effect of the ANS. The ANS then increases its output, principally via sympathetic activation at the vasomotor centers of the brain stem, producing centrally mediated constriction of peripheral vessels. (See Schwartz 10th ed., p. 112.)

3. Chemoreceptors in the aorta and carotid bodies do NOT sense which of the following?
   A. Changes in O_2 tension
   B. H^+ ion concentration
   C. HCO_3^- concentration
   D. Carbon dioxide (CO_2) levels

Answer: C

Chemoreceptors in the aorta and carotid bodies are sensitive to changes in O_2 tension, H^+ ion concentration, and carbon dioxide (CO_2) levels. Stimulation of the chemoreceptors results in vasodilation of the coronary arteries, slowing of the heart rate, and vasoconstriction of the splanchnic and skeletal circulation. In addition, a variety of protein and nonprotein mediators are produced at the site of injury as part of the inflammatory response, and they act as afferent impulses to induce a host response. (See Schwartz 10th ed., p. 112.)

4. Neurogenic shock is characterized by the presence of
   A. Cool, moist skin
   B. Increased cardiac output
   C. Decreased peripheral vascular resistance
   D. Decreased blood volume

Answer: C

Neurogenic shock is caused by loss of arteriolar and venular tone in response to paralysis (such as occurs with high spinal anesthesia), acute gastric dilatation, or sudden pain, or unpleasant sights; as such, it is characterized by a decrease in peripheral vascular resistance. Affected patients usually present with warm, dry skin, a pulse rate that is slower than normal, and hypotension. A normovolemic state usually exists, and urine output is generally well maintained. Although blood volume measurements indicate a normal intravascular volume, because of the greatly increased reservoir capacity of the arterioles and venules, there is a decrease in cardiac output secondary to decreased venous return to the right side of the heart. (See Schwartz 10th ed., p. 129.)

5. When a patient with hemorrhagic shock is resuscitated using an intravenous colloid solution rather than lactated Ringer solution, all of the following statements are true EXCEPT
   A. Circulating levels of immunoglobulins are decreased.
   B. Colloid solutions may bind to the ionized fraction of serum calcium.
   C. Endogenous production of albumin is decreased.
   D. Extracellular fluid volume deficit is restored.

Answer: D

Because of higher osmotic pressure, colloid solutions draw extracellular fluid into the vascular space, increasing the extracellular fluid deficit. In addition, the ionized fraction of serum calcium is decreased, circulating levels of immunoglobulin drop, and reaction to tetanus toxoid given to the patient suffering from major trauma is decreased. Endogenous production of albumin also decreases. Colloid resuscitation is no more effective than crystalloid resuscitation, and it is more expensive. (See Schwartz 10th ed., p. 122.)

6. In hemorrhage, larger arterioles vasoconstrict in response to the sympathetic nervous system. Which categories of shock are associated with vasodilation of larger arterioles?
   A. Septic shock
   B. Cardiogenic shock
   C. Neurogenic shock
   D. A & C

Answer: D

The microvascular circulation plays an integral role in regulating cellular perfusion and is significantly influenced in response to shock. The microvascular bed is innervated by the sympathetic nervous system and has a profound effect on the larger arterioles. Following hemorrhage, larger arterioles vasoconstrict; however, in the setting of sepsis or neurogenic shock, these vessels vasodilate. Additionally, a host of other vasoactive proteins, including vasopressin, angiotensin II, and endothelin-1, also lead to vasoconstriction to limit organ perfusion to organs such as skin, skeletal muscle, kidneys, and the gastrointestinal (GI) tract to preserve perfusion of the myocardium and central nervous system (CNS). (See Schwartz 10th ed., p. 114.)

7. Which of the following is true about antidiuretic hormone (ADH) production in injured patients?
   A. ADH acts as a potent mesenteric vasoconstrictor.
   B. ADH levels fall to normal within 2 to 3 days of the initial insult.
   C. ADH decreases hepatic gluconeogenesis.
   D. ADH secretion is mediated by the renin-angiotensin system.

Answer: A
The pituitary also releases vasopressin or antidiuretic hormone (ADH) in response to hypovolemia, changes in circulating blood volume sensed by baroreceptors and left atrial stretch receptors, and increased plasma osmolality detected by hypothalamic osmoreceptors. Epinephrine, angiotensin II, pain, and hyperglycemia increase production of ADH. ADH levels remain elevated for about 1 week after the initial insult, depending on the severity and persistence of the hemodynamic abnormalities. ADH acts on the distal tubule and collecting duct of the nephron to increase water permeability, decrease water and sodium losses, and preserve intravascular volume. Also known as arginine vasopressin, ADH acts as a potent mesenteric vasoconstrictor, shunting circulating blood away from the splanchnic organs during hypovolemia. This may contribute to intestinal ischemia and predispose to intestinal mucosal barrier dysfunction in shock states. Vasopressin also increases hepatic gluconeogenesis and increases hepatic glycolysis. (See Schwartz 10th ed., p. 113)

8. Which of following occur as a result of epinephrine and norepinephrine?
   A. Hepatic glycogenolysis
   B. Hypoglycemia
   C. Insulin sensitivity
   D. Lipogenesis

Answer: A
Epinephrine and norepinephrine have a profound impact on cellular metabolism. Hepatic glycogenolysis, gluconeogenesis, ketogenesis, skeletal muscle protein breakdown, and adipose tissue lipolysis are increased by catecholamines. Cortisol, glucagon, and ADH also contribute to the catabolism during shock. Epinephrine induces further release of glucagon, while inhibiting the pancreatic β-cell release of insulin. The result is a catabolic state with glucose mobilization, hyperglycemia, protein breakdown, negative nitrogen balance, lipolysis, and insulin resistance during shock and injury. The relative underuse of glucose by peripheral tissues preserves it for the glucose-dependent organs such as the heart and brain. (See Schwartz 10th ed., p. 115.)

9. A patient has a blood pressure of 70/50 mm Hg and a serum lactate level of 30 mg/100 mL (normal: 6–16). His cardiac output is 1.9 L/min, and his central venous pressure is 2 cm H_2O. The most likely diagnosis is
   A. Congestive heart failure
   B. Cardiac tamponade
   C. Hypovolemic shock
   D. Septic shock

Answer: C
The findings given in the question are characteristic of hypovolemic shock, which can be defined as inadequate tissue perfusion secondary to an extracellular fluid loss. The high lactate level is a result of anaerobic metabolism due to decreased blood flow to tissues. The hemodynamic measurements indicate both low blood flow and low venous return. The total combination is most consistent with a diagnosis of hypovolemic shock. Pulmonary embolus, congestive heart failure, and cardiac tamponade are all associated with a high central venous pressure. Septic shock, particularly in its early phases, is usually hyperdynamic, and affected patients have a greater-than-normal cardiac output. Complete hemodynamic monitoring is vital in hypovolemic shock so that prompt diagnosis and rational therapy can be expeditiously carried out. (See Schwartz 10th ed., p. 119.)

10. Which cytokine is anti-inflammatory and increases after shock and trauma?
    A. Interleukin (IL)-1
    B. IL-2
    C. IL-6
    D. IL-10

Answer: D
Interleukin (IL)-10 is considered an anti-inflammatory cytokine that may have immunosuppressive properties. Its production is increased after shock and trauma, and it has been associated with depressed immune function clinically, as well as an increased susceptibility to infection. IL-10 is secreted by T cells, monocytes, and macrophages, and inhibits pro-inflammatory cytokine secretion, O_2 radical production by phagocytes, adhesion molecule expression, and lymphocyte activation. Administration of IL-10 depresses cytokine production and improves some aspects of immune function in experimental models of shock and sepsis. (See Schwartz 10th ed., p. 118.)

11. Tumor necrosis factor-alpha (TNF-α)
    A. Can be released as a response to bacteria or endotoxin
    B. Increased more in trauma than septic patients
    C. Induces procoagulant activity and peripheral vasoconstriction
    D. Contributes to anemia of chronic illness

Answer: A
Tumor necrosis factor-alpha (TNF-α) was one of the first cytokines to be described, and is one of the earliest cytokines released in response to injurious stimuli. Monocytes, macrophages, and T cells release this potent proinflammatory cytokine. TNF-α levels peak within 90 minutes of stimulation and return frequently to baseline levels within 4 hours. Release of TNF-α may be induced by bacteria or endotoxin, and leads to the development of shock and hypoperfusion, most commonly observed in septic shock. Production of TNF-α also may be induced following other insults, such as hemorrhage and ischemia. TNF-α levels correlate with mortality in animal models of hemorrhage. In contrast, the increase in serum TNF-α levels reported in trauma patients is far less than that seen in septic patients. Once released, TNF-α can produce peripheral vasodilation, activate the release of other cytokines, induce procoagulant activity, and stimulate a wide array of cellular metabolic changes. During the stress response, TNF-α contributes to the muscle protein breakdown and cachexia. (See Schwartz 10th ed., p. 116.)

12. A 70-kg male patient presents to ED following a stab wound to the abdomen. He is hypotensive, markedly tachycardic, and appears confused. What percent of blood volume has he lost?
    A. 5%
    B. 15%
    C. 35%
    D. 55%

Answer: D
The clinical signs of shock may be evidenced by agitation, cool clammy extremities, tachycardia, weak or absent peripheral pulses, and hypotension. Such apparent clinical shock results from at least 25 to 30% loss of the blood volume. However, substantial volumes of blood may be lost before the classic clinical manifestations of shock are evident. Thus, when a patient is significantly tachycardic or hypotensive, this represents both significant blood loss and physiologic decompensation. The clinical and physiologic response to hemorrhage has been classified according to the magnitude of volume loss. Loss of up to 15% of the circulating volume (700–750 mL for a 70-kg patient) may produce little in terms of obvious symptoms, while loss of up to 30% of the circulating volume (1.5 L) may result in mild tachycardia, tachypnea, and anxiety. Hypotension, marked tachycardia (ie, pulse greater than 110–120 beats per minute [bpm]), and confusion may not be evident until more than 30% of the blood volume has been lost; loss of 40% of circulating volume (2 L) is immediately life threatening, and generally requires operative control of bleeding. (See Schwartz 10th ed., p. 119.)

13. Vasodilatory shock
    A. Is characterized by failure of vascular smooth muscle to constrict due to low levels of catecholamines
    B. Leads to suppression of the renin-angiotensin system
    C. Can also be caused by carbon monoxide poisoning
    D. Is similar to early cardiogenic shock

Answer: C

In the peripheral circulation, profound vasoconstriction is the typical physiologic response to the decreased arterial pressure and tissue perfusion with hemorrhage, hypovolemia, or acute heart failure. This is not the characteristic response in vasodilatory shock. Vasodilatory shock is the result of dysfunction of the endothelium and vasculature secondary to circulating inflammatory mediators and cells or as a response to prolonged and severe hypoperfusion. Thus, in vasodilatory shock, hypotension results from failure of the vascular smooth muscle to constrict appropriately. Vasodilatory shock is characterized by peripheral vasodilation with resultant hypotension and resistance to treatment with vasopressors. Despite the hypotension, plasma catecholamine levels are elevated, and the renin-angiotensin system is activated in vasodilatory shock. The most frequently encountered form of vasodilatory shock is septic shock. Other causes of vasodilatory shock include hypoxic lactic acidosis, carbon monoxide poisoning, decompensated and irreversible hemorrhagic shock, terminal cardiogenic shock, and postcardiotomy shock. Thus, vasodilatory shock seems to represent the final common pathway for profound and prolonged shock of any etiology. (See Schwartz 10th ed., p. 124.)

14. A patient in septic shock remains hypotensive despite adequate fluid resuscitation and initiation of norepinephrine. What is often given to patients with hypotension refractory to norepinephrine?
    A. Dopamine
    B. Arginine vasopressin
    C. Dobutamine
    D. Milrinone

Answer: B

After first-line therapy of the septic patient with antibiotics, IV fluids, and intubation if necessary, vasopressors may be necessary to treat patients with septic shock. Catecholamines are the vasopressors used most often, with norepinephrine being the first-line agent followed by epinephrine. Occasionally, patients with septic shock will develop arterial resistance to catecholamines. Arginine vasopressin, a potent vasoconstrictor, is often efficacious in this setting and is often added to norepinephrine. (See Schwartz 10th ed., p. 125.)

15. Tight glucose management in critically ill and septic patients
    A. Requires insulin to keep serum glucose <140
    B. Has no effect on mortality
    C. Has no effect on ventilator support
    D. Decreases length of antibiotic therapy

Answer: D

Hyperglycemia and insulin resistance are typical in critically ill and septic patients, including patients without underlying diabetes mellitus. A recent study reported significant positive impact of tight glucose management on outcome in critically ill patients. The two treatment groups in this randomized, prospective study were assigned to receive intensive insulin therapy (maintenance of blood glucose between 80 and 110 mg/dL) or conventional treatment (infusion of insulin only if the blood glucose level exceeded 215 mg/dL, with a goal between 180 and 200 mg/dL). The mean morning glucose level was significantly higher in the conventional treatment as compared with the intensive insulin therapy group (153 vs 103 mg/dL). Mortality in the intensive insulin treatment group (4.6%) was significantly lower than in the conventional treatment group (8.0%), representing a 42% reduction in mortality. This reduction in mortality was most notable in the patients requiring longer than 5 days in the ICU. Furthermore, intensive insulin therapy reduced episodes of septicemia by 46%, reduced duration of antibiotic therapy, and decreased the need for prolonged ventilatory support and renal replacement therapy. (See Schwartz 10th ed., p. 125.)

16. Cardiogenic shock
    A. Is most commonly caused by exacerbation of congestive heart failure.
    B. Cardiogenic shock following an acute myocardial infarction is typically present on admission.
    C. Cardiogenic shock occurs in 5 to 10% of acute MIs.
    D. Is characterized by hypotension, reduced cardiac index, and reduced pulmonary artery wedge pressure.

Answer: C

Cardiogenic shock is defined clinically as circulatory pump failure leading to diminished forward flow and subsequent tissue hypoxia, in the setting of adequate intravascular volume. Hemodynamic criteria include sustained hypotension (ie, systolic blood pressure [SBP] <90 mm Hg for at least 30 minutes), reduced cardiac index (<2.2 L/min per square meter), and elevated pulmonary artery wedge pressure (>15 mm Hg). Mortality rates for cardiogenic shock are 50 to 80%. Acute, extensive MI is the most common cause of cardiogenic shock; a smaller infarction in a patient with existing left ventricular dysfunction also may precipitate shock. Cardiogenic shock complicates 5 to 10% of acute MIs. Conversely, cardiogenic shock is the most common cause of death in patients hospitalized with acute MI. Although shock may develop early after MI, it typically is not found on admission. Seventy-five percent of patients who have cardiogenic shock complicating acute MIs develop signs of cardiogenic shock within 24 hours after onset of infarction (average 7 hours). (See Schwartz 10th ed., p. 126.)

17. All of the following result from the placement of an intra-aortic balloon pump in a patient with acute myocardial failure EXCEPT
    A. Reduction of systolic afterload
    B. Increased cardiac output
    C. Increased myocardial O_2 demand
    D. Increased diastolic perfusion pressure

Answer: C

Intra-aortic balloon pumping increases cardiac output and improves coronary blood flow by reduction of systolic afterload and augmentation of diastolic perfusion pressure. Unlike vasopressor agents, these beneficial effects occur without an increase in myocardial O_2 demand. An intra-aortic balloon pump can be inserted at the bedside in the ICU via the femoral artery through either a cutdown or using the percutaneous approach. (See Schwartz 10th ed., p. 127.)

18. Which constellation of clinical findings is suggestive of cardiac tamponade?
    A. Hypotension, wide pulse pressure, tachycardia
    B. Tachycardia, hypotension, jugular venous distension
    C. Hypotension, wide pulse pressure, jugular venous distension
    D. Hypotension, muffled heart tones, jugular venous distension

Answer: D

Cardiac tamponade also may be associated with dyspnea, orthopnea, cough, peripheral edema, chest pain, tachycardia, muffled heart tones, jugular venous distention, and elevated central venous pressure. Beck's triad consists of hypotension, muffled heart tones, and neck vein distention. Unfortunately, absence of these clinical findings may not be sufficient to exclude cardiac injury and cardiac tamponade. Muffled heart tones may be difficult to appreciate in a busy trauma center and jugular venous distention and central venous pressure may be diminished by coexistent bleeding. Therefore, patients at risk for cardiac tamponade whose hemodynamic status permits additional diagnostic tests frequently require additional diagnostic maneuvers to confirm cardiac injury or tamponade. (See Schwartz 10th ed., p. 128.)

19. A 43-year-old man is struck by a motor vehicle while crossing the street; he arrives in the ED hypotensive, bradycardic, and unable to move his extremities. What is the most likely cause of his hypotension?
    A. Hypovolemic shock
    B. Obstructive shock
    C. Neurogenic shock
    D. Vasodilatory shock

Answer: A

In a subset of patients with spinal cord injuries from penetrating wounds, most of the patients with hypotension had blood loss as the etiology (74%) rather than neurogenic causes, and few (7%) had the classic findings of neurogenic shock. In the multiply injured patient, other causes of hypotension including hemorrhage, tension pneumothorax, and cardiogenic shock must be sought and excluded. (See Schwartz 10th ed., p. 129.)

20. Corticosteroids in the treatment of septic shock
    A. Improves rates of shock reversal in patients requiring vasopressors
    B. Improves mortality in patients with relative adrenal insufficiency
    C. Is contraindicated in patients with positive bacterial blood cultures
    D. None of the above

Answer: B

The use of corticosteroids in the treatment of sepsis and septic shock has been controversial for decades. The observation that severe sepsis often is associated with adrenal insufficiency or glucocorticoid receptor resistance has generated renewed interest in therapy for septic shock with corticosteroids. A single IV dose of 50 mg of hydrocortisone improved mean arterial blood pressure response relationships to norepinephrine and phenylephrine in patients with septic shock, and was most notable in patients with relative adrenal insufficiency. A more recent study evaluated therapy with hydrocortisone (50 mg IV every 6 hours) and fludrocortisone (50 µg orally once daily) versus placebo for 1 week in patients with septic shock. As in earlier studies, the authors performed corticotropin tests on these patients to document and stratify patients by relative adrenal insufficiency. In this study, the 7-day treatment with low doses of hydrocortisone and fludrocortisone significantly and safely lowered the risk of death in patients with septic shock and relative adrenal insufficiency. In an international, multicenter, randomized trial of corticosteroids in sepsis (CORTICUS study; 499 analyzable patients), steroids showed no benefit in intent to treat mortality or shock reversal. This study suggested that hydrocortisone therapy cannot be recommended as routine adjuvant therapy for septic shock. However, if SBP remains less than 90 mm Hg despite appropriate fluid and vasopressor therapy, hydrocortisone at 200 mg/day for 7 days in four divided doses or by continuous infusion should be considered. (See Schwartz 10th ed., p. 126.)

21. What is FALSE about serum lactate?
    A. Generated from pyruvate in the setting of insufficient O_2.
    B. Metabolized by the liver and kidneys.
    C. Is an indirect measure of the magnitude and severity of shock.
    D. The time to peak lactate from admission predicts rates of survival.

Answer: D

Lactate is generated by conversion of pyruvate to lactate by lactate dehydrogenase in the setting of insufficient O_2. Lactate is released into the circulation and is predominantly taken up and metabolized by the liver and kidneys. The liver accounts for approximately 50% and the kidney for about 30% of whole body lactate uptake. Elevated serum lactate is an indirect measure of the O_2 debt, and therefore an approximation of the magnitude and duration of the severity of shock. The admission lactate level, highest lactate level, and time interval to normalize the serum lactate are important prognostic indicators for survival. For example, in a study of 76 consecutive patients, 100% survival was observed among the patients with normalization of lactate within 24 hours, 78% survival when lactate normalized between 24 and 48 hours, and only 14% survivorship if it took longer than 48 hours to normalize the serum lactate. In contrast, individual variability of lactate may be too great to permit accurate prediction of outcome in any individual case. Base deficit and volume of blood transfusion required in the first 24 hours of resuscitation may be better predictors of mortality than the plasma lactate alone. (See Schwartz 10th ed., p. 130.)

CHAPTER 6

Surgical Infections

1. Transferrin plays a role in host defense by
   A. Sequestering iron, which is necessary for microbial growth
   B. Increasing the ability of fibrinogen to trap microbes
   C. Direct injury to the bacterial cell membrane
   D. Direct injury to the bacterial mitochondria

Answer: A
Once microbes enter a sterile body compartment (eg, pleural or peritoneal cavity) or tissue, additional host defenses act to limit and/or eliminate these pathogens. Initially, several primitive and relatively nonspecific host defenses act to contain the nidus of infection, which may include microbes as well as debris, devitalized tissue, and foreign bodies, depending on the nature of the injury. These defenses include the physical barrier of the tissue itself, as well as the capacity of proteins, such as lactoferrin and transferrin, to sequester the critical microbial growth factor iron, thereby limiting microbial growth. In addition, fibrinogen within the inflammatory fluid has the ability to trap large numbers of microbes during the process in which it polymerizes into fibrin. Within the peritoneal cavity, unique host defenses exist, including a diaphragmatic pumping mechanism whereby particles including microbes within peritoneal fluid are expunged from the abdominal cavity via specialized structures on the undersurface of the diaphragm. Concurrently, containment by the omentum, the so-called "gatekeeper" of the abdomen and intestinal ileus, serves to wall off infection. However, the latter processes and fibrin trapping have a high likelihood of contributing to the formation of an intra-abdominal abscess. (See Schwartz 10th ed., p. 138.)

2. Which is NOT a component of systemic inflammatory response syndrome (SIRS)?
   A. Temperature
   B. White blood cell (WBC) count
   C. Blood pressure
   D. Heart rate

Answer: C
Infection is defined by the presence of microorganisms in host tissue or the bloodstream. At the site of infection the classic findings of rubor, calor, and dolor in areas such as the skin or subcutaneous tissue are common. Most infections in normal individuals with intact host defenses are associated with these local manifestations, plus systemic manifestations such as elevated temperature, elevated white blood cell (WBC) count, tachycardia, or tachypnea. The systemic manifestations noted above comprise the *systemic inflammatory response syndrome* (SIRS). (See Schwartz 10th ed., p. 138.)

3. The best method for hair removal from an operative field is
   A. Shaving the night before
   B. Depilating the night before surgery
   C. Shaving in the operating room
   D. Using hair clippers in the operating room

Answer: D
Hair removal should take place using a clipper rather than a razor; the latter promotes overgrowth of skin microbes in small nicks and cuts. Dedicated use of these modalities clearly has been shown to diminish the quantity of skin microflora. (See Schwartz 10th ed., p. 141.)

4. A patient with necrotizing pancreatitis undergoes computed tomography (CT)-guided aspiration, which results in growth of *Escherichia coli* on culture. The most appropriate treatment is
   A. Culture-appropriate antibiotic therapy
   B. Endoscopic retrograde cholangiopancreatography with sphincterotomy
   C. CT-guided placement of drain(s)
   D. Exploratory laparotomy

Answer: D

The primary precept of surgical infectious disease therapy consists of drainage of all purulent material, debridement of all infected, devitalized tissue, and debris, and/or removal of foreign bodies at the site of infection, plus remediation of the underlying cause of infection. A discrete, walled-off purulent fluid collection (ie, an abscess) requires drainage via percutaneous drain insertion or an operative approach in which incision and drainage take place. An ongoing source of contamination (eg, bowel perforation) or the presence of an aggressive, rapidly spreading infection (eg, necrotizing soft tissue infection) invariably requires expedient, aggressive operative intervention, both to remove contaminated material and infected tissue (eg, radical debridement or amputation) and to remove the initial cause of infection (eg, bowel resection). (See Schwartz 10th ed., p. 141.)

5. Which factor does NOT influence the development of surgical site infections (SSIs)?
   A. Duration of procedure
   B. Degree of microbial contamination of the wound
   C. Malnutrition
   D. General anesthesia

Answer: D

Surgical site infections (SSIs) are infections of the tissues, organs, or spaces exposed by surgeons during performance of an invasive procedure. SSIs are classified into incisional and organ/space infections, and the former are further subclassified into superficial (limited to skin and subcutaneous tissue) and deep incisional categories. The development of SSIs is related to three factors: (1) the degree of microbial contamination of the wound during surgery, (2) the duration of the procedure, and (3) host factors such as diabetes, malnutrition, obesity, immune suppression, and a number of other underlying disease states. (See Schwartz 10th ed., p. 147.)

6. During a laparoscopic appendectomy, a large bowel injury was caused during trochar placement with spillage of bowel contents into the abdomen. What class of surgical wound is this?
   A. Class I (clean)
   B. Class II (clean/contaminated)
   C. Class III (contaminated)
   D. Class IV (dirty)

Answer: C

Surgical wounds are classified based on the presumed magnitude of the bacterial load at the time of surgery. *Clean wounds* (Class I) include those in which no infection is present; only skin microflora potentially contaminate the wound, and no hollow viscus that contains microbes is entered. Class ID wounds are similar except that a prosthetic device (eg, mesh or valve) is inserted. *Clean/contaminated wounds* (Class II) include those in which a hollow viscus, such as the respiratory, alimentary, or genitourinary tracts, with indigenous bacterial flora is opened under controlled circumstances without significant spillage of contents. *Contaminated wounds* (Class III) include open accidental wounds encountered early after injury, those with extensive introduction of bacteria into a normally sterile area of the body due to major breaks in sterile technique (eg, open cardiac massage), gross spillage of viscus contents such as from the intestine, or incision through inflamed, albeit nonpurulent, tissue. *Dirty wounds* (Class IV) include traumatic wounds in which a significant delay in treatment has occurred and in which necrotic tissue is present, those created in the presence of overt infection as evidenced by the presence of purulent material, and those created to access a perforated viscus accompanied by a high degree of contamination. (See Schwartz 10th ed., p. 147.)

7. The most appropriate treatment of a 4-cm hepatic abscess is
   A. Antibiotic therapy alone
   B. Aspiration for culture and antibiotic therapy
   C. Percutaneous drainage and antibiotic therapy
   D. Operative exploration, open drainage of the abscess, and antibiotic therapy

Answer: C

Hepatic abscesses are rare, currently accounting for approximately 15 per 100,000 hospital admissions in the United States. Pyogenic abscesses account for approximately 80% of cases, the remaining 20% being equally divided among parasitic and fungal forms. Formerly, pyogenic liver abscesses were caused by pylephlebitis due to neglected appendicitis or diverticulitis. Today, manipulation of the biliary tract to treat a variety of diseases has become a more common cause, although in nearly 50% of patients no cause is identified. The most common aerobic bacteria identified in recent series include *E. coli*, *Klebsiella pneumoniae*, and other enteric bacilli, enterococci, and *Pseudomonas* spp., while the most common anaerobic bacteria are *Bacteroides* spp., anaerobic streptococci, and *Fusobacterium* spp. *Candida albicans* and other similar yeasts cause the majority of fungal hepatic abscesses. Small (<1 cm), multiple abscesses should be sampled and treated with a 4- to 6-week course of antibiotics. Larger abscesses invariably are amenable to percutaneous drainage, with parameters for antibiotic therapy and drain removal similar to those mentioned above. Splenic abscesses are extremely rare and are treated in a similar fashion. Recurrent hepatic or splenic abscesses may require operative intervention—unroofing and marsupialization or splenectomy, respectively. (See Schwartz 10th ed., p. 150.)

8. Postoperative urinary tract infections (UTIs)
   A. Are usually treated with a 7- to 10-day course of antibiotics.
   B. Initial therapy should be directed by results of urine culture.
   C. Are established by >10⁴ CFU/mL of bacteria in urine culture in asymptomatic patients.
   D. Can be reduced by irrigating indwelling Foley catheters daily.

Answer: B

The presence of a postoperative UTI should be considered based on urinalysis demonstrating WBCs or bacteria, a positive test for leukocyte esterase, or a combination of these elements. The diagnosis is established after $>10^4$ CFU/mL of microbes are identified by culture techniques in symptomatic patients, or $>10^5$ CFU/mL in asymptomatic individuals. Treatment for 3 to 5 days with a single antibiotic directed against the most common organisms (eg, *E. Coli*, *K. pneumoniae*) that achieves high levels in the urine is appropriate. Initial therapy is directed by Gram's stain results and is refined as culture results become available. Postoperative surgical patients should have indwelling urinary catheters removed as quickly as possible, typically within 1 to 2 days, as long as they are mobile, to avoid the development of a UTI. (See Schwartz 10th ed., p. 152.)

9. The first step in the evaluation and treatment of a patient with an infected bug bite on the leg with cellulitis, bullae, thin grayish fluid draining from the wound, and pain out of proportion to the physical findings is
   A. Obtain C-reactive protein
   B. CT scan of the leg
   C. Magnetic resonance imaging (MRI) of the leg
   D. Operative exploration

Answer: D

The diagnosis of necrotizing infection is established solely upon a constellation of clinical findings, not all of which are present in every patient. Not surprisingly, patients often develop sepsis syndrome or septic shock without an obvious cause. The extremities, perineum, trunk, and torso are most commonly affected, in that order. Careful examination should be undertaken for an entry site such as a small break or sinus in the skin from which grayish, turbid semipurulent material ("dishwater pus") can be expressed, as well as for the presence of skin changes (bronze hue or brawny induration), blebs, or crepitus. The patient often develops pain at the site of infection that appears to be out of proportion to any of the physical manifestations. Any of these findings mandates immediate surgical intervention, which should consist of exposure and direct visualization of potentially infected tissue (including deep soft tissue, fascia, and underlying muscle) and radical resection of affected areas. Radiologic studies should be undertaken only in patients in whom the diagnosis is not seriously considered, as they delay surgical intervention and frequently provide confusing information. Unfortunately, surgical extirpation of infected tissue frequently entails amputation and/or disfiguring procedures; however, incomplete procedures are associated with higher rates of morbidity and mortality. (See Schwartz 10th ed., p. 151.)

10. What is FALSE regarding intravascular catheter infections?
    A. Selected low-virulence infections can be treated with a prolonged course of antibiotics.
    B. In high-risk patients, prophylactic antibiotics infused through the catheter can reduce rate of catheter infections.
    C. Bacteremia with gram-negative bacteria or fungi should prompt catheter removal.
    D. Many patients with intravascular catheter infections are asymptomatic.

Answer: B
Many patients who develop intravascular catheter infections are asymptomatic, often exhibiting solely an elevation in the WBC count. Blood cultures obtained from a peripheral site and drawn through the catheter that reveal the presence of the same organism increase the index of suspicion for the presence of a catheter infection. Obvious purulence at the exit site of the skin tunnel, severe sepsis syndrome due to any type of organism when other potential causes have been excluded, or bacteremia due to gram-negative aerobes or fungi should lead to catheter removal. Selected catheter infections due to low-virulence microbes such as *Staphylococcus epidermidis* can be effectively treated in approximately 50 to 60% of patients with a 14- to 21-day course of an antibiotic, which should be considered when no other vascular access site exists. Use of systemic antibacterial or antifungal agents to prevent catheter infection is of no utility and is contraindicated. (See Schwartz 10th ed., p. 154.)

11. Patients with a penicillin allergy are LEAST likely to have a cross-reaction with
    A. Synthetic penicillins
    B. Carbapenems
    C. Cephalosporins
    D. Monobactams

Answer: D
Allergy to antimicrobial agents must be considered prior to prescribing them. First, it is important to ascertain whether a patient has had any type of allergic reaction in association with administration of a particular antibiotic. However, one should take care to ensure that the purported reaction consists of true allergic symptoms and signs, such as urticaria, bronchospasm, or other similar manifestations, rather than indigestion or nausea. Penicillin allergy is quite common, the reported incidence ranging from 0.7 to 10%. Although avoiding the use of any beta-lactam drug is appropriate in patients who manifest significant allergic reactions to penicillins, the incidence of cross-reactivity appears low for all related agents, with 1% cross-reactivity for carbapenems, 5 to 7% cross-reactivity for cephalosporins, and extremely small or nonexistent cross-reactivity for monobactams. (See Schwartz 10th ed., p. 146.)

12. What is the estimated risk of transmission of human immunodeficiency virus (HIV) from a needlestick from a source with HIV-infected blood?
    A. <0.5%
    B. 1%
    C. 5%
    D. 10%

Answer: A
While alarming to contemplate, the risk of human immunodeficiency virus (HIV) transmission from patient to surgeon is low. As of May 2011, there had been six cases of surgeons with HIV seroconversion from a possible occupational exposure, with no new cases reported since 1999. Of the numbers of health care workers with likely occupationally acquired HIV infection ($n = 200$), surgeons were one of the lower risk groups (compared to nurses at 60 cases and nonsurgeon physicians at 19 cases). The estimated risk of transmission from a needlestick from a source with HIV-infected blood is estimated at 0.3%. (See Schwartz 10th ed., p. 156.)

13. Closure of an appendectomy wound in a patient with perforated appendicitis who is receiving appropriate antibiotics will result in a wound infection in what percentage of patients?
    A. 3–4%
    B. 8–12%
    C. 15–18%
    D. 22–25%

Answer: A
Surgical management of the wound is also a critical determinant of the propensity to develop an SSI. In healthy individuals, class I and II wounds may be closed primarily, while skin closure of class III and IV wounds is associated with high rates of incisional SSIs (~25–50%). The superficial aspects of these latter types of wounds should be packed open and allowed to heal by secondary intention, although selective use of delayed primary closure has been associated with a reduction in incisional SSI rates. It remains to be determined whether National Nosocomial Infections Surveillance (NNIS) system type stratification schemes can be employed prospectively in order to target specific subgroups of patients who will benefit from the use of prophylactic antibiotic and/or specific wound management techniques. One clear example based on cogent data from clinical trials is that class III wounds in healthy patients undergoing appendectomy for perforated or gangrenous appendicitis can be primarily closed as long as antibiotic therapy directed against aerobes and anaerobes is administered. This practice leads to SSI rates of approximately 3 to 4%. (See Schwartz 10th ed., p. 149.)

14. A chronic carrier state occurs with hepatitis C infection in what percentage of patients?
    A. 90–99%
    B. 75–80%
    C. 50–60%
    D. 10–30%

Answer: B
Hepatitis C virus (HCV), previously known as non-A, non-B hepatitis, is an RNA flavivirus first identified specifically in the late 1980s. This virus is confined to humans and chimpanzees. A chronic carrier state develops in 75 to 80% of patients with the infection, with chronic liver disease occurring in three-fourths of patients who develop chronic infection. The number of new infections per year has declined since the 1980s due to routine testing of blood donors for this virus. Fortunately, HCV is not transmitted efficiently through occupational exposures to blood, with the seroconversion rate after accidental needlestick approximately 1.8%. (See Schwartz 10th ed., p. 156.)

15. Possible exposure to anthrax should be initially treated with
    A. Colistin
    B. Ciprofloxacin or doxycycline
    C. Amoxicillin
    D. Observation

Answer: B
Inhalational anthrax develops after a 1- to 6-day incubation period, with nonspecific symptoms including malaise, myalgia, and fever. Over a short period of time, these symptoms worsen, with development of respiratory distress, chest pain, and diaphoresis. Characteristic chest roentgenographic findings include a widened mediastinum and pleural effusions. A key aspect in establishing the diagnosis is eliciting an exposure history. Rapid antigen tests are currently under development for identification of this gram-positive rod. Postexposure prophylaxis consists of administration of either ciprofloxacin or doxycycline. If an isolate is demonstrated to be penicillin-sensitive, the patient should be switched to amoxicillin. Inhalational exposure followed by the development of symptoms is associated with a high mortality rate. Treatment options include combination therapy with ciprofloxacin, clindamycin, and rifampin; clindamycin added to blocks production of toxin, while rifampin penetrates into the central nervous system and intracellular locations. (See Schwartz 10th ed., p. 156.)

16. The most effective postexposure prophylaxis for a surgeon stuck with a needle while operating on an HIV-positive patient is
    A. None (no effective treatment is known).
    B. Two- or three-drug therapy started within hours of exposure.
    C. Single drug therapy started within 24 hours of exposure.
    D. Triple drug therapy started within 24 hours of exposure.

Answer: B

Postexposure prophylaxis for HIV has significantly decreased the risk of seroconversion for health care workers with occupational exposure to HIV. Steps to initiate postexposure prophylaxis should be initiated within hours rather than days for the most effective preventive therapy. Postexposure prophylaxis with a two- or three-drug regimen should be initiated for health care workers with significant exposure to patients with an HIV-positive status. If a patient's HIV status is unknown, it may be advisable to begin postexposure prophylaxis while testing is carried out, particularly if the patient is at high risk for infection due to HIV (eg, intravenous narcotic use). Generally, postexposure prophylaxis is not warranted for exposure to sources with unknown status, such as deceased persons or needles from a sharps container. (See Schwartz 10th ed., p. 156.)

17. What is NOT an early goal in treatment of severe sepsis?
    A. Mean arterial pressure >65 mm Hg
    B. Central venous pressure 8 to 2 mm Hg
    C. Urine output >0.5 cc/kg/h
    D. Serum lactate <2 mmol/L

Answer: D

Patients presenting with severe sepsis should receive resuscitation fluids to achieve a central venous pressure target of 8 to 12 mm Hg, with a goal of mean arterial pressure of >65 mm Hg and urine output of >0.5 cc/kg/h. Delaying this resuscitative step for as little as 3 hours until arrival in the ICU has been shown to result in poor outcome. Typically this goal necessitates early placement of central venous catheter. (See Schwartz 10th ed., p. 154.)

18. A patient in the ICU has been on ventilator support for 3 weeks. He has new onset elevated WBC count, fever, and consolidation seen on chest X-ray. What is an appropriate next step?
    A. Exchange endotracheal tube and change respiratory circuit.
    B. Obtain bronchoalveolar lavage.
    C. Start treatment with empiric penicillin G.
    D. Obtain chest CT.

Answer: B

Prolonged mechanical ventilation is associated with nosocomial pneumonia. These patients present with more severe disease, are more likely to be infected with drug-resistant pathogens, and suffer increased mortality compared with patients who develop community-acquired pneumonia. The diagnosis of pneumonia is established by presence of a purulent sputum, elevated leukocyte count, fever, and new chest X-ray abnormalities such as consolidation. The presence of two of the clinical findings, plus chest X-ray findings, significantly increases the likelihood of pneumonia. Consideration should be given to performing bronchoalveolar lavage to obtain samples for Gram stain and culture. Some authors advocate quantitative cultures as a means to identify a threshold for diagnosis. Surgical patients should be weaned from mechanical ventilation as soon as feasible, based on oxygenation and inspiratory effort, as prolonged mechanical ventilation increases the risk of nosocomial pneumonia. (See Schwartz 10th ed., p. 153.)

19. Patients with severe, necrotizing pancreatitis should be treated with
    A. No antibiotics unless CT-guided aspiration of the area yields positive cultures
    B. Empiric cefoxitin or cefotetan
    C. Empiric cefuroxime plus gentamicin
    D. Empiric carbapenems or fluoroquinolones

Answer: D

Current care of patients with severe acute pancreatitis includes staging with dynamic, contrast-enhanced helical CT scan with 3-mm tomographs to determine the extent of pancreatic necrosis, coupled with the use of one of several prognostic scoring systems. Patients who exhibit significant pancreatic necrosis should be carefully monitored in the ICU and undergo follow-up CT examination. The weight of current evidence also favors administration of empiric antibiotic therapy to reduce the incidence and severity of secondary pancreatic infection, which typically occurs several weeks after the initial episode of pancreatitis. Several randomized, prospective trials have demonstrated a decrease in the rate of infection and mortality using agents such as carbapenems or fluoroquinolones that achieve high pancreatic tissue levels. (See Schwartz 10th ed., p. 150.)

20. A patient with a localized wound infection after surgery should be treated with
   A. Antibiotics and warm soaks to the wound
   B. Antibiotics alone
   C. Antibiotics and opening the wound
   D. Incision and drainage alone

Answer: D

Effective therapy for incisional SSIs consists solely of incision and drainage without the addition of antibiotics. Antibiotic therapy is reserved for patients in whom evidence of severe cellulitis is present, or who manifest concurrent sepsis syndrome. The open wound often is allowed to heal by secondary intention, with dressings being changed twice a day. The use of topical antibiotics and antiseptics, to further wound healing, remains unproven, although anecdotal studies indicate their potential utility in complex wounds that do not heal with routine measures. (See Schwartz 10th ed., p. 149.)

21. Which areas likely do NOT contain resident microorganisms?
   A. Terminal ileum
   B. Oropharynx
   C. Main pancreatic duct
   D. Nares

Answer: C

The urogenital, biliary, pancreatic ductal, and distal respiratory tracts do not possess resident microflora in healthy individuals, although microbes may be present if these barriers are affected by disease (eg, malignancy, inflammation, calculi, or foreign body), or if microorganisms are introduced from an external source (eg, urinary catheter or pulmonary aspiration). In contrast, significant numbers of microbes are encountered in many portions of the gastrointestinal tract, with vast numbers being found within the oropharynx and distal colorectum, although the specific organisms differ. (See Schwartz 10th ed., p. 137.)

Trauma

1. Cricothyroidotomy
   A. Should not be performed in children younger than 12 years
   B. Should only be performed in patients who are not good candidates for a tracheostomy
   C. Requires the use of an endotracheal tube smaller than 4 mm in diameter
   D. Is preferable to the use of percutaneous transtracheal ventilation

Answer: A
Patients in whom attempts at intubation have failed or are precluded from intubation due to extensive facial injuries require a surgical airway. Cricothyroidotomy (Fig. 7-1) and percutaneous transtracheal ventilation are preferred over tracheostomy in most emergency situations because of their simplicity and safety. One disadvantage of cricothyroidotomy is the inability to place a tube greater than 6 mm in diameter due to the limited aperture of the cricothyroid space. Cricothyroidotomy is also relatively contraindicated in patients younger than 12 years because of the risk of damage to the cricoid cartilage and the subsequent risk of subglottic stenosis. (See Schwartz 10th ed., p. 163.)

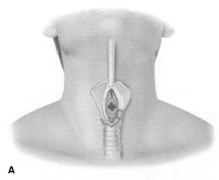
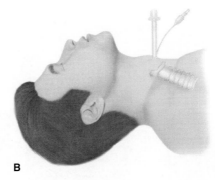

A   B

FIG. 7-1. A&B: Cricothyroidotomy is recommended for emergent surgical establishment of a patent airway. A vertical skin incision avoids injury to the anterior jugular veins, which are located just lateral to the midline. Hemorrhage from these vessels obscures vision and prolongs the procedure. When a transverse incision is made in the cricothyroid membrane, the blade of the knife should be angled inferiorly to avoid injury to the vocal cords. **A.** Use of a tracheostomy hook stabilizes the thyroid cartilage and facilitates tube insertion. **B.** A 6.0-endotracheal tube is inserted after digital confirmation of airway access.

2. Which of the following is NOT a sign of tension pneumothorax?
   A. Tracheal deviation
   B. Decreased breath sounds
   C. Respiratory distress with hypertension
   D. Distended neck veins

Answer: C
The diagnosis of tension pneumothorax is presumed in any patient manifesting respiratory distress and hypotension in combination with any of the following physical signs: tracheal deviation away from the affected side, lack of or decreased breath sounds on the affected side, and subcutaneous emphysema on the affected side. Patients may have distended neck veins due to impedance of venous return, but the neck veins may be flat due to concurrent systemic hypovolemia. Tension pneumothorax and simple pneumothorax have similar signs, symptoms, and examination findings, but hypotension qualifies the pneumothorax as a tension pneumothorax. (See Schwartz 10th ed., p. 163.)

3. Which of the following is a cause of cardiogenic shock in a trauma patient?
   A. Hemothorax
   B. Penetrating injury to the aorta
   C. Air embolism
   D. Iatrogenic increased afterload due to pressors

Answer: C

In trauma patients the differential diagnosis of cardiogenic shock consists of a short list: (1) tension pneumothorax, (2) pericardial tamponade, (3) myocardial contusion or infarction, and (4) air embolism.

Tension pneumothorax is the most frequent cause of cardiac failure. Traumatic pericardial tamponade is most often associated with penetrating injury to the heart. As blood leaks out of the injured heart, it accumulates in the pericardial sac. Because the pericardium is not acutely distensible, the pressure in the pericardial sac rises to match that of the injured chamber. Since this pressure is usually greater than that of the right atrium, right atrial filling is impaired and right ventricular preload is reduced. This leads to decreased right ventricular output and increased central venous pressure (CVP). Increased intrapericardial pressure also impedes myocardial blood flow, which leads to subendocardial ischemia and a further reduction in cardiac output. This vicious cycle may progress insidiously with injury of the vena cava or atria, or precipitously with injury of either ventricle. With acute tamponade, as little as 100 mL of blood within the pericardial sac can produce life-threatening hemodynamic compromise. Patients usually present with a penetrating injury in proximity to the heart, and they are hypotensive and have distended neck veins or an elevated CVP. The classic findings of Beck's triad (hypotension, distended neck, and muffled heart sounds) and pulsus paradoxus are not reliable indicators of acute tamponade. Ultrasonography (US) in the emergency department (ED) using a subxiphoid or parasternal view is extremely helpful if the findings are clearly positive (Fig. 7-2); however, equivocal findings are common. Early in the course of tamponade, blood pressure (BP) and cardiac output will transiently improve with fluid administration. This may lead the surgeon to question the diagnosis or be lulled into a false sense of security. (See Schwartz 10th ed., Figure 7-5, pp. 165 and 171.)

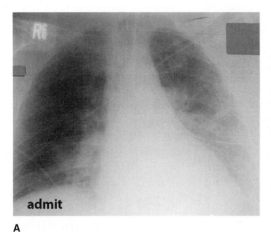

admit

A

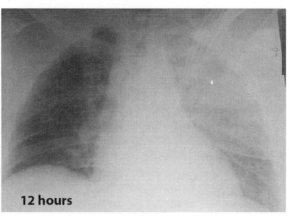

12 hours

B

FIG. 7-2. A. Admission chest film may not show the full extent of the patient's pulmonary parenchymal injury. **B.** This patient's left pulmonary contusion blossomed 12 hours later, and its associated opacity is noted on repeat chest radiograph.

4. A trauma patient arrives following a stab wound to the left chest with systolic blood pressure (SBP) 85 mm Hg, which improves slightly with intravenous (IV) fluid resuscitation. Chest X-ray demonstrates clear lung fields. What is the most appropriate next step?
   A. Computed tomography (CT) scan of the chest
   B. Pelvic X-ray
   C. Focused abdominal sonography for trauma (FAST) examination
   D. Tube thoracostomy of the left chest

Answer: C
During the circulation section of the primary survey, four life-threatening injuries must be identified promptly: (1) massive hemothorax, (2) cardiac tamponade, (3) massive hemoperitoneum, and (4) mechanically unstable pelvic fractures with bleeding.

In this patient hemothorax is unlikely given normal chest X-ray; thus, hemoperitoneum and cardiac tamponade should be suspected. Cardiac tamponade occurs most commonly after penetrating thoracic wounds, although occasionally blunt rupture of the heart, particularly the atrial appendage, is seen. Acutely, <100 mL of pericardial blood may cause pericardial tamponade. The classic Beck's triad—dilated neck veins, muffled heart tones, and a decline in arterial pressure—is usually not appreciated in the trauma bay because of the noisy environment and associated hypovolemia. Diagnosis is best achieved by bedside ultrasound of the pericardium, which is one of the four views of the FAST examination. (See Schwartz 10th ed., p. 166.)

5. Primary repair of the trachea should be carried out with
   A. Wire suture
   B. Absorbable monofilament suture
   C. Nonabsorbable monofilament suture
   D. Absorbable braided suture

Answer: B
Injuries of the trachea are repaired with a running 3-0 absorbable monofilament suture. Tracheostomy is not required in most patients. Esophageal injuries are repaired in a similar fashion. If an esophageal wound is large or if tissue is missing, a sternocleidomastoid muscle pedicle flap is warranted, and a closed suction drain is a reasonable precaution. The drain should be near but not in contact with the esophageal or any other suture line. It can be removed in 7 to 10 days if the suture line remains secure. Care must be taken when exploring the trachea and esophagus to avoid iatrogenic injury to the recurrent laryngeal nerve. (See Schwartz 10th ed., p. 202.)

6. In which patient is emergency department thoracotomy contraindicated?
   A. Motor vehicle accident victim, cardiac tamponade seen on ultrasound, SBP decreasing to 50 mm Hg.
   B. Motor vehicle accident victim, became asystolic during transport with 5 minutes of cardiopulmonary resuscitation (CPR) with no signs of life.
   C. Patient with chest stab wound, SBP decreasing to 50 mm Hg.
   D. Patient with chest stab wound, became asystolic during transport with 20 minutes of CPR with no signs of life.

Answer: D
The utility of resuscitative thoracotomy (RT) has been debated for decades. Current indications are based on 30 years of prospective data, supported by a recent multicenter prospective study. RT is associated with the highest survival rate after isolated cardiac injury; 35% of patients presenting in shock and 20% without vital signs (ie, no pulse or obtainable BP) are salvaged after isolated penetrating injury to the heart. For all penetrating wounds, survival rate is 15%. Conversely, patient outcome is poor when RT is done for blunt trauma, with 2% survival among patients in shock and <1% survival among those with no vital signs. Thus, patients undergoing cardiopulmonary resuscitation (CPR) upon arrival to the ED should undergo RT selectively based on injury and transport time. (See Schwartz 10th ed., p. 167.)

7. A patient with spontaneous eye opening, who is confused and localizes pain has a Glasgow Coma Score (GCS) of
   A. 9
   B. 11
   C. 13
   D. 15

Answer: C
The Glasgow Coma Score (GCS) should be determined for all injured patients (Table 7-1). It is calculated by adding the scores of the best motor response, best verbal response, and eye opening. Scores range from 3 (the lowest) to 15 (normal). Scores of 13 to 15 indicate mild head injury, 9 to 12 moderate injury, and less than 9 severe injury. The GCS is useful for both triage and prognosis. (See Schwartz 10th ed., Table 7-3, pp. 168 and 170.)

TABLE 7-1		Glasgow Coma Scale[a]	
		Adults	**Infants/Children**
Eye opening	4	Spontaneous	Spontaneous
	3	To voice	To voice
	2	To pain	To pain
	1	None	None
Verbal	5	Oriented	Alert, normal vocalization
	4	Confused	Cries, but consolable
	3	Inappropriate words	Persistently irritable
	2	Incomprehensible words	Restless, agitated, moaning
	1	None	None
Motor response	6	Obeys commands	Spontaneous, purposeful
	5	Localizes pain	Localizes pain
	4	Withdraws	Withdraws
	3	Abnormal flexion	Abnormal flexion
	2	Abnormal extension	Abnormal extension
	1	None	None

[a]Score is calculated by adding the scores of the best motor response, best verbal response, and eye opening. Scores range from 3 (the lowest) to 15 (normal).

8. Neck injuries
   A. Less than 15% penetrating injuries require neck exploration, a majority can be managed conservatively.
   B. Divided into three zones, with zone I above the angle of the mandible, zone II between the thoracic outlet and angle of mandible, and zone III inferior to the clavicles.
   C. All patients with neck injury should receive computed tomography angiogram (CTA) of the neck.
   D. Patients with dysphagia, hoarseness, hematoma, venous bleeding, hemoptysis, or subcutaneous emphysema should undergo neck exploration.

Answer: A
Zone I is inferior to the clavicles encompassing the thoracic outlet structures, zone II is between the thoracic outlet and the angle of the mandible, and zone III is above the angle of the mandible. Patients with symptomatic zone I and III injuries should ideally undergo diagnostic imaging before operation if they remain hemodynamically stable. Specific symptoms which indicate further imaging include dysphagia, hoarseness, hematoma, venous bleeding, minor hemoptysis, and subcutaneous emphysema. Symptomatic patients should undergo CTA with further evaluation or operation based upon the imaging findings; less than 15% of penetrating cervical trauma requires neck exploration. Asymptomatic patients are typically observed for 6 to 12 hours. The one caveat is asymptomatic patients with a transcervical gunshot wound; these patients should undergo CTA to determine the track of the bullet. CTA of the neck and chest determines trajectory of the injury tract; further studies are performed based on proximity to major structures. Angiographic diagnosis, particularly of zone III injuries, can then be managed by selective angioembolization. (See Schwartz 10th ed., p. 177.)

9. Appropriate surgical management of a through-and-through gunshot wound to the lung with minimal bleeding and some air leak is
   A. Chest tube only
   B. Oversewing entrance and exit wounds to decrease the air leak
   C. Pulmonary tractotomy with a stapler and oversewing of vessels or bronchi
   D. Wedge resection of the injured lung

Answer: C
Pulmonary injuries requiring operative intervention usually result from penetrating injury. Formerly the entrance and exit wounds were oversewn to control hemorrhage. This set the stage for air embolism, which occasionally caused sudden death in the operating room or in the immediate postoperative period. A recent development, pulmonary tractotomy, has been employed to reduce this problem as well as the need for pulmonary resection. Linear stapling devices are inserted directly into the injury tract and positioned to cause the least degree of devascularization. Two staple lines are created and the lung is divided between. This allows direct access to the bleeding vessels and leaking bronchi. No effort is made to close the defect. Lobectomy or pneumonectomy is rarely necessary. Lobectomy is only indicated for a completely devascularized

or destroyed lobe. Parenchymal injuries severe enough to require pneumonectomy are rarely survivable, and major pulmonary hilar injuries necessitating pneumonectomy are usually lethal in the field. (See Schwartz 10th ed., p. 202.)

Answer: B

The presence of abdominal rigidity and hemodynamic compromise is an undisputed indication for prompt surgical exploration. Blunt abdominal trauma is evaluated initially by FAST examination in most major trauma centers, and this has largely supplanted diagnostic peritoneal lavage (DPL). FAST is not 100% sensitive, however, so diagnostic peritoneal aspiration is warranted in hemodynamically unstable patients without a defined source of blood loss to rule out abdominal hemorrhage. This method is exquisitely sensitive for detecting intraperitoneal fluid of >250 mL. Patients with fluid on FAST examination, considered a "positive FAST," who do not have immediate indications for laparotomy and are hemodynamically stable undergo CT scanning to quantify their injuries. CT also is indicated for hemodynamically stable patients for whom the physical examination is unreliable. Despite the increasing diagnostic accuracy of multidetector CT scanners, identification of intestinal injuries remains a limitation. Patients with free intra-abdominal fluid without solid organ injury are closely monitored for evolving signs of peritonitis; if patients have a significant closed head injury or cannot be serially examined, DPL should be performed to exclude bowel injury. After placement of the catheter, a 10-mL syringe is connected and the abdominal contents aspirated (termed a *diagnostic peritoneal aspiration*). The aspirate is considered to show positive findings if >10 mL of blood is aspirated. If <10 mL is withdrawn, a liter of normal saline is instilled. The effluent is withdrawn via siphoning and sent to the laboratory for red blood cell (RBC) count, white blood cell (WBC) count, and determination of amylase, bilirubin, and alkaline phosphatase levels. See Table 7-2 for values representing positive findings. (See Schwartz 10th ed., Table 7-6, pp. 179 and 181.)

10. What is true regarding the evaluation of blunt abdominal trauma?
    A. Patients with abdominal wall rigidity and negative abdominal CT should undergo diagnostic peritoneal lavage (DPL) to rule out small bowel injury.
    B. If FAST examination is negative in a hemodynamically unstable patient then DPL is indicated to rule out abdominal bleeding.
    C. FAST examination cannot detect intraperitoneal fluid if the total volume is <1000 mL.
    D. Bowel injury can be ruled out in hemodynamically stable patients with abdominal CT scanning.

TABLE 7-2	Criteria for "positive" finding on diagnostic peritoneal lavage	
	Abdominal Trauma	**Thoracoabdominal Stab Wounds**
Red blood cell count	>100,000/mL	>10,000/mL
White blood cell count	>500/mL	>500/mL
Amylase level	>19 IU/L	>19 IU/L
Alkaline phosphatase level	>2 IU/L	>2 IU/L
Bilirubin level	>0.01 mg/dL	>0.01 mg/dL

11. After an automobile accident, a 30-year-old woman is discovered to have a posterior pelvic fracture. Hypotension and tachycardia respond marginally to volume replacement. Once it is evident that her major problem is free intraperitoneal bleeding and a pelvic hematoma in association with the fracture, appropriate management would be
   A. Application of medical antishock trousers with inflation of the extremity and abdominal sections.
   B. Arterial embolization of the pelvic vessels.
   C. Celiotomy and ligation of the internal iliac arteries bilaterally.
   D. Celiotomy and pelvic packing.
   E. External fixation application to stabilize the pelvis.

12. Which is true of vascular injuries of the extremities?
   A. In the absence of hard signs of vascular injury, if the difference between SBP in an injured limb is within 15% of the uninjured limb, no further evaluation is needed.
   B. Occult profunda femoris injuries can result in compartment syndrome and limb loss.
   C. All patients with significant hematoma should be surgically explored.
   D. Vascular injury repair should be performed prior to realignment of bony fractures or dislocations.

Answer: D

Severe pelvic bleeding is a major problem in the trauma patient. Neither external fixation nor the use of medical antishock trousers control free intra-abdominal hemorrhage regardless of its source. In the unstable patient, celiotomy is mandatory. If there is a ruptured retroperitoneal hematoma bleeding into the peritoneal cavity, control is a major problem. Internal iliac artery ligation has been abandoned as it is rarely effective. Angiography and arterial embolization may be effective with an arterial bleeding problem, but most severe pelvic hemorrhage is venous in origin. If the hematoma is stable, it is best to leave it undisturbed. However, if the hematoma has ruptured into the peritoneal cavity, pelvic packing offers the best hope of control. (See Schwartz 10th ed., p. 181.)

Answer: B

Physical examination often identifies arterial injuries, and findings are classified as either hard signs or soft signs of vascular injury (Table 7-3). In general, hard signs constitute indications for operative exploration, whereas soft signs are indications for further testing or observation. Bony fractures or knee dislocations should be realigned before definitive vascular examination. In management of vascular trauma, controversy exists regarding the treatment of patients with soft signs of injury, particularly those with injuries in proximity to major vessels. It is known that some of these patients will have arterial injuries that require repair. The most common approach has been to measure SBP using Doppler ultrasonography and compare the value for the injured side with that for the uninjured side, termed the *A-A index*. If the pressures are within 10% of each other, a significant injury is unlikely and no further evaluation is performed. If the difference is >10%, CTA or arteriography is indicated. Others argue that there are occult injuries, such as pseudoaneurysms or injuries of the profunda femoris or peroneal arteries, which may not be detected with this technique. If hemorrhage occurs from these injuries, compartment syndrome and limb loss may occur. Although busy trauma centers continue to debate this issue, the surgeon who is obliged to treat the occasional injured patient may be better served by performing CTA in selected patients with soft signs. (See Schwartz 10th ed., Table 7-8, pp. 181 and 185.)

TABLE 7-3	Signs and symptoms of peripheral arterial injury	
Hard Signs (Operation Mandatory)	**Soft Signs (Further Evaluation Indicated)**
Pulsatile hemorrhage	Proximity to vasculature
Absent pulses	Significant hematoma
Acute ischemia	Associated nerve injury
	A-A index of <0.9
	Thrill or bruit

A-A index = systolic blood pressure on the injured side compared with that on the uninjured side.

13. Which of the following statements about blunt carotid injuries is true?
    A. Magnetic resonance imaging is the diagnostic modality of choice in patients at risk.
    B. Approximately 50% of patients have a delayed diagnosis.
    C. The mechanism of injury is usually cervical flexion and rotation.
    D. Such injuries are always treated operatively when identified.

Answer: B

Blunt injury to the carotid or vertebral arteries may cause dissection, thrombosis, or pseudoaneurysm. More than one half of patients have a delayed diagnosis. Facial contact resulting in hypertension and rotation appears to be the mechanism. To reduce delayed recognition, the authors employ CTA in patients at risk, to identify these injuries before neurologic symptoms develop. The injuries frequently occur at or extend into the base of the skull and are usually not surgically accessible. Currently accepted treatment for thrombosis and dissection is anticoagulation with heparin followed by warfarin for 3 months. Pseudoaneurysms also occur near the base of the skull. If they are small, they can be followed with repeat angiography. If enlargement occurs, consideration should be given to the placement by an interventional radiologist of a stent across the aneurysm. Another possibility is to approach the intracranial portion of the carotid by removing the overlying bone and performing a direct repair. This method has only recently been described and has been performed in a limited number of patients. (See Schwartz 10th ed., p. 198.)

14. Massive transfusion protocols
    A. Should include transfusion of plasma and platelets in addition to packed RBCs
    B. Should only be initiated after blood typing, but cross-match is not needed
    C. Should be initiated in patients with tachycardia despite administration of 3.5 L of crystalloid fluids
    D. Should include testing for coagulopathies, present in 5% of patients requiring massive transfusion

Answer: A

In the critically injured patient requiring large amounts of blood component therapy, a massive transfusion protocol should be followed. This approach calls for administration of various components in a specific ratio during transfusion to achieve restoration of blood volume and correction of coagulopathy. Although the optimal ratio is yet to be determined, current scientific evidence indicates a presumptive 1:2 RBC: plasma ratio in patients at risk for massive transfusion. Because complete typing and cross-matching takes up to 45 minutes, patients requiring emergent transfusions are given type O, type-specific, or biologically compatible RBCs. Blood typing, and to a lesser extent cross-matching, is essential to avoid life-threatening intravascular hemolytic transfusion reactions (Fig. 7-3).

Injured patients with life-threatening hemorrhage develop an acute coagulopathy of trauma (ACOT). Activated protein C is a key element, although the complete mechanism remains to be elucidated. Fibrinolysis is an important component of the ACOT; present in only 5% of injured patients requiring hospitalization, but 20% in those requiring massive transfusion. (See Schwartz 10th ed., Figure 7-32, pp. 184 and 186.)

Massive Transfusion Protocol

Trigger: Uncontrolled hemorrhage
- eg, SBP <90 mm Hg Despite 3½ L Crystalloid (50 mL/kg)
- eg, EBL >150 mL/min
- eg, pH<7.1; body temperature <34°C; ISS >25

Surgery & Anesthesia Response

Continued Treatment of Shock
Hemorrhage Control
Correct Hypothermia
Correct Acidosis
Normalize Ca^{++}
Check labs q30 min as needed

Ongoing Component Therapy
PT, PTT >1.5 control ➔ 2 units thawed plasma
rapidTEG-ACT >110 sec ➔ 2 units thawed plasma

Platelet count <50,000/mcL ➔ 1 unit of apheresis platelets
rapidTEG-MA <55mm ➔ 1 unit of apheresis platelets

Fibrinogen <100 mg/dL ➔ 10 units pooled cryoprecipitate
rapidTEG-angle <63 degrees ➔ 10 units pooled cryoprecipitate

rapidTEG EPL >15% ➔ 5 g amicar

Blood Bank Response

Shipment	PRBCs	FFP	Platelets	Cryo
1	4	2		
2	4	2	1	10
3	4	2		
4	4	2	1	10

Shipments are delivered every 30 min until Massive Transfusion Protocol is terminated. Each shipment's quantity can be doubled at the request of Surgery or Anesthesia. Shipments >4 are determined by patient's clinical course and lab values.

FIG. 7-3. Denver Health Medical Center's Massive Transfusion Protocol. ACT = activated clotting time; Cryo = cryoprecipitate; EPL = estimated percent lysis; FFP = fresh frozen plasma; INR = international normalized ratio; MA = maximum amplitude; PRBCs = packed red blood cells; PT = prothrombin time; PTT = partial thromboplastin time; SBP = systolic blood pressure; TEG = thromboelastography.

15. The most appropriate treatment for a duodenal hematoma that occurs from blunt trauma is
    A. Exploratory laparotomy and bypass of the duodenum.
    B. Exploratory laparotomy and evacuation of the hematoma.
    C. Exploratory laparotomy to rule out associated injuries.
    D. Observation.

Answer: D
Duodenal hematomas are caused by a direct blow to the abdomen and occur more often in children than adults. Blood accumulates between the seromuscular and submucosal layers, eventually causing obstruction. The diagnosis is suspected by the onset of vomiting following blunt abdominal trauma; barium examination of the duodenum reveals either the coiled spring sign or obstruction. Most duodenal hematomas in children can be managed nonoperatively with nasogastric suction and parenteral nutrition. Resolution of the obstruction occurs in the majority of patients if this therapy is continued for 7 to 14 days. If surgical intervention becomes necessary, evacuation of the hematoma is associated with equal success but fewer complications than bypass procedures. Despite few existing data on adults, there is no reason to believe that their hematomas should be treated differently from those of children. A new approach is laparoscopic evacuation if the obstruction persists more than 7 days. (See Schwartz 10th ed., p. 207.)

16. Damage control surgery (DCS)
    A. Limits enteric spillage by rapid repair of partial small bowel injuries with whipstitch, and complete transection with a GIA stapling device.
    B. Aims to control surgical bleeding and identify injuries that can be managed conservatively or with interventional radiology.
    C. Is indicated when patients develop intraoperative refractory hypothermia, serum pH >7.6, or refractory coagulopathy.
    D. Abdominal wall should be closed with penetrating towel clips.

Answer: A

The goal of damage control surgery (DCS) is to control surgical bleeding and limit gastrointestinal (GI) spillage. The operative techniques used are temporary measures, with definitive repair of injuries delayed until the patient is physiologically replete. Small GI injuries (stomach, duodenum, small intestine, and colon) may be controlled using a rapid whipstitch of 2-0 polypropylene. Complete transection of the bowel or segmental damage is controlled using a GIA stapler, often with resection of the injured segment. Before the patient is returned to the surgical intensive care unit (SICU), the abdomen must be temporarily closed. Originally, penetrating towel clips were used to approximate the skin; however, the ensuing bowel edema often produces a delayed abdominal compartment syndrome. Instead, the bowel is covered with a fenestrated subfascial sterile drape (45 × 60 cm Steri-Drape 3M Health Care), and two Jackson-Pratt drains are placed along the fascial edges; this is then covered using an Ioban drape, which allows closed suction to control reperfusion-related ascitic fluid egress while providing adequate space for bowel expansion to prevent abdominal compartment syndrome. (See Schwartz 10th ed., p. 193.)

17. Therapy for increased intracranial pressure (ICP) in a patient with a closed head injury is instituted when the ICP is greater than
    A. 10
    B. 20
    C. 30
    D. 40

Answer: B

In patients with abnormal findings on CT scans and GCS scores of ≤8, intracranial pressure (ICP) should be monitored using fiberoptic intraparenchymal devices or intraventricular catheters. Although an ICP of 10 mm Hg is believed to be the upper limit of normal, therapy generally is not initiated until ICP is >20 mm Hg. Indications for operative intervention to remove space-occupying hematomas are based on the clot volume, amount of midline shift, location of the clot, GCS score, and ICP. A shift of >5 mm typically is considered an indication for evacuation, but this is not an absolute rule. (See Schwartz 10th ed., p. 195.)

18. Cerebral perfusion pressure (CPP)
    A. Equals the SBP minus ICP
    B. Should be targeted to be greater than 100 mm Hg
    C. Is lowered with sedation, osmotic diuresis, paralysis, ventricular drainage, and barbiturate coma
    D. Can be increased by lowering ICP and avoiding hypotension

Answer: D

The goal of resuscitation and management in patients with head injuries is to avoid hypotension (SBP of <100 mm Hg) and hypoxia (partial pressure of arterial oxygen of <60 or arterial oxygen saturation of <90). Attention, therefore, is focused on maintaining cerebral perfusion rather than merely lowering ICP. Resuscitation efforts aim for a euvolemic state and an SBP of >100 mm Hg. Cerebral perfusion pressure (CPP) is equal to the mean arterial pressure minus the ICP, with a target range of >50 mm Hg. CPP can be increased by either lowering ICP or raising mean arterial pressure. Sedation, osmotic diuresis, paralysis, ventricular drainage, and barbiturate coma are used in sequence, with coma induction being the last resort. (See Schwartz 10th ed., p. 195.)

19. An 18-year-old man is admitted to the ED shortly after being involved in an automobile accident. He is in a coma (GCS = 7). His pulse is barely palpable at a rate of 140 beats per minute, and BP is 60/0. Breathing is rapid and shallow, aerating both lung fields. His abdomen is moderately distended with no audible peristalsis. There are closed fractures of the right forearm and the left lower leg. After rapid IV administration of 2 L of lactated Ringer solution in the upper extremities, his pulse is 130 and BP 70/0. The next immediate step should be to
    A. Obtain cross-table lateral X-rays of the cervical spine.
    B. Obtain head and abdominal CT scans.
    C. Obtain supine and lateral decubitus X-rays of the abdomen.
    D. Obtain an arch aortogram.
    E. Explore the abdomen.

Answer: E

Ideally, a patient seriously injured in an automobile accident should undergo X-rays of the cervical spine, the chest, and the abdomen. When he has a GCS of 7, CT scans of the head are certainly desirable. If the chest X-ray shows a widened mediastinum, arch aortograms are indicated. However, this patient has had no response to a rapid fluid challenge, and if he is to survive, bleeding must be controlled immediately. The head injury, although severe, is not responsible for his hypotension and tachycardia. The most likely problem is uncontrolled abdominal hemorrhage. Immediate abdominal exploration offers the best chance for survival. (See Schwartz 10th ed., p. 164.)

20. A 36-year-old patient arrives in the trauma bay with a stab wound to the left chest. After placement of a left thoracostomy tube and fluid resuscitation, his breathing is stable with BP 160/74 mm Hg and heart rate of 110 beats per minute. CT scanning reveals a descending thoracic pseudoaneurysm and no intracranial or intra-abdominal injury. What is the most appropriate next step?
    A. Open repair with partial left heart bypass
    B. Endovascular repair with stent
    C. Esmolol drip
    D. Admission to SICU with repeat CT in 24 hours

Answer: C

Descending thoracic aortic injuries may require urgent if not emergent intervention. However, operative intervention for intracranial or intra-abdominal hemorrhage or unstable pelvic fractures takes precedence. To prevent aortic rupture, pharmacologic therapy with a selective β_1 antagonist, esmolol, should be instituted in the trauma bay, with a target SBP of <100 mm Hg and heart rate of <100 beats per minute. Endovascular stenting is now the mainstay of treatment, but open operative reconstruction is warranted, or necessary, in select patients. Endovascular techniques are particularly appropriate in patients who cannot tolerate single lung ventilation, patients older than 60 years who are at risk for cardiac decompensation with aortic clamping, or patients with uncontrolled intracranial hypertension. (See Schwartz 10th ed., p. 200.)

21. A patient with penetrating injury to the chest should undergo thoracotomy if
    A. There is more than 500 mL of blood which drains from the chest tube when placed.
    B. There is more than 200 mL/h of blood for 3 hours from the chest tube.
    C. There is an air leak that persists for >48 hours.
    D. There is documented lung injury on CT scan.

Answer: B

The most common injuries from both blunt and penetrating thoracic trauma are hemothorax and pneumothorax. More than 85% of patients can be definitively treated with a chest tube. The indications for thoracotomy include significant initial or ongoing hemorrhage from the tube thoracostomy and specific imaging-identified diagnoses. One caveat concerns the patient who presents after a delay. Even when the initial chest tube output is 1.5 L, if the output ceases and the lung is re-expanded, the patient may be managed nonoperatively, if hemodynamically stable (Table 7-4). (See Schwartz 10th ed., Table 7-10, p. 200.)

TABLE 7-4	Indications for operative treatment of thoracic injuries
• Initial tube thoracostomy drainage of >1000 mL (penetrating injury) or >1500 mL (blunt injury)
• Ongoing tube thoracostomy drainage of >200 mL/h for 3 consecutive hours in noncoagulopathic patients
• Caked hemothorax despite placement of two chest tubes
• Selected descending torn aortas
• Great vessel injury (endovascular techniques may be used in selected patients)
• Pericardial tamponade
• Cardiac herniation
• Massive air leak from the chest tube with inadequate ventilation
• Tracheal or main stem bronchial injury diagnosed by endoscopy or imaging
• Open pneumothorax
• Esophageal perforation
• Air embolism

22. After sustaining a gunshot wound to the right upper quadrant of the abdomen, the patient has no signs of peritonitis. Her vital signs are stable, and CT scan shows a grade III liver injury. What is the next step in management?
    A. Exploratory laparotomy with control of hepatic parenchymal hemorrhage.
    B. Admission to SICU with serial complete blood count.
    C. Admission to SICU with repeat CT in 24 hours.
    D. Hepatic angiography.

Answer: B

The liver's large size makes it the organ most susceptible to blunt trauma, and it is frequently involved in upper torso penetrating wounds. Nonoperative management of solid organ injuries is pursued in hemodynamically stable patients who do not have overt peritonitis or other indications for laparotomy. Patients with more than grade II injuries should be admitted to the SICU with frequent hemodynamic monitoring, determination of hemoglobin, and abdominal examination. The only absolute contraindication to nonoperative management is hemodynamic instability. Factors such as high injury grade, large hemoperitoneum, contrast extravasation, or pseudoaneurysms may predict complications or failure of nonoperative management. Angioembolization and endoscopic retrograde cholangiopancreatography (ERCP) are useful adjuncts that can improve the success rate of nonoperative management. The indication for angiography to control hepatic hemorrhage is transfusion of 4 units of RBCs in 6 hours or 6 units of RBCs in 24 hours without hemodynamic instability. (See Schwartz 10th ed., p. 203.)

23. A 25-year-old man has multiple intra-abdominal injuries after a gunshot wound. Celiotomy reveals multiple injuries to small and large bowel and major bleeding from the liver. After repair of the bowel injuries, the abdomen is closed with towel clips, leaving a large pack in the injured liver. Within 12 hours, there is massive abdominal swelling with edema fluid, and intra-abdominal pressure exceeds 35 mm Hg. The immediate step in managing this problem is to
    A. Administer albumin intercavernously
    B. Give an IV diuretic
    C. Limit IV fluid administration
    D. Open the incision to decompress the abdomen

Answer: D

Cardiac, pulmonary, and renal problems develop when invasive ascites compresses the diaphragm and the inferior vena cava. Dialysis, diuresis, and increasing serum oncotic pressure will not correct this problem rapidly enough to save the patient's life. Opening the incision relieves the intra-abdominal pressure. There are few reports of sudden hypotension after this maneuver, but volume loading has largely eliminated this problem. (See Schwartz 10th ed., p. 217.)

24. Which of the following statements is correct regarding traumatic spleen injury?
    A. An elevation in WBC to 20,000/mm³ and platelets to 300,000/mm³ on postoperative day 7 is a common benign finding in postsplenectomy patients.
    B. Delayed rebleeding or rupture will typically occur within 48 hours of injury.
    C. Common complications after splenectomy include subdiaphragmatic abscess, pancreatic tail injury, and gastric perforation.
    D. Postsplenectomy vaccines against encapsulated bacteria is optimally administered preoperatively or immediately postoperative.

Answer: C

Unlike hepatic injuries, which usually rebleed within 48 hours, delayed hemorrhage or rupture of the spleen can occur up to weeks after injury. Indications for early intervention include initiation of blood transfusion within the first 12 hours and hemodynamic instability. After splenectomy or splenorrhaphy, postoperative hemorrhage may be due to loosening of a tie around the splenic vessels, an improperly ligated or unrecognized short gastric artery, or recurrent bleeding from the spleen if splenic repair was used. An immediate postsplenectomy increase in platelets and WBCs is normal; however, beyond postoperative day 5, a WBC count above 15,000/mm³ and a platelet/WBC ratio of <20 are strongly associated with sepsis and should prompt a thorough search for underlying infection. A common infectious complication after splenectomy is a subphrenic abscess, which should be managed with percutaneous drainage. Additional sources of morbidity include a concurrent but unrecognized iatrogenic injury to the pancreatic tail during rapid splenectomy resulting in pancreatic ascites or fistula, and a gastric perforation during short gastric ligation. Enthusiasm for splenic salvage was driven by the rare, but often fatal, complication of overwhelming postsplenectomy sepsis. Overwhelming postsplenectomy sepsis is caused by encapsulated bacteria, *Streptococcus pneumoniae*, *Haemophilus influenzae*, and *Neisseria meningitidis,* which are resistant to antimicrobial treatment. In patients undergoing splenectomy, prophylaxis against these bacteria is provided via vaccines administered optimally at 14 days. (See Schwartz 10th ed., p. 206.)

25. The most appropriate treatment for a duodenal hematoma that occurs from blunt trauma is
    A. Exploratory laparotomy and bypass of the duodenum
    B. Exploratory laparotomy and evacuation of the hematoma
    C. Exploratory laparotomy to rule out associated injuries
    D. Observation

Answer: D
Duodenal hematomas are caused by a direct blow to the abdomen and occur more often in children than adults. Blood accumulates between the seromuscular and submucosal layers, eventually causing obstruction. The diagnosis is suspected by the onset of vomiting following blunt abdominal trauma; barium examination of the duodenum reveals either the coiled spring sign or obstruction. Most duodenal hematomas in children can be managed nonoperatively with nasogastric suction and parenteral nutrition. Resolution of the obstruction occurs in the majority of patients if this therapy is continued for 7 to 14 days. If surgical intervention becomes necessary, evacuation of the hematoma is associated with equal success but fewer complications than bypass procedures. Despite few existing data on adults, there is no reason to believe that their hematomas should be treated differently from those of children. A new approach is laparoscopic evacuation if the obstruction persists more than 7 days. (See Schwartz 10th ed., p. 207.)

26. A 19-year-old man fell off his skateboard, reporting blunt injury to his upper abdomen. Abdominal CT and magnetic resonance cholangiopancreatography (MRCP) confirmed he suffered transection of the main pancreatic duct at the middle of the pancreatic body. Which of the following would be the most appropriate next step in management?
    A. Nonoperative treatment
    B. Endoscopic retrograde cholangiopancreatography (ERCP) with stenting of pancreatic duct
    C. Distal pancreatectomy with splenic preservation
    D. Primary repair of pancreatic duct with closed suction drainage

Answer: C
Optimal management of pancreatic trauma is determined by where the parenchymal damage is located and whether the intrapancreatic common bile duct and main pancreatic duct remain intact. Patients with pancreatic contusions (defined as injuries that leave the ductal system intact) can be treated nonoperatively or with closed suction drainage if undergoing laparotomy for other indications. Patients with proximal pancreatic injuries, defined as those that lie to the right of the superior mesenteric vessels, are also managed with closed suction drainage. In contrast, distal pancreatic injuries are managed based upon ductal integrity. Pancreatic duct disruption can be identified through direct exploration of the parenchymal laceration, operative pancreatography, endoscopic retrograde pancreatography (ERCP), or magnetic resonance cholangiopancreatography (MRCP). Patients with distal ductal disruption undergo distal pancreatectomy, preferably with splenic preservation. An alternative, which preserves both the spleen and distal transected end of the pancreas, is either a Roux-en-Y pancreaticojejunostomy or pancreaticogastrostomy. If the patient is physiologically compromised, distal pancreatectomy with splenectomy is the preferred approach. (See Schwartz 10th ed., p. 207.)

27. The most appropriate treatment for a gunshot wound to the hepatic flexure of the colon that cannot be repaired primarily is
    A. End colostomy and mucous fistula.
    B. Loop colostomy.
    C. Exteriorized repair.
    D. Resection of the right colon with ileocolostomy.

Answer: D
Numerous large retrospective and several prospective studies have now clearly demonstrated that primary repair is safe and effective in the majority of patients with penetrating injuries. Colostomy is still appropriate in a few patients, but the current dilemma is how to select them. Exteriorized repair is probably no longer indicated since most patients who were once candidates for this treatment are now successfully managed by primary repair. Two methods have been advocated that result in 75 to 90% of penetrating colonic injuries

being safely treated by primary repair. The first is to repair all perforations not requiring resection. If resection is required due to the local extent of the injury, and it is proximal to the middle colic artery, the proximal portion of the right colon up to and including the injury is resected and an ileocolostomy performed. If resection is required distal to the middle colic artery, an end colostomy is created and the distal colon oversewn and left within the abdomen. The theory behind this approach is that an ileocolostomy heals more reliably than colocolostomy, because in the trauma patient who has suffered shock and may be hypovolemic, assessing the adequacy of the blood supply of the colon is much less reliable than in elective procedures. The blood supply of the terminal ileum is never a problem. The other approach is to repair all injuries regardless of the extent and location (including colocolostomy), and reserve colostomy for patients with protracted shock and extensive contamination. The theory used to support this approach is that systemic factors are more important than local factors in determining whether a suture line will heal. Both of these approaches are reasonable and result in the majority of patients being treated by primary repairs. When a colostomy is required, regardless of the theory used to reach that conclusion, performing a loop colostomy proximal to a distal repair should be avoided because a proximal colostomy does not protect a distal suture line. All suture lines and anastomoses are performed with the running single-layer technique. (See Schwartz 10th ed., p. 209.)

28. Which of the following statements is FALSE regarding traumatic genitourinary injury?
    A. If exploratory laparotomy is performed for trauma, all blunt and penetrating wounds to the kidneys should be explored.
    B. Renal vascular injuries are common after penetrating trauma, and can be deceptively tamponaded by surrounding fascia.
    C. Success of renal artery repair after blunt trauma is slim, but can be attempted if injury occurred within 5 hours or patient does not have any reserve renal function (solitary kidney or bilateral injury).
    D. Suspected ureteral injuries in patients with penetrating trauma or pelvic fractures can be evaluated intraoperatively with methylene blue or indigo carmine administered intravenously.
    E. Bladder injuries with extraperitoneal extravasation can be managed with Foley decompression for 2 weeks.

Answer: A
When undergoing laparotomy for trauma, the best policy is to explore all penetrating wounds to the kidneys. However, over 90% of blunt injuries are treated nonoperatively; the indications for surgery include parenchymal injuries leading to hypotension and evidence of renovascular injury. If laparotomy is performed in the setting of blunt kidney injury for other reasons, expanding or pulsatile perinephric hematomas should be explored. Injuries to the ureters are uncommon but may occur in patients with pelvic fractures and penetrating trauma. An injury may not be identified until a complication (ie, a urinoma) becomes apparent. If an injury is suspected during operative exploration but is not clearly identified, methylene blue or indigo carmine is administered IV with observation for extravasation. Bladder injuries are subdivided into those with intraperitoneal extravasation and those with extraperitoneal extravasation. Extraperitoneal ruptures are treated nonoperatively with bladder decompression for 2 weeks, whereas injuries with intraperitoneal extravasation can be closed primarily. Urethral injuries are managed by bridging the defect with a Foley catheter, with or without direct suture repair. Strictures are not uncommon but can be managed electively. (See Schwartz 10th ed., p. 211.)

29. At what pressure is operative decompression of a compartment mandatory?
    A. 15 mm Hg
    B. 25 mm Hg
    C. 35 mm Hg
    D. 45 mm Hg

Answer: D

In comatose or obtunded patients, the diagnosis is more difficult to secure. A compatible history, firmness of the compartment to palpation, and diminished mobility of the joint are suggestive. The presence or absence of a pulse distal to the affected compartment is notoriously unreliable in the diagnosis of a compartment syndrome. A frozen joint and myoglobinuria are late signs and suggest a poor prognosis. As in the abdomen, compartment pressure can be measured. The small, hand-held Stryker device is a convenient tool for this purpose. Pressures greater than 45 mm Hg usually require operative intervention. Patients with pressures between 30 and 45 mm Hg should be carefully evaluated and closely watched. (See Schwartz 10th ed., p. 215.)

30. Which is true regarding trauma in geriatric patients?
    A. Admission GCS score after severe head injury is a good predictor of outcome.
    B. Rib fractures are associated with pulmonary contusion in 35% of patients, and complicated by pneumonia in 10 to 30% of patients.
    C. Approximately 10% of patients older than 65 years will sustain a rib fracture from a fall <6 ft.
    D. Chronologic age older than 65 years is associated with higher morbidity and mortality after trauma.

Answer: B

Mortality in patients with severe head injury more than doubles after the age of 55 years. Moreover, 25% of patients with a normal GCS score of 15 had intracranial bleeding, with an associated mortality of 50%. Just as there is no absolute age that predicts outcome, admission GCS score is a poor predictor of individual outcome. Therefore, the majority of trauma centers advocate an initial aggressive approach with reevaluation at the 72-hour mark to determine subsequent care. Secondly, one of the most common sequelae of blunt thoracic trauma is rib fractures. In fact, in one study, 50% of patients older than 65 years sustained rib fractures from a fall of <6 ft, compared with only 1% of patients younger than 65 years. Concurrent pulmonary contusion is noted in up to 35% of patients, and pneumonia complicates the injuries in 10 to 30% of patients with rib fractures. (See Schwartz 10th ed., p. 221.)

1. A 22-year-old man is brought to the emergency room after a house fire. He has burns around his mouth and his voice is hoarse, but breathing is unlabored. What most appropriate next step in management?
   A. Immediate endotracheal intubation.
   B. Examination of oral cavity and pharynx, with fiberoptic laryngoscope if available.
   C. Place on supplemental oxygen.
   D. Placement of two large-bore intravenous (IV) catheters with fluid resuscitation.

Answer: B
With direct thermal injury to the upper airway or smoke inhalation, rapid and severe airway edema is a potentially lethal threat. Anticipating the need for intubation and establishing an early airway is critical. Perioral burns and singed nasal hair are signs that the oral cavity and pharynx should be further evaluated for mucosal injury, but these physical findings alone do not indicate an upper airway injury. Signs of impending respiratory compromise may include a hoarse voice, wheezing, or stridor; subjective dyspnea is a particularly concerning symptom, and should trigger prompt elective endotracheal intubation. In patients with combined multiple trauma, especially oral trauma, nasotracheal intubation may be useful but should be avoided if oral intubation is safe and easy. (See Schwartz 10th ed., p. 227.)

2. What percentage burn does a patient have who has suffered burns to one leg (circumferential), one arm (circumferential), and the anterior trunk?
   A. 18%
   B. 27%
   C. 36%
   D. 45%

Answer: D
A general idea of the burn size can be made by using the rule of nines. Each upper extremity accounts for 9% of the total body surface area (TBSA), each lower extremity accounts for 18%, the anterior and posterior trunk each accounts for 18%, the head and neck account for 9%, and the perineum accounts for 1%. Although the rule of nines is reasonably accurate for adults, a number of more precise charts have been developed that are particularly helpful in assessing pediatric burns. Most emergency rooms have such a chart. A diagram of the burn can be drawn on the chart, and more precise calculations of the burn size made from the accompanying TBSA estimates given.

Children younger than 4 years have much larger heads and smaller thighs in proportion to total body size than do adults. In infants the head accounts for nearly 20% of the TBSA; a child's body proportions do not fully reach adult percentages until adolescence. Even when using precise diagrams, interobserver variation may vary by as much as ±20%. An observer's experience with burned patients, rather than educational level, appears to be the best predictor of the accuracy of burn size estimation. For smaller burns, an accurate assessment of size can be made by using the patient's palmar hand surface, including the digits, which amounts for approximately 1% of TBSA. (See Schwartz 10th ed., p. 229.)

3. A 40-year-old woman is admitted to the burn unit after an industrial fire at a plastics manufacturing plant with burns to the face and arms. Her electrocardiogram (ECG) shows S-T elevation, and initial chemistry panel and arterial blood gas reveal an anion gap metabolic acidosis with normal arterial carboxyhemoglobin. What is the most appropriate next step?
   A. Correction of acidosis by adding sodium bicarbonate to IV fluids.
   B. Administration of 100% oxygen and hydroxocobalamin.
   C. Transthoracic echocardiogram.
   D. Blood culture with IV antibiotics.

4. Which of the following is a common sequelae of electrical injury?
   A. Cardiac arrhythmias
   B. Paralysis
   C. Brain damage
   D. Cataracts

Answer: B

Hydrogen cyanide toxicity may also be a component of smoke inhalation injury. Afflicted patients may have a persistent lactic acidosis or S-T elevation on ECG. Cyanide inhibits cytochrome oxidase, which is required for oxidative phosphorylation. Treatment consists of sodium thiosulfate, hydroxocobalamin, and 100% oxygen. Sodium thiosulfate works by transforming cyanide into a nontoxic thiocyanate derivative, but it works slowly and is not effective for acute therapy. Hydroxocobalamin quickly complexes with cyanide and is excreted by the kidney, and is recommended for immediate therapy. In the majority of patients, the lactic acidosis will resolve with ventilation and sodium thiosulfate treatment becomes unnecessary. (See Schwartz 10th ed., p. 228.)

Answer: D

Myoglobinuria frequently accompanies electrical burns, but the clinical significance appears to be trivial. Disruption of muscle cells releases cellular debris and myoglobin into the circulation to be filtered by the kidney. If this condition is untreated, the consequence can be irreversible renal failure. However, modern burn resuscitation protocols alone appear to be sufficient treatment for myoglobinuria.

Cardiac damage, such as myocardial contusion or infarction, may be present. More likely, the conduction system may be deranged. Household current at 110 V either does no damage or induces ventricular fibrillation. If there are no electrocardiographic rhythm abnormalities present upon initial emergency department evaluation, the likelihood that they will appear later is minuscule. Even with high-voltage injuries, a normal cardiac rhythm on admission generally means that subsequent dysrhythmia is unlikely. Studies confirm that commonly measured cardiac enzymes bear little correlation to cardiac dysfunction, and elevated enzymes may be from skeletal muscle damage. Mandatory ECG monitoring and cardiac enzyme analysis in an ICU setting for 24 hours following injury is unnecessary in patients with electrical burns, even those resulting from high-voltage current, in patients who have stable cardiac rhythms on admission.

The nervous system is exquisitely sensitive to electricity. The most devastating injury with frequent brain damage occurs when current passes through the head, but spinal cord damage is possible whenever current has passed from one side of the body to the other. Schwann cells are quite susceptible, and delayed transverse myelitis can occur days or weeks after injury. Conduction initially remains normal through existing myelin, but as myelin wears out, it is not replaced and conduction ceases. Anterior spinal artery syndrome from vascular dysregulation can also precipitate spinal cord dysfunction. Damage to peripheral nerves is common and may cause permanent functional impairment. Every patient with an electrical injury must have a thorough neurologic examination as part of the initial assessment. Persistent neurologic symptoms may lead to chronic pain syndromes, and posttraumatic stress disorders are apparently more common after electrical burns than thermal burns.

Cataracts are a well-recognized sequela of high-voltage electrical burns. They occur in 5 to 7% of patients, frequently are bilateral, occur even in the absence of contact points on the head, and typically manifest within 1 to 2 years of injury. Electrically injured patients should undergo a thorough ophthalmologic examination early during their acute care. (See Schwartz 10th ed., p. 229.)

5. An 8-year-old boy is brought to the emergency room after accidentally touching a hot iron with his forearm. On examination, the burned area has weeping blisters and is very tender to the touch. What is the burn depth?
   A. First degree
   B. Second degree
   C. Third degree
   D. Fourth degree

Answer: B

Burn wounds are commonly classified as superficial (first degree), partial thickness (second degree), full thickness (third degree), and fourth degree burns, which affect underlying soft tissue. Partial thickness burns are classified as either superficial or deep partial thickness burns by depth of involved dermis. Clinically, first-degree burns are painful but do not blister, second-degree burns have dermal involvement and are extremely painful with weeping and blisters, and third-degree burns are leathery, painless, and nonblanching. (See Schwartz 10th ed., p. 229.)

6. Three hours after a burn injury that consisted of circumferential, third-degree burns at the wrist and elbow of the right arm, a patient loses sensation to light touch in his fingers. Motor function of his digits, however, remains intact. The most appropriate treatment for this patient now would consist of
   A. Elevation of the extremity, Doppler ultrasonography every 4 hours, and if distal pulses are absent 8 hours later, immediate escharotomy.
   B. Palpation for distal pulses and immediate escharotomy if pulses are absent.
   C. Doppler ultrasonography for assessment of peripheral flow and immediate escharotomy if flow is decreased.
   D. Immediate escharotomy under general anesthesia from above the elbow to below the wrist on both medial and lateral aspects of the arm.

Answer: C

Third-degree burn injuries are characterized by almost complete loss of elasticity of the skin. Thus, as soft tissue swelling progresses, neurovascular compromise may occur. Failure to recognize this problem may result in the loss of distal extremities. The most reliable signs of decreased peripheral blood flow in burned patients are slow capillary refill as observed in the nail beds, the onset of neurologic deficits, and decreased or absent Doppler ultrasonic pulse detection. When vascular impairment is diagnosed, immediate escharotomies are indicated. Anesthesia is not required for escharotomy—the burn area is insensate because skin nerve endings are destroyed by third-degree burns. (See Schwartz 10th ed., p. 234.)

7. What is the fluid requirement of a 50-kg man with first-degree burns to his left arm and leg, circumferential second-degree burn to his right arm, and third-degree burns to his torso and right leg. What is the rate of initial fluid resuscitation?
   A. 4.5 L over 8 hours, followed by 4.5 L over 16 hours
   B. 4.5 L over 8 hours, followed by 6 L over 16 hours
   C. 6 L over 8 hours, followed by 6 L over 16 hours
   D. 6 L over 8 hours, followed by 9 L over 16 hours

Answer: A

The most commonly used formula, the Parkland or Baxter formula, consists of 3 to 4 mL/kg/% burn of lactated Ringer solution, of which half is given during the first 8 hours postburn, and the remaining half over the subsequent 16 hours. The concept behind continuous fluid requirements is simple. The burn (and/or inhalation injury) drives an inflammatory response that leads to capillary leak; as plasma leaks into the extravascular space, crystalloid administration maintains the intravascular volume. Therefore, if a patient receives a large fluid bolus in a prehospital setting or emergency department that fluid has likely leaked into the interstitium and the patient still requires ongoing burn resuscitation according to the estimates. Continuation of fluid volumes should depend on the time since injury, urine output, and mean arterial pressure. As the leak closes, the patient will require less volume to maintain these two resuscitation end points. (See Schwartz 10th ed., p. 230.)

8. A patient with a 90% burn encompassing the entire torso develops an increasing Pco_2 and peak inspiratory pressure. Which of the following is most likely to resolve this problem?
   A. Increase the delivered tidal volume.
   B. Increase the respiratory rate.
   C. Increase the Fio_2.
   D. Perform a thoracic escharotomy.

Answer: D

The adequacy of respiration must be monitored continuously throughout the resuscitation period. Early respiratory distress may be due to the compromise of ventilation caused by chest wall inelasticity related to a deep circumferential burn wound of the thorax. Pressures required for ventilation increase and arterial Pco_2 rises. Inhalation injury, pneumothorax, or other causes can also result in respiratory distress and should be appropriately treated.

Thoracic escharotomy is seldom required, even with a circumferential chest wall burn. When required, escharotomies are performed bilaterally in the anterior axillary lines. If there is significant extension of the burn onto the adjacent abdominal wall, the escharotomy incisions should be extended to this area by a transverse incision along the costal margins. (See Schwartz 10th ed., p. 230.)

9. Which of the following is FALSE regarding silver sulfadiazine?
   A. Used as prophylaxis against burn wound infections with a wide range of antimicrobial activity.
   B. Safe to use on full and partial thickness burn wounds, as well as skin grafts.
   C. Has limited systemic absorption.
   D. May inhibit epithelial migration in partial thickness wound healing.

Answer: B
Silver sulfadiazine is one of the most widely used in clinical practice. Silver sulfadiazine has a wide range of antimicrobial activity, primarily as prophylaxis against burn wound infections rather than treatment of existing infections. It has the added benefits of being inexpensive and easily applied, and has soothing qualities. It is not significantly absorbed systemically and thus has minimal metabolic derangements. Silver sulfadiazine has a reputation for causing neutropenia, but this association is more likely due to neutrophil margination from the inflammatory response. True allergic reactions to the sulfa component of silver sulfadiazine are rare, and at-risk patients can have a small test patch applied to identify a burning sensation or rash. Silver sulfadiazine destroys skin grafts and is contraindicated on burns or donor sites in proximity to newly grafted areas. Also, silver sulfadiazine may retard epithelial migration in healing partial thickness wounds. (See Schwartz 10th ed., p. 232.)

10. Successful antibiotic penetration of a burn eschar can be achieved with
    A. Mafenide acetate
    B. Neomycin
    C. Silver nitrate
    D. Silver sulfadiazine

Answer: A
Mafenide acetate is the antibiotic agent that penetrates burn eschar to reach the interface with the patient's viable tissue. This agent has the disadvantages that it is quite painful on any partial thickness areas, and it is a carbonic anhydrase inhibitor that interferes with renal buffering mechanisms. Chloride is retained, and metabolic acidosis results. For these reasons, silver sulfadiazine is more commonly used in burn centers unless a major problem with burn wound sepsis is present. (See Schwartz 10th ed., p. 232.)

11. Which of the following is true regarding nutritional needs of burn patients?
    A. The hypermetabolic response to burn wounds typically raises the basic metabolic rate by 120%.
    B. Oxandrolone, an anabolic steroid, can improve lean body mass but can be associated with hyperglycemia and clinically significant rise in hepatic transaminitis.
    C. Early enteral feeding is safe when burns are less than 20% TBSA, otherwise enteral feeding should await return of bowel function to avoid feeding a patient with gastric ileus.
    D. For patients with greater than 40% TBSA, caloric needs are estimated to be 25 kcal/kg/day plus 40 kcal/%TBSA/day.

Answer: D
The hypermetabolic response in burn injury may raise baseline metabolic rates by as much as 200%. This can lead to catabolism of muscle proteins and decreased lean body mass that may delay functional recovery. Early enteral feeding for patients with burns larger than 20% TBSA is safe, and may reduce loss of lean body mass, slow the hypermetabolic response, and result in more efficient protein metabolism.

Calculating the appropriate caloric needs of the burn patient can be challenging. A commonly used formula in nonburned patients is the Harris-Benedict equation, which calculates caloric needs using factors such as gender, age, height, and weight. This formula uses an activity factor for specific injuries, and for burns, the basal energy expenditure is multiplied by two. The Harris-Benedict equation may be inaccurate in burns of less than 40% TBSA, and in these patients the Curreri formula may be more appropriate. This formula estimates caloric needs to be 25 kcal/kg/day plus 40 kcal/%TBSA/day.

The anabolic steroid oxandrolone has been extensively studied in pediatric patients as well, and has demonstrated improvements in lean body mass and bone density in severely burned children. The weight gain and functional improvements seen with oxandrolone may persist even after stopping administration of the drug. A recent double-blinded, randomized study of oxandrolone showed decreased length of stay, improved hepatic protein synthesis, and no adverse effects on the endocrine function, though the authors noted a rise in transaminases with unclear clinical significance. (See Schwartz 10th ed., p. 232.)

12. A 14-year-old girl sustains a steam burn measuring 6 by 7 inches over the ulnar aspect of her right forearm. Blisters develop over the entire area of the burn wound, and by the time the patient is seen 6 hours after the injury, some of the blisters have ruptured spontaneously. All of the following therapeutic regimens might be considered appropriate for this patient EXCEPT
A. Application of silver sulfadiazine cream (Silvadene) and daily washes, but no dressing.
B. Application of mafenide acetate cream (Sulfamylon), but no daily washes or dressing.
C. Homograft application without sutures to secure it in place, but no daily washes or dressing.
D. Heterograft (pigskin) application with sutures to secure it in place and daily washes, but no dressing.

Answer: D
A number of different acceptable regimens exist for treating small, superficial second-degree burn injuries. In all cases, the necrotic epithelium is first debrided. Topical antibacterial agents then may be applied and the wounds treated open or closed with dressings changed daily or every other day. Biologic dressings (homografts or heterografts) may be applied to superficial second-degree burns at the time of initial debridement. Typically, these dressings quickly adhere to the wounds, relieve pain, and promote rapid epithelialization. These dressings should not be sutured in place, however, because suturing creates the potential for a closed-space infection and for conversion of a second degree to a full-thickness injury. If a biologic dressing does not adhere, it should be removed immediately, and the wound should then be treated with topical antibacterial agents. (See Schwartz 10th ed., p. 234.)

13. Which is FALSE concerning surgical treatment of burn wounds?
A. Tangential excision consists of tangential slices of burn tissue until bleeding tissue is encountered. Thus, excision can be associated with potentially significant blood loss.
B. Human cadaveric allograft is a permanent alternative to split-thickness skin grafts when there are insufficient donor sites.
C. Bleeding from tangential excision can be helped with injection of epinephrine tumescence solution, pneumatic tourniquets, epinephrine soaked compresses, and fibrinogen and thrombin spray sealant.
D. Meshed split thickness skin grafts allow serosanguinous drainage to prevent graft loss and provide a greater area of wound coverage.

Answer: B
The strategy of early excision and grafting in burned patients revolutionized survival outcomes in burn care. Excision is performed with repeated tangential slices using a Watson or Goulian blade until viable, diffusely bleeding tissue remains. The downside of tangential excision is a high blood loss, though this may be ameliorated using techniques such as instillation of an epinephrine tumescence solution underneath the burn. Pneumatic tourniquets are helpful in extremity burns, and compresses soaked in a dilute epinephrine solution are necessary adjuncts after excision. A fibrinogen and thrombin spray sealant (Tisseel Fibrin Sealant; Baxter, Deerfield, IL) also has beneficial effects on both hemostasis and graft adherence to the wound bed.

Since full thickness burns are impractical for most burn wounds, split-thickness sheet autografts harvested with a power dermatome make the most durable wound coverings, and have a decent cosmetic appearance. In larger burns, meshed autografted skin provides a larger area of wound coverage. This also allows drainage of blood and serous fluid to prevent accumulation under the skin graft with subsequent graft loss. Areas of cosmetic importance, such as the face, neck, and hands, should be grafted with nonmeshed sheet grafts to ensure optimal appearance and function. Options for temporary wound coverage include human cadaveric allograft, which is incorporated into the wound but is rejected by the immune system and must be eventually replaced.(See Schwartz 10th ed., p. 234.)

14. A 45-year-old woman is admitted to a hospital because of a third-degree burn injury to 40% of her TBSA, and her wounds are treated with topical silver sulfadiazine cream (Silvadene). Three days after admission, a burn wound biopsy semiquantitative culture shows 10^4 *Pseudomonas* organisms per gram of tissue. The patient's condition is stable at this time. The most appropriate management for this patient would be to
   A. Repeat the biopsy and culture in 24 hours.
   B. Start subeschar clysis with antibiotics.
   C. Administer systemic antibiotics.
   D. Surgically excise the burn wounds.

Answer: B
Bacterial proliferation in a burn wound may occur despite topical antibacterial agents. When bacterial proliferation has escaped control, as proved by quantitative burn wound biopsy, administration of antibiotics by needle clysis beneath the eschar is indicated. This therapy is most effective if initiated early, before invasive burn wound sepsis has developed or wound colonization has reached greater than 10^4 organisms per gram of tissue. Systemic antibiotics usually are ineffective at this point because by the third day after a burn, blood flow to a burn wound is markedly decreased. Thus, adequate levels of antibiotic are not achieved at the eschar-viable tissue interface where the bacterial proliferation is occurring. Before the use of subeschar antibiotics, *Pseudomonas* sepsis of burn wounds accompanied by ecthyma gangrenosum was uniformly fatal in children. Once colonization of a burn wound has occurred, surgical excision is extremely dangerous, as systemic seeding will occur. (See Schwartz 10th ed., p. 232.)

15. Fourteen days after admission to the hospital for a 30% partial thickness burn and hemodynamic instability requiring central venous access, a patient develops a spiking temperature curve. On physical examination, the central venous catheter insertion site was red, tender, and warm. The best treatment for this complication is to
   A. Exchange of central venous catheter over guidewire, culture tip of previous catheter.
   B. Treat patient with IV antibiotics until blood cultures drawn from catheter are negative.
   C. Removal of central venous catheter, culture tip, and placement of new catheter on contralateral site.
   D. Removal of catheter and treat patient with oral antibiotics and pain medication as needed.

Answer: C
Burn patients often require central venous access for fluid resuscitation and hemodynamic monitoring. Because of the anatomic relation of their burns to commonly used access sites, burn patients may be at higher risk for catheter-related bloodstream infections. The 2009 CDC NHSN report (http://www.cdc.gov/nhsn/dataStat.html) indicates that American burn centers have higher infectious complication rates than any other ICUs. Because burn patients may commonly exhibit leukocytosis with a documented bloodstream infection, practice has been to rewire lines over a guidewire and to culture the catheter tip. However, this may increase the risk of catheter-related infections in burned patients and a new site should be used if at all possible. (See Schwartz 10th ed., p. 233.)

CHAPTER 9

Wound Healing

1. Which of the following is FALSE regarding polymorpho-nuclear neutrophils (PMNs) and their role in wound healing?
   A. PMNs release proteases that degrade ground substance within the wound site.
   B. Neutrophils use fibrin clot generated at the wound site as scaffolding for migration into the wound.
   C. Neutrophil migration is stimulated by local prosta-glandins, complement factors, interleukin-1 (IL-1), tumor necrosis factor-α (TNF-α), transforming growth factor-β (TGF-β), platelet factor 4, or bacterial products.
   D. PMNs are the first cells to infiltrate the wound, peaking at 24 to 48 hours.
   E. Neutrophils release cytokines that later assist with col-lagen deposition and epithelial closure.

Answer: E

Polymorphonuclear neutrophils (PMNs) are the first infiltrating cells to enter the wound site, peaking at 24 to 48 hours. Increased vascular permeability, local prostaglandin release, and the pres-ence of chemotactic substances such as complement factors, interleukin-1 (IL-1), tumor necrosis factor-α (TNF-α), trans-forming growth factor-β (TGF-β), platelet factor 4, or bacterial products all stimulate neutrophil migration.

The postulated primary role of neutrophils is phagocytosis of bacteria and tissue debris. PMNs are also a major source of cytokines early during inflammation, especially TNF-α, which may have a significant influence on subsequent angio-genesis and collagen synthesis. PMNs also release proteases such as collagenases, which participate in matrix and ground substance degradation in the early phase of wound healing. Other than their role in limiting infections, these cells do not appear to play a role in collagen deposition or acquisition of mechanical wound strength. On the contrary, neutrophil fac-tors have been implicated in delaying the epithelial closure of wounds. (See Schwartz 10th ed., p. 243.)

2. The proliferative phase of wound healing occurs how long after the injury?
   A. 1 day
   B. 2 days
   C. 7 days
   D. 14 days

Answer: C

Normal wound healing follows a predictable pattern that can be divided into overlapping phases defined by the cel-lular populations and biochemical activities: (1) hemostasis and inflammation, (2) proliferation, and (3) maturation and remodeling.

The proliferative phase is the second phase of wound heal-ing and roughly spans days 4 through 12. It is during this phase that tissue continuity is reestablished. Fibroblasts and endothelial cells are the last cell populations to infiltrate the healing wound, and the strongest chemotactic factor for fibroblasts is platelet-derived growth factor (PDGF). Upon entering the wound environment, recruited fibroblasts first need to proliferate, and then become activated, to carry out their primary function of matrix synthesis remodeling. This activation is mediated mainly by the cytokines and growth factors released from wound macrophages. (See Schwartz 10th ed., p. 241.)

3. Which of the following is true regarding the fibroblastic phase of wound healing?
   A. Early during wound healing, the predominant composititon of the matrix is fibronectin and type II collagen.
   B. After complete replacement of the scar with type III collagen, the mechanical strength will equal that of uninjured tissue approximately 6 to 12 months postinjury.
   C. Even though the tensile strength of a wound reaches a plateau after several weeks, the tensile strength will increase over another 6 to 12 months due to fibril formation and cross-linking.
   D. As the scar matures, matrix metalloproteinases (MMPs) break down type I collagen and replace it with type III collagen.

Answer: C

The maturation and remodeling of the scar begins during the fibroblastic phase, and is characterized by a reorganization of previously synthesized collagen. Collagen is broken down by matrix metalloproteinases (MMPs), and the net wound collagen content is the result of a balance between collagenolysis and collagen synthesis. There is a net shift toward collagen synthesis and eventually the reestablishment of extracellular matrix composed of a relatively acellular collagen-rich scar.

Wound strength and mechanical integrity in the fresh wound are determined by both the quantity and quality of the newly deposited collagen. The deposition of matrix at the wound site follows a characteristic pattern: fibronectin and collagen type III constitute the early matrix scaffolding; glycosaminoglycans and proteoglycans represent the next significant matrix components; and collagen type I is the final matrix. By several weeks postinjury the amount of collagen in the wound reaches a plateau, but the tensile strength continues to increase for several more months. Fibril formation and fibril cross-linking result in decreased collagen solubility, increased strength, and increased resistance to enzymatic degradation of the collagen matrix. Fibrillin, a glycoprotein secreted by fibroblasts, is essential for the formation of elastic fibers found in connective tissue. Scar remodeling continues for many (6–12) months postinjury, gradually resulting in a mature, avascular, and acellular scar. The mechanical strength of the scar never achieves that of the uninjured tissue. (See Schwartz 10th ed., p. 245.)

4. Which of the following is commonly seen in Ehlers-Danlos syndrome (EDS)?
   A. Small bowel obstructions.
   B. Spontaneous thrombosis.
   C. Direct or recurrent hernias in children.
   D. Abnormal scarring of the hands with contractures.

Answer: C

Ehlers-Danlos syndrome (EDS) is a group of 10 disorders that present as a defect in collagen formation. Over half of the affected patients manifest genetic defects encoding alpha chains of collagen type V, causing it to be either quantitatively or structurally defective. These changes lead to "classic" EDS with phenotypic findings that include thin, friable skin with prominent veins, easy bruising, poor wound healing, atrophic scar formation, recurrent hernias, and hyperextensible joints. Gastrointestinal (GI) problems include bleeding, hiatal hernia, intestinal diverticula, and rectal prolapse. Small blood vessels are fragile, making suturing difficult during surgery. Large vessels may develop aneurysms, varicosities, arteriovenous fistulas, or may spontaneously rupture. (See Schwartz 10th ed., p. 246.)

5. Patients with Marfan syndrome are associated with what genetic decect?
   A. *MFN-1* gene deletion
   B. Type I collagen gene mutation
   C. *COL7A1* gene mutation
   D. *FBN-1* gene mutation

Answer: D

Patients with Marfan's syndrome have tall stature, arachnodactyly, lax ligaments, myopia, scoliosis, pectus excavatum, and aneurysm of the ascending aorta. Patients who suffer from this syndrome are also prone to hernias. Surgical repair of a dissecting aneurysm is difficult, as the soft connective tissue fails to hold sutures. Skin may be hyperextensible, but shows no delay in wound healing.

The genetic defect associated with Marfan's syndrome is a mutation in the *FBN-1* gene which encodes for fibrillin. Previously, it was thought that structural alteration of the microfibrillar system was responsible for the phenotypic changes seen with the disease. However, recent research indicates an intricate relationship that *FBN-1* gene products play in TGF-β signaling. (See Schwartz 10th ed., p. 246.)

6. When a long bone fracture is repaired by internal fixation with plates and screws
   A. Callus at the fracture site forms more rapidly.
   B. Delayed union is prevented.
   C. Direct bone-to-bone healing occurs without soft callus formation.
   D. Endochondral ossification is more complete.

7. Which of the following is FALSE regarding healing of full-thickness injuries of the GI tract?
   A. Serosal healing is essential to form a water-tight barrier to the lumen of the bowel.
   B. Extraperitoneal segments of bowel that lack serosa have higher rates of anastomotic failure.
   C. There is an early decrease in marginal strength due to an imbalance of greater collagenolysis versus collagen synthesis.
   D. Collagen synthesis is done by fibroblast and smooth muscle cells.
   E. The greatest tensile strength of the GI tract is provided by the serosa.

8. Steroids impair wound healing by
   A. Decreasing angiogenesis and macrophage migration
   B. Decreasing platelet plug integrity
   C. Increasing release of lysosomal enzymes
   D. Increasing fibrinolysis

Answer: C

Precise fracture reduction and fixation allows the fracture to heal bone-to-bone without the soft callus formation and endochondral ossification, which are characteristic of closed fracture management. However, internal reduction does not prevent delayed union, especially when infection or poor blood supply are present. (See Schwartz 10th ed., p. 249.)

Answer: E

The submucosa lies radially and circumferentially outside of these layers, is composed of abundant collagenous and elastic fibers, and supports neural and vascular structures. The submucosa is the layer that imparts the greatest tensile strength and greatest suture-holding capacity, a characteristic that should be kept in mind during surgical repair of the GI tract. Additionally, serosal healing is essential for quickly achieving a watertight seal from the luminal side of the bowel. The importance of the serosa is underscored by the significantly higher rates of anastomotic failure observed clinically in segments of bowel that are extraperitoneal and lack serosa (ie, the esophagus and rectum).

The early integrity of the anastomosis is dependent on formation of a fibrin seal on the serosal side, which achieves watertightness, and on the suture-holding capacity of the intestinal wall, particularly the submucosal layer. There is a significant decrease in marginal strength during the first week due to an early and marked collagenolysis. The lysis of collagen is carried out by collagenase derived from neutrophils, macrophages, and intraluminal bacteria. Collagenase activity occurs early in the healing process, and during the first 3 to 5 days collagen breakdown far exceeds collagen synthesis. The integrity of the anastomosis represents equilibrium between collagen lysis, which occurs early, and collagen synthesis, which takes a few days to initiate. Collagen synthesis in the GI tract is carried out by both fibroblasts and smooth muscle cells. (See Schwartz 10th ed., p. 249.)

Answer: A

The major effect of steroids is to inhibit the inflammatory phase of wound healing (angiogenesis, neutrophil and macrophage migration, and fibroblast proliferation) and the release of lysosomal enzymes. The stronger the anti-inflammatory effect of the steroid compound used, the greater the inhibitory effect on wound healing. Steroids used after the first 3 to 4 days postinjury do not affect wound healing as severely as when they are used in the immediate postoperative period. Therefore if possible, their use should be delayed or, alternatively, forms with lesser anti-inflammatory effects should be administered.

In addition to their effect on collagen synthesis, steroids also inhibit epithelialization and contraction and contribute to increased rates of wound infection, regardless of the time of administration. Steroid-delayed healing of cutaneous wounds can be stimulated to epithelialize by topical application of vitamin A. Collagen synthesis of steroid-treated wounds also can be stimulated by vitamin A. (See Schwartz 10th ed., p. 253.)

9. What type of nerve injury involves disruption of axonal continuity with preserved Schwann cell basal lamina?
   A. Neurapraxia
   B. Axonotemesis
   C. Neurotmesis
   D. Axonolysis

Answer: B

There are three types of nerve injuries: neurapraxia (focal demyelination), axonotmesis (interruption of axonal continuity but preservation of Schwann cell basal lamina), and neurotmesis (complete transection). Following all types of injury, the nerve ends progress through a predictable pattern of changes involving three crucial steps: (1) survival of axonal cell bodies; (2) regeneration of axons that grow across the transected nerve to reach the distal stump; and (3) migration and connection of the regenerating nerve ends to the appropriate nerve ends or organ targets.

Phagocytes remove the degenerating axons and myelin sheath from the distal stump (Wallerian degeneration). Regenerating axonal sprouts extend from the proximal stump and probe the distal stump and the surrounding tissues. Schwann cells ensheathe and help in remyelinating the regenerating axons. Functional units are formed when the regenerating axons connect with the appropriate end targets. (See Schwartz 10th ed., p. 251.)

10. The major cause of impaired wound healing is
    A. Anemia
    B. Diabetes mellitus
    C. Local tissue infection
    D. Malnutrition

Answer: C

All the factors listed impair wound healing, but local infection is the major problem. The surgeon should make every effort to remove all devitalized tissue and leave a clean wound for closure. (See Schwartz 10th ed., p. 252.)

11. How does diabetes mellitus impair wound healing?
    A. Local hypoxemia, reduced angiogenesis, and inflammation due to vascular disease.
    B. Glycosylation of proteoglycans and collagen in wound bed due to hyperglycemia.
    C. Decreased collagen accretion noted in patients with type II diabetes mellitus.
    D. Increased bacterial load to due to hyperglycemia.

Answer: A

Uncontrolled diabetes results in reduced inflammation, angiogenesis, and collagen synthesis. Additionally, the large and small vessel disease that is the hallmark of advanced diabetes contributes to local hypoxemia. Defects in granulocyte function, capillary ingrowth, and fibroblast proliferation all have been described in diabetes. Obesity, insulin resistance, hyperglycemia, and diabetic renal failure contribute significantly and independently to the impaired wound healing observed in diabetics. (See Schwartz 10th ed., p. 253.)

12. Supplementation of which of the following micronutrients improves wound healing in patients without micronutrient deficiency?
    A. Vitamin C
    B. Vitamin A
    C. Selenium
    D. Zinc

Answer: B

The vitamins most closely involved with wound healing are vitamin C and vitamin A. There is no evidence that excess vitamin C is toxic; however, there is no evidence that supertherapeutic doses of vitamin C are of any benefit.

Vitamin A deficiency impairs wound healing, while supplemental vitamin A benefits wound healing in nondeficient humans and animals. Vitamin A increases the inflammatory response in wound healing, probably by increasing the lability of lysosomal membranes. There is an increased influx of macrophages, with an increase in their activation and increased collagen synthesis. Vitamin A directly increases collagen production and epidermal growth factor receptors when it is added in vitro to cultured fibroblasts. As mentioned before, supplemental vitamin A can reverse the inhibitory effects of corticosteroids on wound healing. Vitamin A also can restore wound healing that has been impaired by diabetes, tumor formation, cyclophosphamide, and radiation. Serious injury or stress leads to increased vitamin A requirements. In the severely injured patient, supplemental doses of vitamin A have been recommended. Doses ranging from 25,000 to 100,000 IU/day have been advocated.

Zinc is the most well-known element in wound healing and has been used empirically in dermatologic conditions for centuries. To date, no study has shown improved wound healing with zinc supplementation in patients who are not zinc deficient. (See Schwartz 10th ed., p. 255.)

13. Which type of collagen is most important in wound healing?
   A. Type III
   B. Type V
   C. Type VII
   D. Type XI

Answer: A

Although there are at least 18 types of collagen described, the main ones of interest to wound repair are types I and III. Type I collagen is the major component of extracellular matrix in skin. Type III, which is also normally present in skin, becomes more prominent and important during the repair process. (See Schwartz 10th ed., p. 244.)

14. What is FALSE regarding healing of cartilage?
   A. Cartilage is avascular and depends on diffusion of nutrients.
   B. Superficial cartilage wounds are not associated with an inflammatory response.
   C. Cartilage injuries often heal slowly and result in permanent structural defects.
   D. A major source of nutrients to cartilage is from nearby periosteum.

Answer: D

Cartilage consists of cells (chondrocytes) surrounded by an extracellular matrix made up of several proteoglycans, collagen fibers, and water. Unlike bone, cartilage is very avascular and depends on diffusion for transmittal of nutrients across the matrix. Additionally, the hypervascular perichondrium contributes substantially to the nutrition of the cartilage. Therefore, injuries to cartilage may be associated with permanent defects due to the meager and tenuous blood supply.

The healing response of cartilage depends on the depth of injury. In a superficial injury, there is disruption of the proteoglycan matrix and injury to the chondrocytes. There is no inflammatory response, but an increase in synthesis of proteoglycan and collagen dependent entirely on the chondrocyte. Unfortunately, the healing power of cartilage is often inadequate and overall regeneration is incomplete. Therefore, superficial cartilage injuries are slow to heal and often result in persistent structural defects. (See Schwartz 10th ed., p. 251.)

15. Signs of malignant transformation in a chronic wound include
   A. Persistent granulation tissue with bleeding
   B. Overturned wound edges
   C. Nonhealing after 2 weeks of therapy
   D. Distal edema

Answer: B

Malignant transformation of chronic ulcers can occur in any long-standing wound (Marjolin ulcer). Any wound that does not heal for a prolonged period of time is prone to malignant transformation. Malignant wounds are differentiated clinically from nonmalignant wounds by the presence of overturned wound edges. In patients with suspected malignant transformations, biopsy of the wound edges must be performed to rule out malignancy. Cancers arising de novo in chronic wounds include both squamous and basal cell carcinomas. (See Schwartz 10th ed., p. 259.)

16. What is the difference between hypertrophic scars (HTS) and keloids?
   A. Keloids are an overabundance of fibroplasia as a result of healing, hypertrophic scars are a failure of collagen remodeling.
   B. Hypertrophic scars often regress over time, whereas keloids rarely regress.
   C. Hypertrophic scars are more common in darker-pigmented ethnicities.
   D. Hypertropic scars extend beyond the border of the original wound.

Answer: B

Hypertrophic scars (HTS) and keloids represent an overabundance of fibroplasia in the dermal healing process. HTS rise above the skin level but stay within the confines of the original wound and often regress over time. Keloids rise above the skin level as well, but extend beyond the border of the original wound and rarely regress spontaneously (Fig. 9-1). Both HTS and keloids occur after trauma to the skin, and may be tender, pruritic, and cause a burning sensation. Keloids are 15 times more common in darker-pigmented ethnicities, with individuals of African, Spanish, and Asian ethnicities being especially susceptible. Men and women are equally affected. Genetically, the predilection to keloid formation appears to be autosomal dominant with incomplete penetration and variable expression. (See Schwartz 10th ed., Figure 9-11, p. 261.)

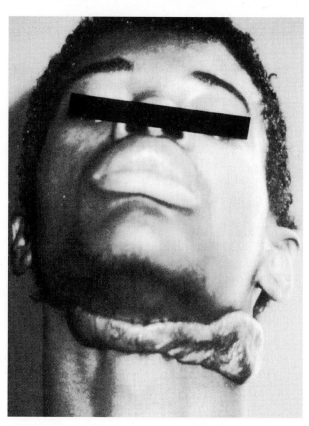

FIG. 9-1. Recurrent keloid on the neck of a 17-year-old patient that had been revised several times. (Reproduced with permission from Murray JC, Pinnell SR: Keloids and excessive dermal scarring, in Cohen IK, Diegelmann RF, Lindblad WJ (eds): *Wound Healing: Biochemical and Clinical Aspects.* Philadelphia: WB Saunders, 1993. Copyright Elsevier.)

17. The treatment of choice for keloids is
    A. Excision alone
    B. Excision with adjuvant therapy (eg, radiation)
    C. Pressure treatment
    D. Intralesional injection of steroids

Answer: B

Excision alone of keloids is subject to a high recurrence rate, ranging from 45 to 100%. There are fewer recurrences when surgical excision is combined with other modalities such as intralesional corticosteroid injection, topical application of silicone sheets, or the use of radiation or pressure. Surgery is recommended for debulking large lesions or as second-line therapy when other modalities have failed. Silicone application is relatively painless and should be maintained for 24 hours a day for about 3 months to prevent rebound hypertrophy. It may be secured with tape or worn beneath a pressure garment. The mechanism of action is not understood, but increased hydration of the skin, which decreases capillary activity, inflammation, hyperemia, and collagen deposition, may be involved. Silicone is more effective than other occlusive dressings and is an especially good treatment for children and others who cannot tolerate the pain involved in other modalities. (See Schwartz 10th ed., p. 262.)

18. What is FALSE about peritoneal adhesions?
    A. Most peritoneal adhesions are a result of intra-abdominal surgery.
    B. Intra-abdominal adhesions are the most common cause of small bowel obstruction.
    C. Operations in the upper abdomen have a higher chance of causing adhesions that cause small bowel obstruction, especially involving the jejunum.
    D. Adhesions are a leading cause of secondary infertility in women.

Answer: C

Peritoneal adhesions are fibrous bands of tissues formed between organs that are normally separated and/or between organs and the internal body wall. Most intra-abdominal adhesions are a result of peritoneal injury, either by a prior surgical procedure or due to intra-abdominal infection. Postmortem examinations demonstrate adhesions in 67% of patients with prior surgical procedures and in 28% with a history of intra-abdominal infection. Intra-abdominal adhesions are the most common cause (65–75%) of small bowel obstruction, especially in the ileum. Operations in the lower abdomen have a higher chance of producing small bowel obstruction. Following rectal surgery, left colectomy, or total colectomy, there is an 11% chance of developing small bowel obstruction within 1 year, and this rate increases to 30% by 10 years. Adhesions also are a leading cause of secondary infertility in women and can cause substantial abdominal and pelvic pain. Adhesions account for 2% of all surgical admissions and 3% of all laparotomies in general surgery. (See Schwartz 10th ed., p. 263.)

19. Which growth factor has been formulated and approved for treatment of diabetic foot ulcers?
    A. PDGF
    B. IGF-1
    C. IL-8
    D. Keritinocyte growth factor
    E. Laminin-5

Answer: A

At present, only platelet-derived growth factor BB (PDGF-BB) is currently approved by the FDA for treatment of diabetic foot ulcers. Application of recombinant human PDGF-BB in a gel suspension to these wounds increases the incidence of total healing and decreases healing time. Several other growth factors have been tested clinically and show some promise, but currently none are approved for use (See Schwartz 10th ed., p. 267.)

CHAPTER 10

Oncology

1. The annual age-adjusted cancer incidence rates among men and women are decreasing for all of the following EXCEPT
   A. Colorectal
   B. Oropharynx
   C. Lung
   D. Thyroid

Answer: D

Incidence rates are declining for most cancer sites, but they are increasing among both men and women for melanoma of the skin, cancers of the liver and thyroid. Incidence rates are decreasing for all four major cancer sites except for breast cancer in women. (See Schwartz 10th ed., p. 274.)

2. Which of the following is NOT a hallmark of cancer?
   A. Ability to invade and metastasize
   B. Ability to evade apoptosis
   C. Ability to evade autophagy
   D. Ability to evade immune destruction

Answer: C

There are six essential alterations in cell physiology that dictate malignant growth: self-sufficiency of growth signals, insensitivity to growth-inhibitory signals, evasion of apoptosis (programmed cell death), potential for limitless replication, angiogenesis, and invasion and metastasis. Recently two additional hallmarks have emerged—reprogramming of energy metabolism and evading immune destruction. (See Schwartz 10th ed., p. 277.)

3. Characteristics of tumorigenic transformation of cells include which of the following?
   A. Enhanced surface adherence
   B. Monolayer confluence inhibition
   C. Acquisition of chemoresistance
   D. Immortalization

Answer: D

Abnormally proliferating, transformed cells outgrow normal cells in the culture dish (ie, in vitro) and commonly display several abnormal characteristics. These include loss of contact inhibition (ie, cells continue to proliferate after a confluent monolayer is formed); an altered appearance and poor adherence to other cells or to the substratum; loss of anchorage dependence for growth; immortalization; and gain of tumorigenicity (ie, the ability to give rise to tumors when injected into an appropriate host). (See Schwartz 10th ed., p. 277.)

4. The cell cycle includes all of the following phases EXCEPT
   A. S phase
   B. G1 phase
   C. G2 phase
   D. G3 phase

Answer: D

The cell cycle is divided into four phases. During the synthetic or S phase, the cell generates a single copy of its genetic material, whereas in the mitotic or M phase, the cellular components are partitioned between two daughter cells. The G1 and G2 phases represent gap phases during which the cells prepare themselves for completion of the S and M phases, respectively. When cells cease proliferation, they exit the cell cycle and enter the quiescent state referred to as G. (See Schwartz 10th ed., p. 279.)

5. Which of the following factors are suggestive of a hereditary cancer?
   A. Tumor development at a younger than normal age.
   B. Presence of bilateral disease.
   C. Association with paraneoplastic syndrome.
   D. Presence of multiple primary malignancies.

Answer: C

The following factors may suggest the presence of a hereditary cancer:

1. Tumor development at a much younger age than usual.
2. Presence of bilateral disease.
3. Presence of multiple primary malignancies.
4. Presentation of a cancer in the less affected sex (eg, male breast cancer).
5. Clustering of the same cancer type in relatives.
6. Occurrence of cancer in association with other conditions such as mental retardation or pathognomonic skin lesions. (See Schwartz 10th ed., p. 287.)

6. Which of the following are associated with familial adenomatous polyposis (FAP)
   A. Osteomas
   B. Glioblastoma multiforme
   C. Meckel diverticulum
   D. Esophageal atresia

Answer: A

Familial adenomatous polyposis (FAP) is associated with benign extracolonic manifestations that may be useful in identifying new cases, including congenital hypertrophy of the retinal pigment epithelium, epidermoid cysts, and osteomas. In addition to colorectal cancer, patients with FAP are at risk for upper intestinal neoplasms (gastric and duodenal polyps, duodenal and periampullary cancer), hepatobiliary tumors (hepatoblastoma, pancreatic cancer, and cholangiocarcinoma), thyroid carcinomas, desmoid tumors, and medulloblastomas. (See Schwartz 10th ed., p. 291.)

7. Which mutated gene malignant disease association is correct
   A. *PTEN* and Li-Fraumeni syndrome
   B. *RET* and MEN2 syndrome
   C. *P16* and synovial sarcoma
   D. *BRCA1* and adrenocortical carcinoma

Answer: B

MEN2 syndrome is caused by gain of function mutations in the RET gene. Li-Fraumeni syndrome is associated with mutation of TP53. Mutations in p16 is associated with melanomas, as well as cancers of the pancreas, esophagus, head and neck, stomach, breast, and colon. BRCA1 is associated with breast and ovarian carcinoma. (See Schwartz 10th ed., pp. 291-293.)

8. Risk for invasive breast cancer development is increased for each factor EXCEPT
   A. Age at menarche <12.
   B. Age at first live birth >30.
   C. Biopsy-proven atypical hyperplasia.
   D. No previous breast biopsy.

Answer: D

Risk factors for the development of breast cancer is summarized in Table 10-1. Previous breast biopsies are associated with an increase in risk of invasive breast cancer. No previous breast biopsy confers the baseline risk. (See Schwartz 10th ed., Table 10-8, p. 297.)

TABLE 10-1	Assessment of risk for invasive breast cancer
Risk Factor	**Relative Risk (%)**
Age at menarche (years)	
>14	1.00
12–13	1.10
<12	1.21
Age at first live birth (years)	
Patients with no first-degree relatives with cancer	
<20	1.00
20–24	1.24
25–29 or nulliparous	1.55
≥30	1.93
Patients with one first-degree-relative with cancer	
<20	1.00
20–24	2.64
25–29 or nulliparous	2.76
≥30	2.83

(Continued)

TABLE 10-1	Assessment of risk for invasive breast cancer (continued)	
Risk Factor (years)		**Relative Risk (%)**
Patients with ≥2 first-degree relatives with cancer		
<20		6.80
20–24		5.78
25–29 or nulliparous		4.91
≥30		4.17
Breast biopsies (number)		
Patients aged <50 at counseling		
0		1.00
1		1.70
≥2		2.88
Patients aged ≥50 at counseling		
0		1.00
1		1.27
≥2		1.62

Source: Modified from Gail MH, Brinton LA, Byar DP, Corle DK, Green SB, Schairer C, et al. Projecting individualized probabilities of developing breast cancer for white females who are being examined annually. *Journal of the National Cancer Institute.* 1989;81:1879-1886.

9. Routine ongoing cancer screening is recommended for which of the following malignancies?
   A. Ovary
   B. Leukemia
   C. Carcinoma of the kidney
   D. Sarcoma

Answer: A
On the occasion of a periodic health examination, the cancer related checkup should include examination for cancers of the thyroid, testicles, ovaries, lymph nodes, oral cavity, and skin, as well as health counseling about tobacco, sun exposure, diet and nutrition, risk factors, sexual practices, and environmental and occupational exposures. (See Schwartz 10th ed., p. 299.)

10. Depending on the tumor, acceptable approaches to biopsy include any of the following EXCEPT
    A. Fine-needle aspiration
    B. Core needle biopsy
    C. Incisional biopsy
    D. Morcellation

Answer: D
A sample of a lesion can be obtained with a needle or with an open incisional or excisional biopsy specimen. Core biopsy specimen, such as fine-needle aspiration, is relatively safe and can be performed either by direct palpation (eg, a breast mass or a soft tissue mass) or can be guided by an imaging study (eg, stereotactic core biopsy specimen of the breast). Open biopsy specimens have the advantage of providing more tissue for histologic evaluation and the disadvantage of being an operative procedure. Incisional biopsy specimens are reserved for very large lesions in which a definitive diagnosis cannot be made by needle biopsy specimen. Excisional biopsy specimens are performed for lesions for which either core biopsy specimen is not possible or the results are nondiagnostic. (See Schwartz 10th ed., p. 300.)

11. Anticancer chemotherapy agents include all of the following EXCEPT
    A. Alkylating agents
    B. Antitumor antibiotics
    C. Prometabolites
    D. Plant alkaloids

Answer: C
Anticancer agents include alkylating agents, antitumor antibiotics, antimetabolites, and plant alkaloids. Antimetabolites are cell-cycle specific agents that have their major activity in the S phase of the cell cycle. These drugs are most effective in tumors that have a high growth fraction, and include folate antagonists, purine antagonists, and pyrimidine antagonists. (See Schwartz 10th ed., p. 307.)

12. Approved strategies for cancer chemoprevention include all of the following EXCEPT
    A. Neurontin for malignant peripheral nerve sheath tumor
    B. Tamoxifen for breast cancer
    C. Celecoxib for FAP syndrome
    D. 13-cis-retinoic acid for oral leukoplakia

Answer: A

The systemic or local administration of therapeutic agents to prevent the development of cancer, called *chemoprevention*, is being actively explored for several cancer types. In breast cancer, the NSABP Breast Cancer Prevention Trial demonstrated that tamoxifen administration reduces the risk of breast cancer by one-half and reduces the risk of estrogen receptor-positive tumors by 69% in high-risk patients. Therefore, tamoxifen has been approved by the FDA for breast cancer chemoprevention. The subsequent NSABP P-2 trial demonstrated that raloxifene is as effective as tamoxifen in reducing the risk of invasive breast cancer and is associated with a lower risk of thromboembolic events and cataracts but a nonstatistically significant higher risk of noninvasive breast cancer; these findings led the FDA to approve raloxifene for prevention as well. Several other agents are also under investigation. Celecoxib has been shown to reduce polyp number and polyp burden in patients with FAP, which led to its approval by the FDA for these patients. In head and neck cancer, 13-cis-retinoic acid has been shown both to reverse oral leukoplakia and to reduce second primary tumor development. (See Schwartz 10th ed., p. 315.)

CHAPTER 11

Transplantation

1. Hyperacute rejection is caused by
   A. Preformed antibodies
   B. B-cell–generated antidonor antibodies
   C. T-cell–mediated allorejection
   D. Nonimmune mechanism

Answer: A

Hyperacute rejection, a very rapid type of rejection, results in irreversible damage and graft loss within minutes to hours after organ reperfusion. It is triggered by preformed antibodies against the donor's human leukocyte antigen (HLA) or ABO blood group antigens. These antibodies activate a series of events that result in diffuse intravascular coagulation, causing ischemic necrosis of the graft. Fortunately, pretransplant blood group typing and cross-matching (in which the donor's cells are mixed with the recipient's serum, and then destruction of the cells is observed) have virtually eliminated the incidence of hyperacute rejection. (See Schwartz 10th ed., p. 324.)

2. The mechanism of action of azathioprine (AZA) is
   A. Inhibition of calcineurin
   B. Interference with DNA synthesis
   C. Binding of FK-506 binding proteins
   D. Inhibition of P7056 kinase

Answer: B

An antimetabolite, azathioprine (AZA) is converted to 6-mercaptopurine and inhibits both the de novo purine synthesis and salvage purine synthesis. AZA decreases T-lymphocyte activity and decreases antibody production. It has been used in transplant recipients for more than 40 years, but became an adjunctive agent after the introduction of cyclosporine. With the development of newer agents such as mycophenolate mofetil (MMF), the use of AZA has decreased significantly. However, it is preferred in recipients who are considering conceiving a child, because MMF is teratogenic in females and can cause birth defects. AZA might be an option for recipients who cannot tolerate the gastrointestinal (GI) side effects of MMF.

The most significant side effect of AZA, often dose-related, is bone marrow suppression. Leukopenia is often reversible with dose reduction or temporary cessation of the drug. Other significant side effects include hepatotoxicity, pancreatitis, neoplasia, anemia, and pulmonary fibrosis. Its most significant drug interaction is with allopurinol, which blocks AZA's metabolism, increasing the risk of pancytopenia. Recommendations are to not use AZA and allopurinol together, or if doing so is unavoidable, to decrease the dose of AZA by 75%. (See Schwartz 10th ed., p. 326.)

3. Which of the following is NOT a side effect of cyclosporine?
   A. Interstitial fibrosis of the renal parenchyma
   B. Gingival hyperplasia
   C. Hirsutism
   D. Pancreatitis

Answer: D
(See Schwartz 10th ed., Table 11-4, p. 327.)

TABLE 11–1	Side effects and drug interactions of the main immunosuppressive drugs			
	COMMON SIDE EFFECTS	**OTHER MEDICATIONS THAT INCREASE BLOOD LEVELS**	**OTHER MEDICATIONS THAT DECREASE BLOOD LEVELS**	**OTHER MEDICATIONS THAT POTENTIATE TOXICITY**
Cyclosporine (CSA)	Hypertension, nephrotoxicity, hirsutism, neurotoxicity, gingival hyperplasia, hypomagnesemia, hyperkalemia	Verapamil, diltiazem, clarithromycin, azithromycin, erythromycin, azole antifungals, protease inhibitors, grapefruit juice	Isoniazid, carbamazepine, phenobarbital, phenytoin, rifampin, St. John's Wort	Nephrotoxicity: ganciclovir, aminoglycosides, NSAIDs, ACE-Is, and ARBs
Tacrolimus (FK506)	Hypertension, nephrotoxicity, alopecia, hyperglycemia, neurotoxicity, hypomagnesemia, hyperkalemia	Verapamil, diltiazem, clarithromycin, azithromycin, erythromycin, azole antifungals, protease inhibitors, grapefruit juice	Isoniazid, carbamazepine, phenobarbital, phenytoin, rifampin, St. John's wort	Nephrotoxicity: ganciclovir, aminoglycosides, NSAIDs, ACE-Is, and ARBs
Sirolimus	Thrombocytopenia and neutropenia, elevated cholesterol, extremity edema, impaired wound healing	Verapamil, diltiazem, clarithromycin, azithromycin, erythromycin, azole antifungals, protease inhibitors, grapefruit juice	Isoniazid, carbamazepine, phenobarbital, phenytoin, rifampin, St. John's wort	—
Mycophenolate mofetil	Leukopenia, thrombocytopenia, GI upset	—	Cholestyramine, antacids	Bone marrow suppression: valganciclovir, ganciclovir, TMP-SMX
Corticosteroids	Hyperglycemia, osteoporosis, cataracts, myopathy, weight gain	—	—	—
Azathioprine	Leukopenia, anemia, thrombocytopenia, neoplasia, hepatitis, cholestasis	—	—	Bone marrow suppression: allopurinol, sulfonamides

ACE-I = angiotensin-converting enzyme inhibitor; ARB = angiotensin receptor blocker; NSAID = nonsteroidal anti-inflammatory drug; TMP-SMX = trimethoprim-sulfamethoxazole

4. Postrenal transplant graft thrombosis usually occurs
   A. Within 2 to 3 days
   B. Within 2 weeks
   C. Within 1 month
   D. Within 3 months

Answer: A
One of the most devastating postoperative complications in kidney recipients is graft thrombosis. It is rare, occurring in fewer than 1% of recipients. The recipient risk factors include a history of recipient hypercoagulopathy and severe peripheral vascular disease; donor-related risk factors include the use of en bloc or pediatric donor kidneys, procurement damage, technical factors such as intimal dissection or torsion of vessels, and hyperacute rejection. Graft thrombosis usually occurs within the first several days posttransplant. Acute cessation of urine output in recipients with brittle posttransplant diuresis and the sudden onset of hematuria or graft pain should arouse suspicion of graft thrombosis. Doppler ultrasound may help confirm the diagnosis. In cases of graft thrombosis, an urgent thrombectomy is indicated; however, it rarely results in graft salvage. (See Schwartz 10th ed., p. 339.)

5. The 1-year graft survival after renal transplantation is
   A. 35–40%
   B. 50–55%
   C. 75–80%
   D. 92–96.5%

Answer: D
According to the 2010 Scientific Registry of Transplant Recipients (SRTR) annual report, a total of 84,614 adult patients were on the kidney transplant waiting list, including 33,215 added just that year. Yet in 2009, only 15,964 adult kidney transplants were performed in the United States (9912 with a deceased donor and 6052 with a living donor). Of note, the number of patients added to the kidney transplant waiting list has increased every year, but the number of kidney transplants performed has been declining since 2006. On the positive side, posttransplant outcomes have continued to improve: in 2009, the 1-year graft survival rate with a living donor kidney was 96.5%; with a deceased donor kidney, the rate was 92.0%. (See Schwartz 10th ed., p. 334.)

6. After completion of the vascular anastomoses, drainage of a transplanted pancreas is accomplished by anastomosis to
   A. Right colon
   B. Left colon
   C. Duodenum
   D. Bladder or small bowel

Answer: D
Over the years, different surgical techniques have been described for (1) the management of exocrine pancreatic secretions and (2) the type of venous drainage. For the secretions, the two most common techniques are drainage of the duodenal segment to the bladder (bladder drainage) or to the small bowel (enteric drainage) (Figs. 11-1 and 11-2). For venous drainage, systemic venous drainage is preferred over portal venous drainage. (See Schwartz 10th ed., Figures 11-12 and 11-13, pp. 341–343.)

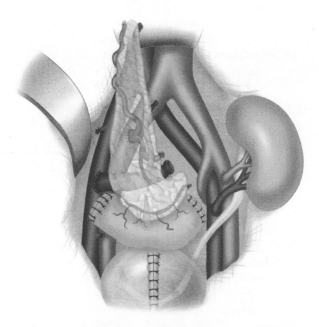

FIG. 11-1. Whole-organ transplant with systemic vein and bladder exocrine drainage. (Reproduced from Gruessner RWG, Sutherland DER, eds. *Transplantation of the Pancreas.* New York: Springer, 2004; Color Plate XIV, Figure 8.2.2.2[B]. With kind permission of Springer Science + Business Media.)

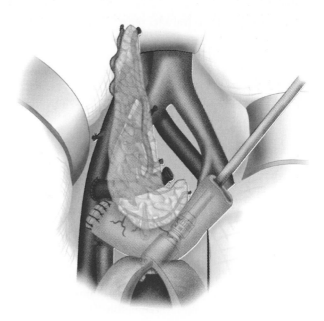

FIG. 11-2. Whole-organ transplant with systemic vein and bladder exocrine drainage. (Reproduced from Gruessner RWG, Sutherland DER, eds. *Transplantation of the Pancreas.* New York: Springer, 2004; Color Plate XIV, Figure 8.2.2.2[A]. With kind permission of Springer Science + Business Media.)

7. All of the following are absolute contraindications in considering a candidate for orthotopic cardiac transplantation EXCEPT
    A. Active infection
    B. Age over 65 years
    C. History of medical noncompliance
    D. Severe pulmonary hypertension

Answer: B

In general terms, contraindications to a liver transplant include insufficient cardiopulmonary reserve, uncontrolled malignancy or infection, and refractory noncompliance. Older age is only a relative contraindication: carefully selected recipients older than 70 years can achieve satisfactory outcomes. Patients with reduced cardiopulmonary reserve are unlikely to survive a liver transplant. Candidates should have a normal ejection fraction. If coronary arterial disease is present, they should undergo revascularization pretransplant. Severe chronic obstructive pulmonary disease (COPD) with oxygen dependence is a contraindication. Severe pulmonary hypertension with a mean pulmonary artery pressure greater than 35 mm Hg that is refractory to medical therapy is also a contraindication. Candidates with pulmonary hypertension should be evaluated with a right heart catheterization. (See Schwartz 10th ed., p. 348.)

8. Heart transplant donors and recipients are matched using the following criteria EXCEPT
    A. Status on the UNOS waiting list
    B. Gender
    C. Blood type
    D. Size

Answer: B

Once a potential deceased donor is identified, the surgeon reviews the status report and screening examination results. The donor is initially matched to the recipient per the recipient's status on the UNOS waiting list, the size match, and the blood type. Results of the donor's serologic testing, echocardiography, chest X-ray, hemodynamic testing, and possibly coronary artery evaluation are assessed, in order to determine whether or not the donor's heart can withstand up to 4 hours of cold ischemic time during procurement, transport, and surgery. (See Schwartz 10th ed., p. 355.)

9. Required laboratory tests in evaluation of a patient under consideration for heart transplantation include all of the following EXCEPT
   A. Psychosocial evaluation
   B. Cardiac catheterization
   C. Dental examination
   D. All of the above

Answer: D
Pretransplant, both candidates and potential donors are evaluated to ensure their suitability for the procedure. Transplant candidates undergo echocardiography, right and left heart catheterization, evaluation for any undiagnosed malignancies, laboratory testing to assess the function of other organs (such as the liver, kidneys, and endocrine system), a dental examination, psychosocial evaluation, and appropriate screening (such as mammography, colonoscopy, and prostate-specific antigen testing). Once the evaluation is complete, the selection committee determines, at a multidisciplinary conference, whether or not a heart transplant is needed and is likely to be successful. Transplant candidates who meet all of the center's criteria are added to the waiting list, according to the UNOS criteria, which are based on health status. (See Schwartz 10th ed., p. 355.)

10. Immunologic rejection is mediated by the recipient's
    A. Eosinophils
    B. Lymphocytes
    C. Neutrophils
    D. Plasma cells

Answer: B
Transplants between genetically nonidentical persons lead to recognition and rejection of the organ by the recipient's immune system, if no intervention is undertaken. The main antigens responsible for this process are part of the major histocompatibility complex (MHC). In humans, these antigens make up the HLA system. The antigen-encoding genes are located on chromosome 6. Two major classes of HLAs are recognized. They differ in their structure, function, and tissue distribution. Class I antigens (HLA-A, HLA-B, and HLA-C) are expressed by all nucleated cells. Class II antigens (HLA-DR, HLA-DP, and HLA-DQ) are expressed by antigen presenting cells (APCs) such as B lymphocytes, dendritic cells, macrophages, and other phagocytic cells.

The principal function of HLAs is to present the fragments of foreign proteins to T lymphocytes. This leads to recognition and elimination of the foreign antigen with great specificity. HLA molecules play a crucial role in transplant recipients as well. They can trigger rejection of a graft via two different mechanisms. The most common mechanism is cellular rejection, in which the damage is done by activated T lymphocytes. (See Schwartz 10th ed., p. 324.)

11. In the prevention of graft rejection, cyclosporine
    A. Blocks transcription of interleukin-1 (IL-1) and tumor necrosis factor-α (TNF-α)
    B. Inhibits lymphocyte nucleic acid metabolism
    C. Results in rapid decrease in the number of circulatory T lymphocytes
    D. Selectively inhibits T-cell activation

Answer: D
The introduction of cyclosporine in the early 1980s dramatically altered the field of transplantation by significantly improving outcomes after kidney transplantation. Cyclosporine binds with its cytoplasmic receptor protein, cyclophilin, which subsequently inhibits the activity of calcineurin, thereby decreasing the expression of several critical T-cell activation genes, the most important being for IL-2. As a result, T-cell activation is suppressed. (See Schwartz 10th ed., p. 328.)

12. The most common cause of renal failure in the United States is
    A. Chronic glomerulonephritis
    B. Chronic pyelonephritis
    C. Diabetes mellitus
    D. Obstructive uropathy

Answer: C
Diabetes and hypertension are the leading causes of chronic renal disease. Concomitant cardiovascular disease (CVD) is a common finding in this population. An estimated 30% to 42% of deaths with a functioning kidney graft are due to CVD. Therefore, assessment of the potential kidney transplant candidate's cardiovascular status is an important part of the pretransplant evaluation. (See Schwartz 10th ed., p. 335.)

13. The best method of monitoring the development of acute rejection in a patient after cardiac transplantation is
    A. Dipyridamole thallium study
    B. Electrocardiogram
    C. Endomyocardial biopsy
    D. Ultrasound examination of the heart

Answer: C

The goal of immunosuppression is to prevent rejection, which is assessed by immunosuppressive levels and, early on, by endomyocardial biopsy. Both T-cell–mediated (cellular) and B-cell–mediated (antibody-mediated) rejection are monitored. (See Schwartz 10th ed., p. 356.)

14. Absolute contraindications to renal transplantation for a patient with chronic renal failure include all of the following EXCEPT
    A. Chronic active hepatitis
    B. Colorectal cancer
    C. Psychiatric illness
    D. Sickle cell disease

Answer: D

Active infection or the presence of a malignancy, active substance abuse, and poorly controlled psychiatric illness are the few absolute contraindications to a kidney transplant. Studies have demonstrated the overwhelming benefits of kidney transplants in terms of patient survival, quality of life, and cost-effectiveness, so most patients with end stage renal disease (ESRD) are referred to for consideration of a kidney transplant. However, to achieve optimal transplant outcomes, the many risks (such as the surgical stress to the cardiovascular system, the development of infections or malignancies with long-term immunosuppression, and the psychosocial and financial impacts on compliance) must be carefully balanced. (See Schwartz 10th ed., p. 334.)

15. All of the following is true for living renal transplant EXCEPT
    A. Donor's kidneys with multiple renal arteries should be avoided.
    B. The donor's left kidney is preferable.
    C. There is no medical benefit to the donor.
    D. The intraperitoneal approach is most often used for harvest.

Answer: B

The kidney, the first organ to be transplanted from living donors, is still the most common organ donated by these individuals. The donor's left kidney is usually preferable because of the long vascular pedicle. Use of living donor kidneys with multiple renal arteries should be avoided, in order to decrease the complexity of the vascular reconstruction and to help avoid graft thrombosis. Most donor nephrectomies are now performed via minimally invasive techniques, that is, laparoscopically, whether hand-assisted or not. With laparoscopic techniques, an intraperitoneal approach is most common: it involves mobilizing the colon, isolating the ureter and renal vessels, mobilizing the kidney, dividing the renal vessels and the distal ureter [C6], and removing the kidney (Fig. 11-3). Extensive dissection around the ureter should be avoided, and the surgeon should strive to preserve as much length of the renal artery and vein as possible. (See Schwartz 10th ed., Figure 11-4, pp. 332–333.)

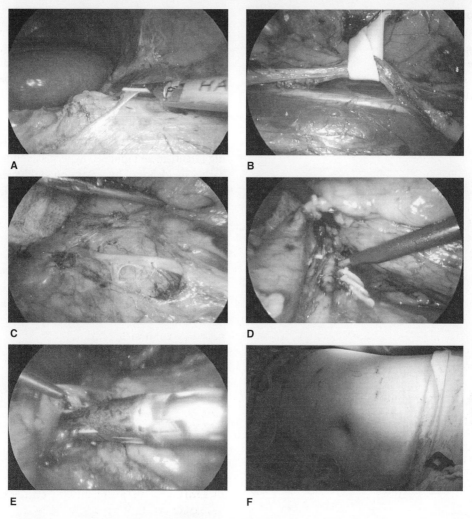

FIG. 11-3. Laparoscopic left donor nephroureterectomy. **A.** Take down of splenic flexure of colon to expose the left renal hilum. **B.** Dissection of left ureter off the psoas muscle. **C.** Dissection of left renal vein and gonadal vein. Left ureter was seen lateral to the dissection. **D.** Dissection of left renal artery. Lumbar veins were clipped and divided. **E.** Endo-TA stapler to transect the left renal artery. **F.** Placement of ports and Pfannenstiel incision for the donor kidney extraction.

16. The single most important factor in determining whether to perform a transplant between a specific donor and recipient is
    A. Mixed lymphocyte culture assays of the donor and recipient
    B. HLA types of the donor and recipient
    C. ABO blood types of the donor and recipient
    D. Peripheral T-cell count of the recipient

Answer: C
ABO blood typing and HLA typing (HLA-A, -B, and -DR) are required before a kidney transplant. The method of screening for preformed antibodies against HLAs (because of prior transplants, blood transfusions, or pregnancies) is evolving. The panel-reactive antibody (PRA) assay is a screening test that examines the ability of serum from a kidney transplant candidate to lyse lymphocytes from a panel of HLA-typed donors. A numeric value, expressed as a percentage, indicates the likelihood of a positive cross-match with a donor. A higher PRA level identifies patients at high risk for a positive cross-match and therefore serves as a surrogate marker to measure the difficulty of finding a suitable donor and the risk of graft rejection. (See Schwartz 10th ed., p. 336.)

17. The most common diagnosis leading to a heart transplant is
    A. COPD
    B. Congenital heart disease
    C. Ischemic dilated cardiomyopathy
    D. Idiopathic dilated myopathy

Answer: C
The most common diagnosis leading to a heart transplant is ischemic dilated cardiomyopathy, which stems from coronary artery disease, followed by idiopathic dilated myopathy and congenital heart disease. About 3000 patients are added to the waiting list each year. (See Schwartz 10th ed., p. 355.)

18. All of the following are side effects of cyclosporine administration for prevention of organ rejection EXCEPT
    A. Hyperkalemia
    B. Hirsutism
    C. Tremor
    D. Bone marrow depression

Answer: D

The metabolism of cyclosporine is via the cytochrome P450 system, resulting in many significant drug interactions (see Table 11-1). Calcineurin inhibitors are nephrotoxic and constrict the afferent arteriole in a dose-dependent, reversible manner (Table 11-2). They can also cause hyperkalemia and hypomagnesemia. Several neurologic complications, including headaches, tremor, and seizures, also have been reported. Cyclosporine has several undesirable cosmetic effects, including hirsutism and gingival hyperplasia. It is associated with a higher incidence of hypertension and hyperlipidemia than is tacrolimus. (See Schwartz 10th ed., Table 11-5, p. 328.)

TABLE 11–2	Drug interactions and side effects associated with calcineurin inhibitors
INTERACTIONS	**MEDICATIONS**
Inhibition of metabolism	Clarithromycin, erythromycin, azole antifungals, diltiazem, verapamil, nicardipine, amiodarone, grapefruit juice, ritonavir, azithromycin
Induction of metabolism	Nevirapine, rifampin, St. John's wort, carbamazepine, phenobarbital, phenytoin, caspofungin
Hyperkalemia	Potassium-sparing diuretics, angiotensinconverting enzyme inhibitors (ACE-Is), angiotensin receptor blockers (ARBs), β-blockers, trimethoprim-sulfamethoxazole
Nephrotoxicity	Nonsteroidal anti-inflammatory drugs, aminoglycosides, amphotericin, ACE-Is, ARBs

19. All of the following are true of extracorporeal membrane oxygenation (ECMO) EXCEPT
    A. Cannulation occurs after withdrawal of life support.
    B. Minimizes ischemic injury to organs of cardiac death donors.
    C. Organs are perfused with warm oxygenated blood after declaration of cardiac death.
    D. Cannulation occurs before withdrawal of life support.

Answer: A

A new development to minimize ischemic injury to organs procured after cardiac death has been the application of declaration of cardiac death (DCD) differs in two key ways: (1) cannulation occurs before withdrawal of life support and (2) organs are perfused via ECMO with warm oxygenated blood after declaration of cardiac death. The initial experience with organs procured using ECMO has been encouraging. (See Schwartz 10th ed., p. 331.)

20. The most significant side effect of sirolimus is
    A. Anemia
    B. Leukopenia
    C. Impaired wound healing
    D. Hypertriglyceridemia

Answer: D

One of the most significant side effects of sirolimus is hypertriglyceridemia, a condition that may be resistant to statins and fibrates. Impaired wound healing (immediately posttransplant in particular), thrombocytopenia, leukopenia, and anemia also are associated with sirolimus, and these problems are exacerbated when it is used in combination with MMF. (See Schwartz 10th ed., p. 328.)

CHAPTER 12

Patient Safety

1. The Donabedian model of measuring quality identifies all of the following as main types of improvements EXCEPT
   A. Changes to structure
   B. Changes to process
   C. Changes to culture
   D. Changes to outcomes

Answer: C

The Donabedian model of measuring quality identifies three main types of improvements: changes to structure, process, and outcome (Fig. 12-1). (See Schwartz 10th ed., p. 367.)

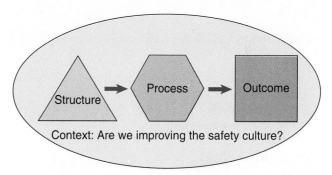

FIG. 12-1. Donabedian model for measuring quality. (From Makary MA, Sexton JB, Freischlag JA, et al, *Patient safety in surgery.* Ann Surg 243:628, 2006. With Permission.)

2. The most common delayed complication following carotid endarterectomy is
   A. Arteriovenous fistulae
   B. Myocardial infarction
   C. Expanding neck hematoma
   D. Localized neurologic deficit

Answer: B

Complications of carotid endarterectomy include central or regional neurologic deficits or bleeding with an expanding neck hematoma. An acute change in mental status or the presence of localized neurologic deficit requires an immediate return to the operating room (OR). An expanding hematoma may warrant emergent airway intubation and subsequent transfer to the OR for control of hemorrhage. Intraoperative anticoagulation with heparin during carotid surgery makes bleeding a postoperative risk. Other complications include arteriovenous fistulae, pseudoaneurysms, and infection, all of which are treated surgically.

Intraoperative hypotension during manipulation of the carotid bifurcation can occur and is related to increased tone from baroreceptors that reflexly cause bradycardia. Should hypotension occur when manipulating the carotid bifurcation, an injection of 1% lidocaine solution around this structure should attenuate this reflexive response. The most common delayed complication following carotid endarterectomy remains myocardial infarction. The possibility of a postoperative myocardial infarction should be considered a cause of labile blood pressure and arrhythmias in high-risk patients. (See Schwartz 10th ed., p. 384.)

3. The most appropriate treatment for a seroma after a soft-tissue biopsy is
   A. Multiple attempts of aspiration with application of pressure dressings.
   B. Immediate return to the OR for drainage.
   C. Single attempt at aspiration with return to the OR if it recurs.
   D. Observation.

Answer: A

Lymph node biopsies have direct and indirect complications that include bleeding, infection, lymph leakage, and seromas. Measures to prevent direct complications include proper surgical hemostasis, proper skin preparation, and a single preoperative dose of antibiotic to cover skin flora 30 to 60 minutes before incision. Bleeding at a biopsy site usually can be controlled with direct pressure. Infection at a biopsy site will appear 5 to 10 days postoperatively and may require opening of the wound to drain the infection. Seromas or lymphatic leaks resolve with aspiration of seromas and the application of pressure dressings, but may require repeated treatments or even placement of a vacuum drain. (See Schwartz 10th ed., p. 383.)

4. Prophylaxis using low-dose unfractionated heparin reduces the incidence of fatal pulmonary embolisms (PE) by
   A. 45%
   B. 50%
   C. 60%
   D. 35%

Answer: B

Deep vein thrombosis (DVT) occurs after approximately 25% of all major surgical procedures performed without prophylaxis, and pulmonary embolism (PE) occurs after 7%. Despite the well-established efficacy and safety of preventive measures, studies show that prophylaxis often is underused or used inappropriately. Both low-dose unfractionated heparin and low-molecular-weight heparin have similar efficacy in DVT and PE prevention. Prophylaxis using low-dose unfractionated heparin has been shown to reduce the incidence of fatal PEs by 50%. (See Schwartz 10th ed., p. 374.)

5. Which of the following is the best test to predict successful extubation of a patient?
   A. Respiratory rate
   B. Negative inspiratory pressure
   C. Tobin index
   D. Minute ventilation

Answer: C

Protocol-driven ventilator weaning strategies are successful and have become part of the standard of care. The use of a weaning protocol for patients on mechanical ventilation greater than 48 hours reduces the incidence of ventilator-associated pneumonia (VAP) and the overall length of time on mechanical ventilation. Unfortunately, there is still no reliable way of predicting which patient will be successfully extubated after a weaning program, and the decision for extubation is based on a combination of clinical parameters and measured pulmonary mechanics. The Tobin index (frequency [breaths per minute]/tidal volume [L]), also known as the *rapid shallow breathing index,* is perhaps the best negative predictive instrument. If the result equals less than 105, then there is nearly a 70% chance the patient will pass extubation. If the score is greater than 105, the patient has an approximately 80% chance of failing extubation. Other parameters such as the negative inspiratory force, minute ventilation, and respiratory rate are used, but individually have no better predictive value than the rapid shallow breathing index. (See Schwartz 10th ed., p. 385.)

6. The root cause of the majority of wrong-site surgeries result from
   A. Communication errors
   B. Emergency surgery
   C. Multiple procedures
   D. Multiple surgeons

Answer: A

The risk of performing wrong-site surgery increases when there are multiple surgeons involved in the same operation or multiple procedures are performed on the same patient, especially if the procedures are scheduled or performed on different areas of the body. Time pressure, emergency surgery, abnormal patient anatomy, and morbid obesity are also thought to be risk factors. Communication errors are the root cause in more than 70% of the wrong-site surgeries reported to The Joint Commission. Other risk factors include receiving an incomplete preoperative assessment; having inadequate procedures in place to verify the correct surgical site; or having an organizational culture that lacks teamwork or reveres the surgeon as someone whose judgment should never be questioned. (See Schwartz 10th ed., p. 378.)

7. Which of the following have been shown to decrease the time of postoperative ileus?
   A. Cyclooxygenase-1 inhibitors
   B. Morphine patient-controlled analgesia
   C. Nasogastric drainage until full return of bowel function
   D. Erythromycin

Answer: D
Pharmacologic agents commonly used to stimulate bowel function include metoclopramide and erythromycin. Metoclopramide's action is limited to the stomach and duodenum, and it may help primarily with gastroparesis. Erythromycin is a motilin agonist that works throughout the stomach and bowel. Several studies demonstrate significant benefit from the administration of erythromycin in those suffering from an ileus. Alvimopan, a newer agent and a mu-opioid receptor antagonist, has shown some promise in many studies for earlier return of gut function and subsequent reduction in length of stay. Neostigmine has been used in refractory pan-ileus patients (Ogilvie syndrome) with some degree of success. It is recommended for patients receiving this type of therapy to be in a monitored unit. (See Schwartz 10th ed., p. 386.)

8. In order to reduce the overall risk of stress gastritis in ICU patients mechanically ventilated for >48 hours, their gastric pH level should be kept greater than
   A. 3
   B. 5
   C. 2
   D. 4

Answer: D
When patients in the ICU have a major bleed from stress gastritis, the mortality risk is as high as 50%. It is important to keep the gastric pH greater than 4 to decrease the overall risk for stress gastritis in patients mechanically ventilated for 48 hours or greater and patients who are coagulopathic. Proton pump inhibitors, H_2-receptor antagonists, and intragastric antacid installation are all effective measures. However, patients who are not mechanically ventilated or who do not have a history of gastritis or peptic ulcer disease should not be placed on gastritis prophylaxis postoperatively because it carries a higher risk of causing pneumonia. (See Schwartz 10th ed., p. 387.)

9. The treatment of choice for a biloma after laparoscopic cholecystectomy is
   A. Reoperation, closure of the leak, and drainage
   B. Percutaneous drainage
   C. Biliary stent
   D. Observation

Answer: C
A bile leak due to an unrecognized injury to the ducts may present after cholecystectomy as a biloma. These patients may present with abdominal pain and hyperbilirubinemia. The diagnosis of a biliary leak can be confirmed by computed tomography (CT) scan, endoscopic retrograde cholangiopancreaticogram (ERCP), or radionuclide scan. Once a leak is confirmed, a retrograde biliary stent and external drainage are the treatment of choice. (See Schwartz 10th ed., p. 387.)

10. The most frequent nosocomial infection is
    A. Urinary tract infection (UTI)
    B. Sepsis
    C. Pneumonia
    D. Fungal infection

Answer: A
The most frequent nosocomial infection is urinary tract infection (UTI). These infections are classified into complicated and uncomplicated forms. The uncomplicated type is a UTI that can be treated with outpatient antibiotic therapy. The complicated UTI usually involves a hospitalized patient with an indwelling catheter whose UTI is diagnosed as part of a fever workup. The interpretation of urine culture results of less than 100,000 CFU/mL is controversial. Before treating such a patient, one should change the catheter and then repeat the culture to see whether the catheter was simply colonized with organisms. Cultures with more than 100,000 CFU/mL

should be treated with the appropriate antibiotics and the catheter should be changed or removed as soon as possible. Under-treatment or misdiagnosis of a UTI can lead to urosepsis and septic shock. (See Schwartz 10th ed., p. 390.)

11. The first step in treating a 70-kg patient with a platelet count of 12,000 due to heparin-induced thrombocytopenia is
    A. Anticoagulation
    B. Transfusion of four units of platelets
    C. Transfusion of eight units of platelets
    D. Transfusion of 12 units of platelets

Answer: D
Thrombocytopenia may require platelet transfusion for a platelet count less than 20,000/mL when invasive procedures are performed, or when platelet counts are low and ongoing bleeding from raw surface areas persists. One unit of platelets will increase the platelet count by 5000 to 7500/mL in adults. It is important to delineate the cause of the low platelet count. Usually there is a self-limiting or reversible condition such as sepsis. Rarely, it is due to heparin-induced thrombocytopenia I and II. Complications of heparin-induced thrombocytopenia II can be serious because of the diffuse thrombogenic nature of the disorder. Simple precautions to limit this hypercoagulable state include saline solution flushes instead of heparin solutions and limiting the use of heparin-coated catheters. The treatment is anticoagulation with synthetic agents such as argatroban. (See Schwartz 10th ed., pp. 388–389.)

12. VAP in ventilated ICU patients reaches a 70% probability at
    A. 5 days
    B. 15 days
    C. 30 days
    D. 45 days

Answer: C
Pneumonia is the second most common nosocomial infection and is the most common infection in ventilated patients. VAP occurs in 15 to 40% of ventilated ICU patients, with a probability rate of 5% per day, up to 70% at 30 days. The 30-day mortality rate of nosocomial pneumonia can be as high as 40% and depends on the microorganisms involved and the timeliness of initiating appropriate antimicrobials Protocol-driven approaches for prevention and treatment of VAP are recognized as beneficial in managing these difficult infectious complications. (See Schwartz 10th ed., pp. 384–385.)

13. Which of the following is the only thing that has been shown to decrease wound infections in surgical patients with contaminated wounds?
    A. Use of iodophor-impregnated polyvinyl drapes.
    B. Saline irrigation of the peritoneum and wound.
    C. Antibiotic irrigation of the peritoneum and wound.
    D. 24 hours of appropriate antibiotics postoperatively (in addition to preoperative dose).

Answer: B
No prospective, randomized, double-blind, controlled studies exist that demonstrate antibiotics used beyond 24 hours in the perioperative period prevent infections. Prophylactic use of antibiotics should simply not be continued beyond this time. Irrigation of the operative field and the surgical wound with saline solution has shown benefit in controlling wound inoculum. Irrigation with an antibiotic-based solution has not demonstrated significant benefit in controlling postoperative infection. (See Schwartz 10th ed., p. 389.)

14. Tracheostomy may decrease the incidence of VAP, overall length of ventilator time, and the number of ICU patient days when performed
    A. Before the fifth day of ventilator support
    B. Before the 10th day of ventilator support
    C. Before the 15th day of ventilator support
    D. Before the 20th day of ventilator support

Answer: B
Although not without risk, tracheostomy decreases the pulmonary dead space and provides for improved pulmonary toilet. When performed before the 10th day of ventilatory support, tracheostomy may decrease the incidence of VAP, the overall length of ventilator time, and the number of ICU patient days. (See Schwartz 10th ed., p. 385.)

15. Which of the following is a dominant cytokine in the pathogenesis of systemic inflammatory response syndrome (SIRS)?
    A. Interleukin-2 (IL-2)
    B. IL-5
    C. IL-6
    D. IL-7

Answer: C
The systemic inflammatory response syndrome (SIRS) and the multiple organ dysfunction syndrome (MODS) carry significant mortality risks (Table 12-1). Specific criteria have been established for the diagnosis of SIRS (Table 12-2), but two criteria are not required for the diagnosis of SIRS: lowered blood pressure and blood cultures positive for infection. SIRS is the result of proinflammatory cytokines related to tissue malperfusion or injury.

The dominant cytokines implicated in this process include interleukin (IL)-1, IL-6, and tissue necrosis factor (TNF). Other mediators include nitric oxide, inducible macrophage-type nitric oxide synthase, and prostaglandin I2. (See Schwartz 10th ed., Tables 12-17 and 12-18, p. 391.)

TABLE 12-1	Mortality associated with patients exhibiting two or more criteria for systemic inflammatory response syndrome (SIRS)
PROGNOSIS	**MORTALITY (%)**
2 SIRS criteria	5
3 SIRS criteria	10
4 SIRS criteria	15–20

TABLE 12-2	Inclusion criteria for the systemic inflammatory response syndrome
Temperature >38°C or <36°C (>100.4°F or <96.8°F)	
Heart rate >90 beats/min	
Respiratory rate >20 breaths/min or Paco$_2$ <32 mm Hg	
White blood cell count <4000 or >12,000 cells/mm³ or >10% immature forms	

Paco$_2$ = partial pressure of arterial carbon dioxide.

16. The most common cause of postrenal failure is
    A. A clogged urinary catheter
    B. An unintentional ligation of ureters
    C. A large retroperitoneal hematoma
    D. Acute kidney failure

Answer: A
Renal failure can be classified as prerenal failure, intrinsic renal failure, and postrenal failure. Postrenal failure, or obstructive renal failure, should always be considered when low urine output (oliguria) or anuria occurs. The most common cause is a misplaced or clogged urinary catheter. Other, less common causes to consider are unintentional ligation or transection of ureters during a difficult surgical dissection (eg, colon resection for diverticular disease) or a large retroperitoneal hematoma (eg, ruptured aortic aneurysm). (See Schwartz 10th ed., p. 387.)

17. Laryngoscopic findings after a superior laryngeal nerve injury include
    A. Ipsilateral vocal cord in a paramedian position
    B. Ipsilateral vocal cord in a middling position
    C. Asymmetry of the glottic opening
    D. Normal examination

Answer: C
Superior laryngeal nerve injury is less debilitating, as the common symptom is loss of projection of the voice. The glottis aperture is asymmetrical on direct laryngoscopy, and management is limited to clinical observation. (See Schwartz 10th ed., p. 384.)

18. All of the following are true statements regarding wound infection EXCEPT
    A. Irrigation of the operative field and surgical wound with saline solution is beneficial.
    B. Prophylactic use of antibiotics continued beyond 48 hours is beneficial.
    C. Irrigation with an antibiotic-based solution has not been shown to be beneficial.
    D. Antibacterial-impregnated polyvinyl placed over the operative wound area for the duration of the surgical procedure is not beneficial.

Answer: B

No prospective, randomized, double-blind, controlled studies exist that demonstrate antibiotics used beyond 24 hours in the perioperative period prevent infections. Prophylactic use of antibiotics should simply not be continued beyond this time. Irrigation of the operative field and the surgical wound with saline solution has shown benefit in controlling wound inoculum. Irrigation with an antibiotic-based solution has not demonstrated significant benefit in controlling postoperative infection.

Antibacterial-impregnated polyvinyl placed over the operative wound area for the duration of the surgical procedure has not been shown to decrease the rate of wound infection. Although skin preparation with 70% isopropyl alcohol has the best bactericidal effect, it is flammable and could be hazardous when electrocautery is used. The contemporary formulas of chlorhexidine gluconate with isopropyl alcohol remain more advantageous. (See Schwartz 10th ed., p. 389.)

19. The most common cause of an empyema in the postoperative patient is
    A. Pneumonia
    B. Systemic sepsis
    C. Esophageal perforation
    D. Retained hemothorax

Answer: A

One of the most debilitating infections is an empyema, or infection of the pleural space. Frequently, an overwhelming pneumonia is the source of an empyema, but a retained hemothorax, systemic sepsis, esophageal perforation from any cause, and infections with a predilection for the lung (eg, tuberculosis) are potential etiologies as well. (See Schwartz 10th ed., pp. 390–391.)

20. The primary cause of hyperbilirubinemia in the surgical patient is
    A. Sepsis
    B. Hematoma from trauma
    C. Cholestasis
    D. Increased unconjugated bilirubin due to hemolysis

Answer: C

Hyperbilirubinemia in the surgical patient can be a complex problem. Cholestasis makes up the majority of causes for hyperbilirubinemia, but other mechanisms of hyperbilirubinemia include reabsorption of blood (eg, hematoma from trauma), decreased bile excretion (eg, sepsis), increased unconjugated bilirubin due to hemolysis, hyperthyroidism, and impaired excretion due to congenital abnormalities or acquired disease. Errors in surgery that cause hyperbilirubinemia largely involve missed or iatrogenic injuries. (See Schwartz 10th ed., p. 387.)

CHAPTER 13

Physiologic Monitoring of the Surgical Patient

1. The point of critical oxygen delivery (DO_{2crit})
   A. Represents the transition from supply-independent to supply-dependent oxygen uptake and is decreased in sepsis.
   B. Represents the minimal rate of oxygen delivery needed for aerobic metabolism and is decreased in sepsis.
   C. Represents the transition from supply-independent to supply-dependent oxygen uptake and is increased in sepsis.
   D. Represents the minimal rate of oxygen delivery needed for aerobic metabolism and is increased in sepsis.

Answer: C

Under normal conditions when the supply of oxygen is plentiful, aerobic metabolism is determined by factors other than the availability of oxygen. However, in pathologic circumstances when oxygen availability is inadequate, oxygen utilization (VO_2) becomes dependent upon oxygen delivery (DO_2). The relationship of VO_2 to DO_2 over a broad range of DO_2 values is commonly represented as two intersecting straight lines. In the region of higher DO_2 values, the slope of the line is approximately zero, indicating that VO_2 is largely independent of DO_2. In contrast, in the region of low DO_2 values, the slope of the line is nonzero and positive, indicating that VO_2 is supply-dependent. The region where the two lines intersect is called the *point of critical oxygen delivery* (DO_{2crit}), and represents the transition from supply-independent to supply-dependent oxygen uptake. Microcirculatory derangements, such as those seen in sepsis, will shift this point higher. Below a critical threshold of oxygen delivery, increased oxygen extraction cannot compensate for the delivery deficit; hence, oxygen consumption begins to decrease. The slope of the supply-dependent region of the plot reflects the maximal oxygen extraction capability of the vascular bed being evaluated. (See Schwartz 10th ed., p. 400.)

2. Of the following parameters, which is the least influenced by an underdamped or overdamped intra-arterial blood pressure monitoring system?
   A. Systolic blood pressure
   B. Mean arterial blood pressure
   C. Diastolic blood pressure
   D. Pulse pressure

Answer: B

If the system is underdamped, then the inertia of the system, which is a function of the mass of the fluid in the tubing and the mass of the diaphragm, causes overshoot of the points of maximum positive and negative displacement of the pressure transducer diaphragm during systole and diastole, respectively. Thus, in an underdamped system, systolic pressure will be overestimated and diastolic pressure will be underestimated. In an overdamped system, displacement of the diaphragm fails to track the rapidly changing pressure waveform, and systolic pressure will be underestimated and diastolic pressure will be overestimated. It is important to note that even in an underdamped or overdamped system, mean pressure will be accurately recorded, provided the system has been properly calibrated. For these reasons, when using direct measurement of intra-arterial pressure to monitor patients, clinicians should make clinical decisions based primarily on the measured mean arterial blood pressure. (See Schwartz 10th ed., p. 401.)

3. Regarding electrocardiographic (ECG) monitoring in the ICU
   A. A standard 3-lead ECG will detect 95% of ischemia, whereas a 12-lead ECG will detect greater than 98%.
   B. Lead V_4 is the most sensitive for detecting perioperative ischemia.
   C. A standard 3-lead ECG will detect ischemia at the same rate as a12-lead ECG; however, it is inferior at identifying dysrhythmias.
   D. Lead V_2 is the most sensitive for detecting perioperative ischemia.

Answer: B
Continuous monitoring of the 12-lead ECG is now available in many ICUs and is proving to be beneficial in certain patient populations. In a study of 185 vascular surgical patients, continuous 12-lead ECG monitoring was able to detect transient myocardial ischemic episodes in 20.5% of the patients. This study demonstrated that the precordial lead V_4, which is not routinely monitored on a standard 3-lead ECG, is the most sensitive for detecting perioperative ischemia and infarction. To detect 95% of the ischemic episodes, two or more precordial leads were necessary. Thus, continuous 12-lead ECG monitoring may provide greater sensitivity than 3-lead ECG for the detection of perioperative myocardial ischemia, and may become standard for monitoring high-risk surgical patients. (See Schwartz 10th ed., p. 401.)

4. Regarding preload, which of the following is true?
   A. It is approximated by the systemic vascular resistance which is calculated by dividing mean arterial pressure (MAP) by cardiac output.
   B. It is approximated by the right ventricular end-diastolic pressure (EDP) as estimated with pulmonary artery occlusion pressure.
   C. It is approximated by the right ventricular EDP as estimated with central venous pressure (CVP).
   D. It is approximated by the left ventricular EDP as estimated with pulmonary artery occlusion pressure.

Answer: D
For the right ventricle, central venous pressure (CVP) approximates right ventricular end-diastolic pressure (EDP). For the left ventricle, pulmonary artery occlusion pressure (PAOP), which is measured by transiently inflating a balloon at the end of a pressure-monitoring catheter positioned in a small branch of the pulmonary artery, approximates left ventricular EDP. The presence of atrioventricular valvular stenosis may alter this relationship. Left ventricular EDP is the most commonly used proxy for preload. (See Schwartz 10th ed., p. 402.)

5. All of the following are true EXCEPT
   A. The relationship between EDP and preload is linear.
   B. EDP is determined by both volume and compliance of the ventricle.
   C. The relationship between EDP and end-diastolic volume (EDV) can be changed with pharmacologic agents.
   D. EDP is often used as a surrogate for EDV because it is easier to approximate in the clinical setting.

Answer: A
Clinicians frequently use EDP as a surrogate for end-diastolic volume (EDV), but EDP is determined not only by volume but also by the diastolic compliance of the ventricular chamber. Ventricular compliance is altered by various pathologic conditions and pharmacologic agents. Furthermore, the relationship between EDP and true preload is not linear, but rather is exponential. (See Schwartz 10th ed., p. 402.)

6. The end-systolic pressure-volume line
   A. Provides a good estimation of left ventricular compliance.
   B. Uses small changes in preload and afterload between cardiac cycles to determine contractility, which is represented by the x-intercept of the line.
   C. The slope will become steeper if contractility is increased.
   D. Requires preload to be held approximately constant to be measured.

Answer: C
If pressure-volume loops are constructed for each cardiac cycle, small changes in preload and/or afterload will result in shifts of the point defining the end of systole. These end-systolic points on the pressure versus volume diagram describe a straight line, known as the *end-systolic pressure-volume line*. A steeper slope of this line indicates greater contractility. (See Schwartz 10th ed., p. 402.)

7. The thermodilution technique for determining cardiac output
   A. Calculates Q_T with the Fick equation
   B. Underestimates cardiac output at low values
   C. Should be performed with a cold indicator liquid to increase the signal-to-noise ratio
   D. Is influenced by respiratory cycle due to changes in blood temperature and Q_T

Answer: D
The relationship used by the thermodilution technique for calculating Q_T is called the *Stewart-Hamilton equation*:

$$Q_T = [V \times (T_B - T_I) \times K_1 \times K_2] / \int T_B(t)dt$$

where V is the volume of the indicator injected, T_B is the temperature of blood, T_I is the temperature of the indicator, K_1 is a constant that is the function of the specific heats of blood and the indicator, K_2 is an empirically derived constant, and $\int T_B(t)dt$ is the area under the time-temperature curve. Determination of cardiac output by the thermodilution method is generally quite accurate, although it tends to systematically overestimate Q_T at low values. Changes in blood temperature and Q_T during the respiratory cycle can influence the measurement. Therefore, results generally should be recorded as the mean of two or three determinations obtained at random points in the respiratory cycle. Using cold injectate widens the difference between T_B and T_I and thereby increases signal-to-noise ratio. Nevertheless, most authorities recommend using room temperature injectate (normal saline or 5% dextrose in water) to minimize errors resulting from warming of the fluid as it is transferred from its reservoir to a syringe for injection. (See Schwartz 10th ed., p. 404.)

8. All of the following are true regarding the fractional saturation of hemoglobin in mixed venous blood (SVO_2) EXCEPT
   A. It will decrease with worsening heart failure.
   B. It will decrease with increased sedation.
   C. It will decrease with worsening anemia.
   D. It will decrease with fever.

Answer: B
The Fick equation for cardiac output can be rearranged as follows:

$$CVO_2 = Cao_2 - VO_2/Q_T$$

If the small contribution of dissolved oxygen to CVO_2 and Cao_2 is ignored, the rearranged equation can be rewritten as:

$$SVO_2 = Sao_2 - VO_2/(Q_T \times Hgb \times 1.36)$$

where SVO_2 is the fractional saturation of hemoglobin in mixed venous blood, Sao_2 is the fractional saturation of hemoglobin in arterial blood, and Hgb is the concentration of hemoglobin in blood. Thus it can be seen that SVO_2 is a function of VO_2 (ie, metabolic rate), Q_T, Sao_2, and Hgb. Accordingly, subnormal values of SVO_2 can be caused by a decrease in Q_T (eg, due to heart failure or hypovolemia), a decrease in Sao_2 (eg, due to intrinsic pulmonary disease), a decrease in Hgb (ie, anemia), or an increase in metabolic rate (eg, due to seizures or fever). (See Schwartz 10th ed., p. 404.)

9. The Surviving Sepsis Campaign guidelines recommend which of the following regarding the initial resuscitation of sepsis-induced hypoperfusion?
   A. Goal MAP ≥60 mm Hg.
   B. Goal SVO_2 of 80%.
   C. Goal urine output ≥ 1 mL/kg/h.
   D. That goals of resuscitation be met within the first 6 hours of management.

Answer: D
The Surviving Sepsis Campaign guidelines for the management of severe sepsis and septic shock recommends that during the first 6 hours of resuscitation, the goals of initial resuscitation of sepsis-induced hypoperfusion should include all of the following: CVP 8 to 12 mm Hg, MAP ≥65 mm Hg, urine output ≥0.5 mL/kg/h. $ScVO_2$ of 70% or SVO_2 of 65%. (See Schwartz 10th ed., p. 405.)

10. Noninvasive methods of measuring cardiac output
    A. Allow for continuous measurement of Q_T
    B. Show excellent correlation with Q_T as measured by thermodilution
    C. Have rarely been adopted into clinical practice due to the increased training burden
    D. Have similar complication rates as the use of a pulmonary artery catheter

Answer: A
Noninvasive methods of monitoring cardiac output include impedance cardiography and pulse contour analysis among others. Impedance cardiography is attractive because it is noninvasive, provides a continuous readout of Q_T, and does not require extensive training. However, measurements of Q_T obtained by impedance cardiography are not sufficiently reliable to be used for clinical decision-making and have poor correlation with thermodilution. Measurements of Q_T based on pulse contour monitoring are comparable in accuracy to standard PAC thermodilution methods, but are less invasive since transcardiac catheterization is not needed. The use of pulse contour analysis has been applied using noninvasive photoplethysmographic measurements of arterial pressure. However, the accuracy of this technique has been questioned and its clinical utility remains to be determined. (See Schwartz 10th ed., p. 408.)

11. Using pulse pressure variability (PPV) to determine pre-load responsiveness
    A. Is reliable for a patient in rate-controlled atrial fibril-lation, but not for a patient in atrial flutter.
    B. Is a better predictor of preload responsiveness than CVP.
    C. Defines PPV as the difference between the maximal pulse pressure and the minimal pulse pressure observed at different points in the respiratory cycle.
    D. Is unreliable in mechanically ventilated patients due to decreased venous return during inspiration.

Answer: B

When intrathoracic pressure increases during the applica-tion of positive airway pressure in mechanically ventilated patients, venous return decreases and, as a consequence, left ventricular stroke volume also decreases. Therefore, pulse pressure variation (PPV) during a positive pressure episode can be used to predict the responsiveness of cardiac output to changes in preload. PPV is defined as the difference between the maximal pulse pressure and the minimal pulse pressure divided by the average of these two pressures. This approach has been validated by comparing PPV, CVP, PAOP, and sys-tolic pressure variation as predictors of preload responsive-ness in a cohort of critically ill patients. Receiver-operating characteristic curves demonstrated that PPV was the best predictor of preload responsiveness. Although atrial arrhyth-mias can interfere with the usefulness of this technique, PPV remains a useful approach for assessing preload responsive-ness in most patients because of its simplicity and reliability. (See Schwartz 10th ed., p. 408.)

12. Strategies for increasing oxygen delivery in mechanically ventilated, critically ill patients include
    A. Increasing Sao_2 by increasing inspiratory time
    B. Increasing Sao_2 by increasing respiratory rate
    C. Increasing SVO_2 by switching to a reversed inspira-tory to expiratory ratio ventilation strategy
    D. Increasing SVO_2 by increasing positive end-expiratory pressure (PEEP)

Answer: A

Sao_2 in mechanically ventilated patients depends on the mean airway pressure, the fraction of inspired oxygen (Fio_2), and SVO_2. Thus, when Sao_2 is low, the clinician has only a limited number of ways to improve this parameter. The clinician can increase mean airway pressure by increasing positive-end expiratory pressure (PEEP) or inspiratory time. Fio_2 can be increased to a maximum of 1.0 by decreasing the amount of room air mixed with the oxygen supplied to the ventilator. SVO_2 can be increased by increasing Hgb or Q_T or decreasing oxygen utilization (eg, by administering a muscle relaxant and sedation). (See Schwartz 10th ed., p. 409.)

13. All of the following are true regarding airway pressures EXCEPT
    A. Bronchospasm will cause increased peak pressure with a relatively normal plateau pressure.
    B. Pneumothorax will cause increased peak and plateau pressures.
    C. Lobar atelectasis will cause increased plateau pres-sures with relatively normal peak pressures.
    D. Plateau pressure is independent of airway resistance.

Answer: C

The peak airway pressure measured at the end of inspiration (P_{peak}) is a function of the tidal volume, the resistance of the airways, lung/chest wall compliance, and peak inspiratory flow. The airway pressure measured at the end of inspiration when the inhaled volume is held in the lungs by briefly clos-ing the expiratory valve is termed the *plateau airway pressure* ($P_{plateau}$). As a static parameter, plateau airway pressure is inde-pendent of the airway resistance and peak airway flow, and is related to the lung/chest wall compliance and delivered tidal volume. If both P_{peak} and $P_{plateau}$ are increased (and tidal volume is not excessive), then the underlying problem is a decrease in the compliance in the lung/chest wall unit. Common causes of this problem include pneumothorax, hemothorax, lobar atelectasis, pulmonary edema, pneumonia, acute respiratory distress syndrome (ARDS), active contraction of the chest wall or diaphragmatic muscles, abdominal distention, and intrinsic PEEP, such as occurs in patients with bronchospasm and insufficient expiratory times. When P_{peak} is increased but $P_{plateau}$ is relatively normal, the primary problem is an increase in airway resistance, such as occurs with bronchospasm, use of a small-caliber endotracheal tube, or kinking or obstruction of the endotracheal tube. (See Schwartz 10th ed., pp. 409–410.)

14. Causes of an increase in end-tidal-CO_2 include
    A. Massive pulmonary embolism
    B. Reduced cardiac output
    C. Sustained hyperventilation
    D. Reduced minute ventilation

Answer: D

Causes of an *increase* in $Petco_2$ include reduced minute ventilation or increased metabolic rate. Sudden *reduction* in end-tidal-CO_2 ($Petco_2$) suggests either obstruction of the sampling tubing or a catastrophic event such as loss of the airway, airway disconnection or obstruction, ventilator malfunction, or a marked decrease in Q_T. If the airway is connected and patient and the ventilator is functioning properly, then a sudden decrease in $Petco_2$ should prompt efforts to rule out cardiac arrest, massive pulmonary embolism, or cardiogenic shock. $Petco_2$ can be persistently *low* during hyperventilation or with an increase in dead space such as occurs with pulmonary embolization (even in the absence of a change in Q_T). (See Schwartz 10th ed., p. 410.)

15. Which of the following is NOT an indication for intracranial pressure (ICP) monitoring?
    A. Glasgow Coma Scale (GCS) less than or equal to 8 with an abnormal computed tomography (CT) scan.
    B. Severe traumatic brain injury (TBI) in a patient older than 40 years and systolic blood pressure less than 90 mm Hg.
    C. Intracranial hemorrhage without intraventricular blood.
    D. Fulminant hepatic failure with coma and cerebral edema on CT.

Answer: C

Monitoring of intracranial pressure (ICP) currently is recommended in patients with severe TBI, defined as a Glasgow Coma Scale (GCS) score less than or equal to 8 with an abnormal CT scan, and in patients with severe TBI and a normal CT scan if two or more of the following are present: age older than 40 years, unilateral or bilateral motor posturing, or systolic blood pressure less than 90 mm Hg. ICP monitoring is indicated in patients with acute subarachnoid hemorrhage with coma or neurologic deterioration, intracranial hemorrhage with intraventricular blood, ischemic middle cerebral artery stroke, fulminant hepatic failure with coma and cerebral edema on CT scan, and global cerebral ischemia or anoxia with cerebral edema on CT scan. The goal of ICP monitoring is to ensure that cerebral perfusion pressure (CPP) is adequate to support perfusion of the brain. (See Schwartz 10th ed., p. 411.)

16. Currently accepted uses of transcranial Doppler (TCD) include all of the following EXCEPT
    A. Diagnosing vasospasm after subarachnoid hemorrhage
    B. Estimating cerebral perfusion pressure
    C. Confirming brain death after clinical examination in patients under the influence of central nervous system (CNS) depressants.
    D. Confirming brain death after clinical examination in patients with metabolic encephalopathy.

Answer: B

Transcranial Doppler (TCD) measurements of middle and anterior cerebral artery blood flow velocity are useful for the diagnosis of cerebral vasospasm after subarachnoid hemorrhage. Qureshi et al demonstrated that an increase in the middle cerebral artery mean flow velocity as assessed by TCD is an independent predictor of symptomatic vasospasm in a prospective study of patients with aneurysmal subarachnoid hemorrhage. In addition, while some have proposed using TCD to estimate ICP, studies have shown that TCD is not a reliable method for estimating ICP and CPP, and currently cannot be endorsed for this purpose. TCD also is useful to confirm the clinical examination for determining brain death in patients with confounding factors such as the presence of CNS depressants or metabolic encephalopathy. (See Schwartz 10th ed., pp. 411–412.)

17. Regarding jugular venous oximetry in patients with TBI
    A. It requires placement of a catheter in the jugular bulb.
    B. Low jugular venous oxygen saturation (Sjo_2) has not been show to predict poor clinical outcomes.
    C. It is less invasive than placing an intraventricular monitor, but does not allow for continuous monitoring.
    D. It can replace ICP monitoring in patients without evidence of regional variation in cerebral blood flow.

Answer: A

When the arterial oxygen content, hemoglobin concentration, and the oxyhemoglobin dissociation curve are constant, changes in jugular venous oxygen saturation (Sjo_2) reflect changes in the difference between cerebral oxygen delivery and demand. Generally, a decrease in Sjo_2 reflects cerebral hypoperfusion, whereas an increase in Sjo_2 indicates the presence of hyperemia. Sjo_2 monitoring cannot detect decreases in regional cerebral blood flow if overall perfusion is normal or above normal. This technique requires the placement of a catheter in the jugular bulb, usually via the internal jugular vein. Catheters that permit intermittent aspiration of jugular venous blood for analysis or continuous oximetry catheters are available. Low Sjo_2 is associated with poor outcomes after TBI. Nevertheless, the value of monitoring Sjo_2 remains unproven. If it is employed, it should not be the sole monitoring technique, but rather should be used in conjunction with ICP and CPP monitoring. By monitoring ICP, CPP, and Sjo_2, early intervention with volume, vasopressors, and hyperventilation has been shown to prevent ischemic events in patients with TBI. (See Schwartz 10th ed., p. 412.)

18. Monitoring local brain tissue oxygen tension ($PbtO_2$) in patients with severe TBI
    A. Has shown that normal ICP and CPP generally precludes the presence of brain tissue ischemia
    B. Has been shown to lower mortality when compared with ICP monitoring alone
    C. Has not been adopted into routine clinical practice due to additional adverse effects from additional, potentially unnecessary, interventions
    D. Has been shown to increase stroke rate as a complication of catheter placement

Answer: B

While the standard of care for patients with severe TBI includes ICP and CPP monitoring, this strategy does not always prevent secondary brain injury. Growing evidence suggests that monitoring local brain tissue oxygen tension ($PbtO_2$) may be a useful adjunct to ICP monitoring in these patients. Normal values for $PbtO_2$ are 20 to 40 mm Hg, and critical levels are 8 to 10 mm Hg. A recent clinical study sought to determine whether the addition of a $PbtO_2$ monitor to guide therapy in severe TBI was associated with improved patient outcomes. Mortality was significantly lower in the patients who had therapy guided by $PbtO_2$ monitoring in addition to ICP and CPP (25%; $P < 0.05$). The benefits of $PbtO_2$ monitoring may include the early detection of brain tissue ischemia despite normal ICP and CPP. In addition, $PbtO_2$-guided management may reduce potential adverse effects associated with therapies to maintain ICP and CPP. (See Schwartz 10th ed., p. 412.)

CHAPTER 14

Minimally Invasive Surgery

1. The most common arrhythmia seen during laparoscopy is
   A. Atrial fibrilation
   B. Sinus tachycardia
   C. Premature ventricular contractions
   D. Sinus bradycardia

Answer: D
The pressure effects of the pneumoperitoneum on cardiovascular physiology also have been studied. In the hypovolemic individual, excessive pressure on the inferior vena cava and a reverse Trendelenburg position with loss of lower extremity muscle tone may cause decreased venous return and cardiac output. This is not seen in the normovolemic patient. The most common arrhythmia created by laparoscopy is bradycardia. A rapid stretch of the peritoneal membrane often causes a vagovagal response with bradycardia and occasionally hypotension. The appropriate management of this event is desufflation of the abdomen, administration of vagolytic agents (eg, atropine), and adequate volume replacement. (See Schwartz 10th ed., p. 418.)

2. Capacitive coupling
   A. Results when energy bleeds from a port sleeve or laparoscope into adjacent (but not touching) bowel
   B. Is always recognized at the time of surgery
   C. Can result in malfunction of the electrocardiogram monitor
   D. Can result in inaccurate image transmission to the digital monitor

Answer: A
To avoid thermal injury to adjacent structures, the laparoscopic field of view must include all uninsulated portions of the electrosurgical electrode. In addition, the integrity of the insulation must be maintained and assured. Capacitive coupling occurs when a plastic trocar insulates the abdominal wall from the current; in turn the current is bled off a metal sleeve or laparoscope into the viscera (Fig. 14-1). This may result in thermal necrosis and a delayed fecal fistula. Another potential mechanism for unrecognized visceral injury may occur with the direct coupling of current to the laparoscope and adjacent bowel. (See Schwartz 10th ed., Figure 14-7, pp. 427–428.)

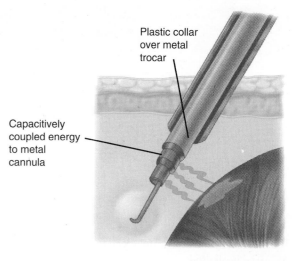

Capacitive coupled
fault condition

Plastic collar
over metal
trocar

Capacitively
coupled energy
to metal
cannula

FIG. 14-1. Capacitive coupling occurs as a result of high current density bleeding from a port sleeve or laparoscope into adjacent bowel. (Reproduced with permission from Odell RC. Laparoscopic electrosurgery, in Hunter JG, Sackier JM, eds. *Minimally Invasive Surgery*. New York: McGraw-Hill, 1993, p 33.)

3. Which of the following are true regarding safe laparoscopic surgery in pregnancy.
   A. The patient should be position in the left lateral position.
   B. Open abdominal access (Hasson) is recommended versus direct puncture laparoscopy (Veress neelde).
   C. The surgery should be performed during the second trimester if possible.
   D. All of the above.

Answer: D

Concerns about the safety of laparoscopic cholecystectomy and appendectomy in the pregnant patient have been thoroughly investigated and readily managed. Access to the abdomen in the pregnant patient should take into consideration the height of the uterine fundus, which reaches the umbilicus at 20 weeks. In order not to damage the uterus or tis blood supply, most surgeons feel that the open (Hasson) approach should be used in favor of direct puncture laparoscopy. The patient should be positioned slightly on the left side to avoid compression of the vena cava by the uterus. Because the pregnancy poses a risk for thromboembolism, sequential compression devices are essential for all procedures. Surgery should be performed in the second trimester, if possible. Protection of the fetus against intraoperative X-rays is imperative. (See Schwartz 10th ed., pp. 435–436.)

4. Systemic effects of CO_2 from pneumoperitoneum can cause all of the following EXCEPT
   A. Hypercarbia
   B. Increased myocardial oxygen demand
   C. Alterations in preload
   D. Increased after load

Answer: C

Alterations in preload are local effects (pressure specific) of CO_2 peritoneum.

The physiologic effects of CO_2 pneumoperitoneum can be divided into two areas (1) gas-specific effects and (2) pressure-specific effects (Fig. 14-2). CO_2 is rapidly absorbed across the peritoneal membrane into the circulation. In the circulation, CO_2 creates a respiratory acidosis by the generation of carbonic acid. Body buffers, the largest reserve of which lies in bone, absorb CO_2 (up to 120 L) and minimize the development of hypercarbia or respiratory acidosis during brief endoscopic procedures. Once the body buffers are saturated, respiratory acidosis develops rapidly, and the respiratory system assumes the burden of keeping up with the absorption of CO_2 and its release from these buffers.

In patients with normal respiratory function, this is not difficult; the anesthesiologist increases the ventilatory rate or

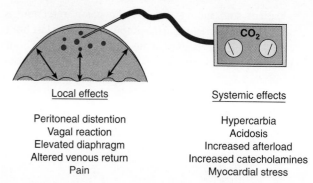

FIG. 14-2. Carbon dioxide gas insufflated into the peritoneal cavity has both local and systemic effects that cause a complex set of hemodynamic and metabolic alterations. (Reproduced with permission from Hunter JG, ed. *Baillière's Clinical Gastroenterology: Laparoscopic Surgery*. London/Philadelphia: Baillière Tindall, 1993, p. 758. Copyright Elsevier.)

vital capacity on the ventilator. If the respiratory rate required exceeds 20 breaths per minute, there may be less efficient gas exchange and increasing hypercarbia. Conversely, if vital capacity is increased substantially, there is a greater opportunity for barotrauma and greater respiratory motion-induced disruption of the upper abdominal operative field. In some situations, it is advisable to evacuate the pneumoperitoneum or reduce the intra-abdominal pressure to allow time for the anesthesiologist to adjust for hypercarbia. Although mild respiratory acidosis probably is an insignificant problem, more severe respiratory acidosis leading to cardiac arrhythmias has been reported. Hypercarbia also causes tachycardia and increased systemic vascular resistance, which elevates blood pressure and increases myocardial oxygen demand. (See Schwartz 10th ed., Figure 14-1, pp. 417–418.)

5. While performing a laparoscopic Nissen fundoplication during the transhiatal dissection the mediastinal pleura is compromised and a CO_2 pneumothorax develops. What is the initial preferred management of the pneumothorax?
   A. Needle thoracostomy over the second intercostal space, mid-clavicular line.
   B. Enlargement of the defect and placement of an 18-French red rubber catheter across the defect.
   C. Abort the procedure and emergent tube thoracostomy with a 28-French chest tube.
   D. No intervention is needed. Continue with the planned procedure.

Answer: B
When a pneumothorax occurs with laparoscopic Nissen fundoplication or Heller myotomy, it is preferable to place an 18-French red rubber catheter with multiple holes cut out of the distal end across the defect. At the end of the procedure, the distal end of the tube is pulled out a 10-mm port side (as the port is removed), and the pneumothorax is evacuated to a primitive water-seal using a bowl of sterile water or saline. (See Schwartz 10th ed., p. 419.)

6. When compared to traditional laparoscopic surgery, the advantages of computer-enhanced surgery are
   A. Natural wrist movements and improved manual dexterity
   B. Ergonomically comfortable workstation with 3-D imaging
   C. Tremor elimination
   D. All of the above

Answer: D
The major revolution in robotic surgery was the development of a master-slave surgical platform that returned the wrist to laparoscopic surgery and improved manual dexterity by developing ergonomically comfortable workstation, with 3-D imaging, tremor elimination, and scaling of movements (eg, large, gross hand movements can be scaled down to allow suturing with microsurgical precision). The most recent iteration of the robotic platform features a second console slave enabling greater assisting and teaching opportunities. (See Schwartz 10th ed., p. 429.)

7. A patient undergoing laparoscopic colon resection is noted to have decreased urine output during the last hour of the case. A bolus is given at the end of the case. One hour later, there is still very poor urine output. The appropriate treatment is
   A. Repeat bolus
   B. Intravenous (IV) furosemide
   C. Check urine electrolytes
   D. None of the above

Answer: D

Low urine output is a normal physiologic response to increased intra-abdominal pressure for up to 1 hour after surgery. Although the effect of the pneumoperitoneum on renal blood flow are immediately reversible, the hormonally mediated changes such as elevated antidiuretic hormone levels decrease urine output for up to 1 hour after the procedure has ended. Intraoperative oliguria is common during laparoscopy, but the urine output is not a reflection of intravascular status; intravenous (IV) fluid administration during an uncomplicated laparoscopic procedure should not be linked to urine output. (See Schwartz 10th ed., p. 418.)

CHAPTER 15

Molecular and Genomic Surgery

1. The process that occurs during translational control of eukaryotic gene expression is
   A. Protein degradation
   B. RNA processing
   C. Posttranslational control
   D. Transcription

Answer: A

Four major steps in the control of eukaryotic gene expression (Fig. 15-1). Transcriptional and posttranscriptional control determine the level of messenger RNA (mRNA) that is available to make a protein, while translational and posttranslational control determine the final outcome of functional proteins. Note that posttranscriptional and posttranslational controls consist of several steps. (See Schwartz 10th ed., Figure 16-6, p. 446.)

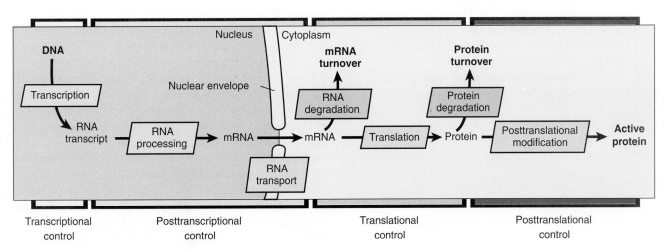

FIG. 15-1. Four major steps in the control of eukaryotic gene expression. Transcriptional and posttranscriptional control determine the level of messenger RNA (mRNA) that is available to make a protein, while translational and posttranslational control determine the final outcome of functional proteins. Note that posttranscriptional and posttranslational controls consist of several steps.

2. All of the following transcription mechanisms occur in eukaryotes EXCEPT
   A. Chromatin structure changes to allow DNA to be accessible to the polymerase.
   B. Three separate RNA polymerases are involved.
   C. Proteins or initiation factors are not required.
   D. Often packaged with histone and nonhistone proteins into chromatins.

Answer: C

Transcription mechanisms in eukaryotes differ from those in prokaryotes. The unique features of eukaryotic transcription are as follows: (1) Three separate RNA polymerases are involved in eukaryotes: RNA polymerase I transcribes the precursor of 5.8S, 18S, and 28S rRNAs; RNA polymerase II synthesizes the precursors of messenger RNA (mRNA) as well as microRNA; and RNA polymerase III makes tRNAs and 5S rRNAs. (2) In eukaryotes, the initial transcript is often the precursor to final mRNAs, tRNAs, and rRNAs. The precursor is then modified and/or processed into its final functional form. RNA splicing is one type of processing to remove the noncoding introns (the region between coding exons) on an mRNA. (3) In contrast to bacterial DNA, eukaryotic DNA often is packaged with histone and nonhistone proteins into chromatins. Transcription will only occur when the chromatin structure changes in such a way that DNA is accessible to the polymerase. (4) RNA is made in the nucleus and transported into cytoplasm, where translation occurs. Therefore, unlike bacteria, eukaryotes undergo uncoupled transcription and translation. (See Schwartz 10th ed., p. 447.)

3. The human genome contains approximately
   A. 35,000 to 40,000 genes
   B. 20,000 to 25,000 genes
   C. 25,000 to 30,000 genes
   D. 30,000 to 35,000 genes

Answer: C

Genome is a collective term for all genes present in one organism. The human genome contains DNA sequences of 3 billion base pairs, carried by 23 pairs of chromosomes. The human genome has an estimated 25,000 to 30,000 genes, and overall, it is 99.9% identical in all people. Approximately 3 million locations where single-base DNA differences exist have been identified and termed *single nucleotide polymorphisms*. Single nucleotide polymorphisms may be critical determinants of human variation in disease susceptibility and responses to environmental factors. (See Schwartz 10th ed., p. 449.)

4. If cyclin-dependent kinase (CDK) is to a cell as an engine is to a car, then cyclins and CKI are
   A. The key and ignition, respectively.
   B. The gas pedal and brakes, respectively.
   C. The distributor and the spark plug, respectively.
   D. The windows and the tires, respectively.

Answer: B

The cell cycle is connected with signal transduction pathways as well as gene expression. Although the S and M phases rarely are subjected to changes imposed by extracellular signals, the G1 and G2 phases are the primary periods when cells decide whether or not to move on to the next phase. During the G1 phase, cells receive green- or red-light signals, S phase entry or G1 arrest, respectively. Growing cells proliferate only when supplied with appropriate mitogenic growth factors. Cells become committed to entry of the cell cycle only toward the end of G1. Mitogenic signals stimulate the activity of early G1 cyclin-dependent kinases (CDKs) (eg, cyclin D/CDK4) that inhibit the activity of pRb protein and activate the transcription factor called *E2F* to induce the expression of batteries of genes essential for G1-S progression. Meanwhile, cells also receive antiproliferative signals such as those from tumor suppressors. These antiproliferative signals also act in the G1 phase to stop cells' progress into the S phase by inducing CKI production. For example, when DNA is damaged, cells will repair the damage before entering the S phase. Therefore, G1 contains one of the most important checkpoints for cell cycle progression. If the analogy is made that CDK is to a cell as an engine is to a car, then cyclins and CKI are the gas pedal and brakes, respectively. Accelerated proliferation or improper cell cycle progression with damaged DNA would be disastrous. Genetic gain-of-function mutations in oncogenes (that often promote expression or activity of the cyclin/CDK complex) or loss-of-function mutations in tumor suppressor (that stimulate production of CKI) are causal factors for malignant transformation. (See Schwartz 10th ed., p. 450.)

5. In cellular apoptosis, the release of cytochrome c activates the
   A. Fas receptor
   B. Death receptor
   C. Tumor necrosis factor receptor
   D. Caspase cascade

Answer: D
A simplified view of the apoptosis pathways (Fig. 15-2). Extracellular death receptor pathways include the activation of Fas and tumor necrosis factor (TNF) receptors, and consequent activation of the caspase pathway. Intracellular death pathway indicates the release of cytochrome c from mitochondria, which also triggers the activation of the caspase cascade. During apoptosis, cells undergo DNA fragmentation, nuclear and cell membrane breakdown, and are eventually digested by other cells. (See Schwartz 10th ed, Figure 15-8, p. 451.)

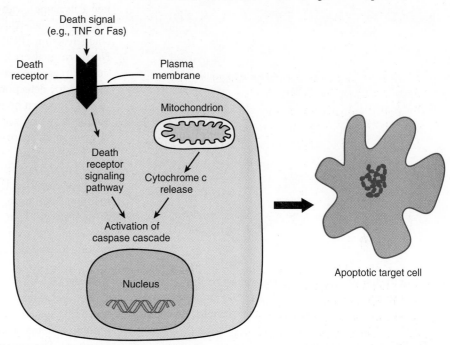

FIG. 15-2. A simplified view of the apoptosis pathways. Extracellular death receptor pathways include the activation of Fas and tumor necrosis factor (TNF) receptors, and consequent activation of the caspase pathway. Intracellular death pathway indicates the release of cytochrome c from mitochondria, which also triggers the activation of the caspase cascade. During apoptosis, cells undergo DNA fragmentation, nuclear and cell membrane breakdown, and are eventually digested by other cells.

6. Dysregulation of transforming growth factor-beta (TGF-β) signaling is associated with all of the following EXCEPT
   A. Cancer
   B. Inguinal hernias
   C. Marfan syndrome
   D. Thoracic aortic aneurysm

Answer: B
Resistance to transforming growth factor-beta's (TGF-β) anticancer action is one hallmark of human cancer cells. TGF-β receptors and SMADs are identified as tumor suppressors. The TGF-β signaling circuit can be disrupted in a variety of ways and in different types of human tumors. Some lose TGF-β responsiveness through downregulation or mutations of their TGF-β receptors. The cytoplasmic SMAD4 protein, which transduces signals from ligand-activated TGF-β receptors to downstream targets, may be eliminated through mutation of its encoding gene. The locus encoding cell cycle inhibitor p15INK4B may be deleted. Alternatively, the immediate downstream target of its actions, CDK4, may become unresponsive to the inhibitory actions of p15INK4B because of mutations that block p15INK4B binding. The resulting cyclin D/CDK4 complexes constitutively inactivate tumor suppressor pRb by hyperphosphorylation. Finally, functional pRb, the end target of this pathway, may be lost through mutation of its gene. For example, in pancreatic and colorectal cancers, 100% of cells derived from these cancers carry genetic defects in the TGF-β signaling pathway. Therefore, the antiproliferative pathway converging onto pRb and the cell division cycle is, in one way or another, disrupted in a majority of human cancer cells. Besides cancer, dysregulation of TGF-β signaling also has been associated with other human diseases such as Marfan syndrome and thoracic aortic aneurysm. (See Schwartz 10th ed., p. 453.)

7. The only gene expression detection method that provides information regarding mRNA size is
   A. Polymerase chain reaction (PCR)
   B. Southern blot hybridization
   C. Northern blot hybridization
   D. Immunoblotting

Answer: C

Northern blotting refers to the technique of size fractionation of RNA in a gel and the transferring of an RNA sample to a solid support (membrane) in such a manner that the relative positions of the RNA molecules are maintained. The resulting membrane then is hybridized with a labeled probe complementary to the mRNA of interest. Signals generated from detection of the membrane can be used to determine the size and abundance of the target RNA. In principle, Northern blot hybridization is similar to Southern blot hybridization (and hence its name), with the exception that RNA, not DNA, is on the membrane. Although reverse-transcriptase polymerase chain reaction (PCR) has been used in many applications, Northern analysis is the only method that provides information regarding mRNA size and has remained a standard method for detection and quantitation of mRNA. The process of Northern hybridization involves several steps, as does Southern hybridization, including electrophoresis of RNA samples in an agarose-formaldehyde gel, transfer to a membrane support, and hybridization to a radioactively labeled DNA probe. Data from hybridization allow quantification of steady-state mRNA levels and, at the same time, provide information related to the presence, size, and integrity of discrete mRNA species. Thus, Northern blot analysis, also termed *RNA gel blot analysis,* commonly is used in molecular biology studies relating to gene expression. (See Schwartz 10th ed., p. 458.)

8. All of the following are cell-surface receptors EXCEPT
   A. Transmitter-gated ion channels
   B. Seven-transmembrane-G-protein–coupled receptors (GPCRs)
   C. Enzyme-linked receptors
   D. Adhesive receptors

Answer: D

There are three major classes of cell-surface receptors: transmitter-gated ion channels, seven-transmembrane-G-protein–coupled receptors (GPCRs), and enzyme-linked receptors. The superfamily of GPCRs is one of the largest families of proteins, representing over 800 genes of the human genome. Members of this superfamily share a characteristic seven-transmembrane configuration. The ligands for these receptors are diverse and include hormones, chemokines, neurotransmitters, proteinases, inflammatory mediators, and even sensory signals such as odorants and photons. Most GPCRs signal through heterotrimeric G proteins, which are guanine nucleotide regulatory complexes. Thus the receptor serves as the receiver, the G protein serves as the transducer, and the enzyme serves as the effector arm. Enzyme-linked receptors possess an extracellular ligand-recognition domain and a cytosolic domain that either has intrinsic enzymatic activity or directly links with an enzyme. Structurally, these receptors usually have only one transmembrane-spanning domain. Of at least five forms of enzyme-linked receptors classified by the nature of the enzyme activity to which they are coupled, the growth factor receptors, such as tyrosine kinase receptor or serine/threonine kinase receptors, mediate diverse cellular events including cell growth, differentiation, metabolism, and survival/apoptosis. Dysregulation (particularly mutations) of these receptors is thought to underlie conditions of abnormal cellular proliferation in the context of cancer. The following sections will further review two examples of growth factor signaling pathways and their connection with human diseases. (See Schwartz 10th ed., p. 452.)

9. The process of decoding information on mRNA to synthe-
   size proteins is called
   A. Transcription
   B. Translation
   C. Replication
   D. Signaling

Answer: B

DNA directs the synthesis of RNA; RNA in turn directs the synthesis of proteins. Proteins are variable-length polypeptide polymers composed of various combinations of 20 different amino acids and are the working molecules of the cell.

The process of decoding information on mRNA to synthe-size proteins is called *translation* (see Fig. 15-3). Translation takes place in ribosomes composed of rRNA and ribosomal proteins. (See Schwartz 10th ed., Figure 15-1, pp. 445 and 447.)

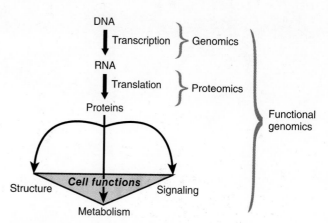

FIG. 15-3. The flow of genetic information from DNA to protein to cell functions. The process of transmission of genetic information from DNA to RNA is called *transcription,* and the process of transmission from RNA to protein is called *translation.* Proteins are the essential controlling components for cell structure, cell signaling, and metabolism. Genomics and proteomics are the study of the genetic composition of a living organism at the DNA and protein level, respectively. The study of the relationship between genes and their cellular functions is called *functional genomics.*

10. The cell cycle period in which DNA is duplicated is
    A. S
    B. G1
    C. M
    D. G2

Answer: A

Figure 15-4. The cell cycle and its control system. M is the mitosis phase, when the nucleus and the cytoplasm divide; S is the phase when DNA is duplicated; G1 is the gap between M and S; G2 is the gap between S and M. A complex of cyclin and cyclin-dependent kinase (CDK) controls specific events of each phase. Without cyclin, CDK is inactive. Different cyclin/CDK complexes are shown around the cell cycle. A, B, D, and E stand for cyclin A, cyclin B, cyclin D, and cyclin E, respectively. (See Schwartz 10th ed., Figure 15-7, p. 450.)

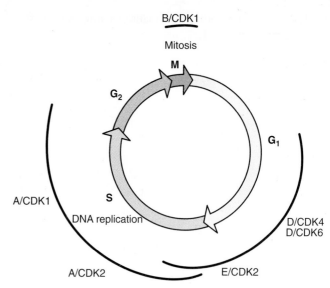

FIG. 15-4. The cell cycle and its control system. M is the mitosis phase, when the nucleus and the cytoplasm divide; S is the phase when DNA is duplicated; G1 is the gap between M and S; G2 is the gap between S and M. A complex of cyclin and cyclin-dependent kinase (CDK) controls specific events of each phase. Without cyclin, CDK is inactive. Different cyclin/CDK complexes are shown around the cell cycle. A, B, D, and E stand for cyclin A, cyclin B, cyclin D, and cyclin E, respectively.

11. In the transcription of prokaryotes, binding of RNA polymerase to the specific promoter region is achieved by
   A. Sigma factors
   B. Operon
   C. Elongation factors
   D. Rho factors

Answer: A

Initiation of transcription in prokaryotes begins with the recognition of DNA sequences by RNA polymerase. First, the bacterial RNA polymerase catalyzes RNA synthesis through loose binding to any region in the double-stranded DNA and then through specific binding to the promoter region with the assistance of accessory proteins called *σ factors* (sigma factors). A promoter region is the DNA region upstream of the transcription initiation site. RNA polymerase binds tightly at the promoter sites and causes the double-stranded DNA structure to unwind. Consequently, few nucleotides can be base-paired with the DNA template to begin transcription. Once transcription begins, the σ factor is released. The growing RNA chain may begin to peel off as the chain elongates. This occurs in such a way that there are always about 10 to 12 nucleotides of the growing RNA chains that are base-paired with the DNA template. (See Schwartz 10th ed., p. 447.)

12. When performing cell culture, cells should be
   A. Maintained in culture indefinitely.
   B. Fed with fresh medium every 2 to 3 days and split when they reach confluency.
   C. Prepared on surfaces wiped with a 50% ethyl alcohol solution.
   D. Maintained in a dehumidified carbon dioxide incubator at 37°F.

Answer: B

Cell culture has become one of the most powerful tools in biomedical laboratories, as cultured cells are being used in a diversity of biologic fields ranging from biochemistry to molecular and cellular biology. Through their ability to be maintained in vitro, cells can be manipulated by the introduction of genes of interest (cell transfection) and be transferred into in vivo biologic receivers (cell transplantation) to study the biologic effect of the interested genes (Fig. 15-5). In the common laboratory settings, cells are cultured either as a monolayer (in which cells grow as one layer on culture dishes) or in suspension. It is important to know the wealth of information concerning cell culturing before attempting the procedure. For example, conditions of culture will depend on the cell types to be cultured (eg, origins of the cells such as epithelial or fibroblasts, or primary versus immortalized/transformed cells). It is also necessary to use cell type-specific culture medium that varies in combination of growth factors and serum concentrations. If primary cells are derived from human patients or animals, some commercial resources have a variety of culture media available for testing. Generally, cells are manipulated in a sterile hood, and the working surfaces are wiped with 70 to 80% ethyl alcohol solution. Cultured cells are usually maintained in a humidified carbon dioxide incubator at 37°C (98.6°F) and need to be examined daily under an inverted microscope to check for possible contamination and confluency (the area cells occupy on the dish). As a general rule, cells should be fed with fresh medium every 2 to 3 days and split when they reach confluency. Depending on the growth rate of cells, the actual time and number of plates required to split cells in two varies from cell line to cell line. Splitting a monolayer requires the detachment of cells from plates by using a trypsin or collagenase treatment, of which concentration and time period vary depending on cell lines. If cultured cells grow continuously in suspension, they are split or subcultured by dilution.

Because cell lines may change their properties when cultured, it is not possible to maintain cell lines in culture indefinitely. (See Schwartz 10th ed., Figure 15-21, p. 462.)

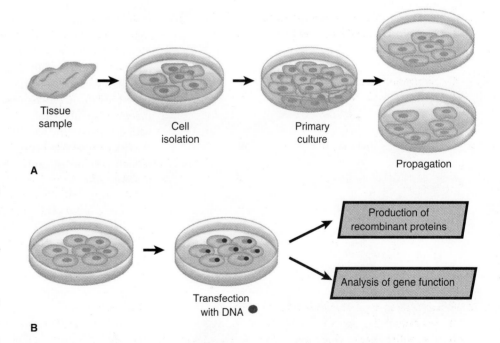

FIG.15-5. Cell culture and transfection. A. Primary cells can be isolated from tissues and cultured in medium for a limited period of time. After genetic manipulations to overcome the cell aging process, primary cells can be immortalized into cell lines for long-term culture. B. DNA can be introduced into cells to produce recombinant gene products or to analyze the biologic functions of the gene.

13. All of the following are involved in gene regulation EXCEPT
    A. Introns
    B. Control of messenger RNA (mRNA) stability
    C. Lack of modification of mRNA
    D. Control of export of mRNA from the nucleus to the cytoplasm

Answer: C

Living cells have the necessary machinery to enzymatically transcribe DNA into RNA and translate the mRNA into protein. This machinery accomplishes the two major steps required for gene expression in all organisms: transcription and translation (see Fig. 15-1). However, gene regulation is far more complex, particularly in eukaryotic organisms. For example, many gene transcripts must be spliced to remove the intervening sequences. The sequences that are spliced off are called *introns,* which appear to be useless, but in fact may carry some regulatory information. The sequences that are joined together, and are eventually translated into protein, are called *exons*. Additional regulation of gene expression includes modification of mRNA, control of mRNA stability, and its nuclear export into cytoplasm (where it is assembled into ribosomes for translation). After mRNA is translated into protein, the levels and functions of the proteins can be further regulated posttranslationally. (See Schwartz 10th ed., p. 446.)

14. Which of the following is a regulator of the cell cycle?
    A. CDK
    B. Tyrosine kinase
    C. Pol II holoenzyme
    D. Caspase

Answer: A

The machinery that drives cell cycle progression is made up of a group of enzymes called *CDKs*. Cyclin expression fluctuates during the cell cycle, and cyclins are essential for CDK activities and form complexes with CDK. The cyclin A/CDK1 and cyclin B/CDK1 drive the progression for the M phase, while cyclin A/CDK2 is the primary S phase complex. Early G1 cyclin D/CDK4/6 or late G1 cyclin E/CDK2 controls the G1-S transition. There also are negative regulators for CDK termed *CDK inhibitors,* which inhibit the assembly or activity of the cyclin-CDK complex. Expression of cyclins and CDK inhibitors often is regulated by developmental and environmental factors. (See Schwartz 10th ed., p. 450.)

15. Which of the following drugs is a monoclonal antibody to an oncogene?
    A. Trastuzumab
    B. Methotrexate
    C. Adriamycin
    D. Gleevec

Answer: A

Patients whose tumors overexpress *HER-2/neu* are candidates for anti–*HER-2/neu* therapy. Trastuzumab (Herceptin) is a recombinant humanized monoclonal antibody directed against *HER-2/neu*. Randomized clinical trials have demonstrated that single-agent trastuzumab therapy is an active and well-tolerated option for first-line treatment of women with *HER-2/neu*–overexpressing metastatic breast cancer. More recently, adjuvant trials demonstrated that trastuzumab also was highly effective in the treatment of women with early-stage breast cancer when used in combination with chemotherapy. Patients who received trastuzumab in combination with chemotherapy had between a 40 and 50% reduction in the risk of breast cancer recurrence and approximately a third reduction in breast cancer mortality. (See Schwartz 10th ed., p. 454.)

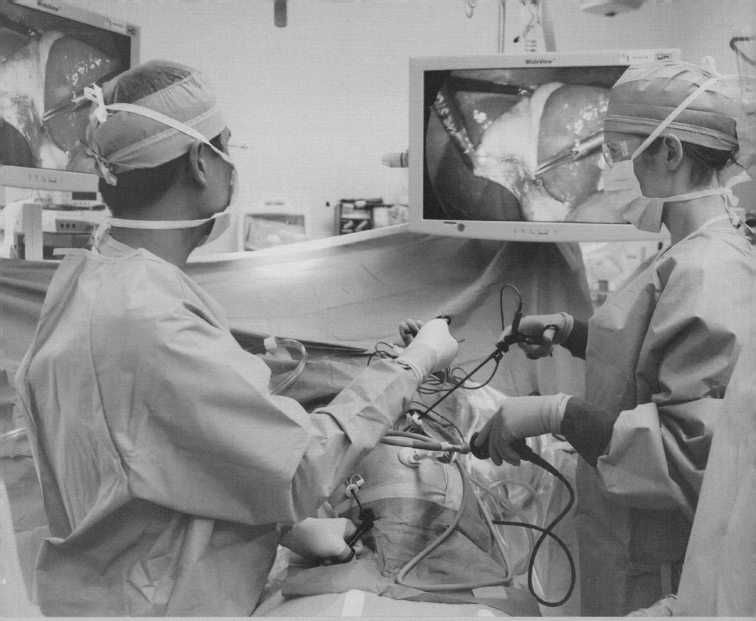

PART II
Specific Consideration

CHAPTER 16

The Skin and Subcutaneous Tissue

1. Following caustic injury to the skin with an alkaline agent the effected area should initially be
   A. Treated with running water or saline for 30 minutes
   B. Treated with running water or saline for 2 hours
   C. Treated with a neutralizing agent
   D. Treated with topical emollients and oral analgesics

Answer: B

The treatment for both types of injuries is based on neutralization of the inciting solution and starts with running distilled water or saline over the affected skin for at least 30 minutes for acidic solutions and 2 hours for alkaline injuries. It should be noted that neutralizing agents do not offer a significant advantage over dilution with water, may delay treatment, and may worsen the injury due to the exothermic reaction that may occur. The clinician observes and treats based on the degree of presentation. Many cases are successfully managed conservatively with topical emollients and oral analgesics, and most cases result in edema, erythema, and induration. If signs of deep second-degree burns develop, local wound care may include debridement, Silvadene, and protective petroleum gauze. In severe cases, injury to the underlying vessels, bones, muscle, and tendon may occur, and these cases may be managed within 24 hours by liposuction through a small catheter and then saline injection. Surgery is indicated for tissue necrosis, uncontrolled pain, or deep-tissue damage. Antibiotics should not be administered unless signs of infection are present. (See Schwartz 10th ed., p. 479.)

2. The treatment of a hydrofluoric acid skin burn is
   A. Application of calcium carbonate gel
   B. Irrigation with sodium bicarbonate
   C. Injection of sodium bicarbonate
   D. Local wound care only

Answer: A

Injuries that have specific additional treatments include hydrofluoride burns. Hydrofluoride is found in air conditioning cleaners and petroleum refineries. Treatment of hydrofluoride burns should include topical or locally injected calcium gluconate to bind fluorine ions. Intra-arterial calcium gluconate can provide pain relief and preserves arteries from necrosis, whereas intravenous (IV) calcium repletes resorbed calcium stores. Topical calcium carbonate gel and quaternary ammonium compounds detoxify fluoride ions. This mitigates the leaching of calcium and magnesium ions by the hydrofluoric acid from the affected tissues and prevents potentially severe hypocalcemia and hypomagnesemia that predispose to cardiac arrhythmias. (See Schwartz 10th ed., pp. 479–480.)

3. The area most amenable to salvage by resuscitative and wound management techniques following thermal injury is called the
   A. Zone of hyperemia
   B. Zone of coagulation
   C. Zone of stasis
   D. Zone of scalding

Answer: C

Exposure of the skin to thermal extremes disrupts its primary function as a barrier to heat loss, evaporation, and microbial invasion. The depth and extent of injury are dependent on the duration and temperature of the exposure. The pathophysiology and management are discussed elsewhere in this book. Briefly, the epicenter of the injury undergoes a varying extent of necrosis (depending on the exposure), otherwise referred to as the *zone of coagulation,* which is surrounded by the zone of stasis, which has marginal perfusion and questionable viability. This is the area of tissue that is most amenable to salvage by appropriate resuscitative and wound management techniques, which would theoretically limit the extent of injury. The outermost area of skin shows characteristics similar to other inflamed tissues and has been designated the zone of hyperemia. The degree of burn corresponds to histologic layers of the affected dermis and correlates with management and prognosis pertaining to timeline of healing and magnitude of scarring. (See Schwartz 10th ed., p. 480.)

4. Tissue ischemia resulting in wounds that are characterized as a partial-thickness injury with a blister is considered
   A. Stage 1
   B. Stage 2
   C. Stage 3
   D. Stage 4

Answer: B

Tissue pressures that exceed the pressure of the microcirculation (30 mm Hg) result in tissue ischemia. Frequent or prolonged ischemic insults will ultimately result in tissue damage. Areas of bony prominence are particularly prone to ischemia, the most common areas being ischial tuberosity (28%), trochanter (19%), sacrum (17%), and heel (9%). Tissue pressures can measure up to 300 mm Hg in the ischial region during sitting and 150 mm Hg over the sacrum while lying supine. Muscle is more susceptible than skin to ischemic insult due to its relatively high metabolic demand. Wounds are staged as follows: stage 1, nonblanching erythema over intact skin; stage 2, partial-thickness injury (epidermis or dermis)—blister or crater; stage 3, full-thickness injury extending down to, but not including, fascia and without undermining of adjacent tissue; and stage 4, full-thickness skin injury with destruction or necrosis of muscle, bone, tendon, or joint capsule. (See Schwartz 10th ed., p. 482.)

5. The presence of sulfur granules in a draining wound should lead to the use of which of the following antibiotics?
   A. Rifampin
   B. Gentamicin
   C. Penicillin
   D. Amphotericin

Answer: C

Actinomycosis should be considered in the differential diagnosis of any acute, subacute, or chronic cutaneous swelling of the head and neck. The cervicofacial form of *Actinomycetes* infection is the most common presentation, typically as an acute pyogenic infection in the submandibular or paramandibular area, but infection could be elsewhere in the mandibular and maxillary regions. The primary skin infection may spread to adjacent structures such as the scalp, orbit, ears, and other areas. Oral infection may spread to the hypopharynx, larynx, trachea, salivary glands, and sinuses. Actinomycosis can spread beyond boundaries of tissue planes and may also mimic chronic osteomyelitis. Treatment consists of a combination of penicillin therapy and surgical debridement. Debulking and debriding infected tissue arising from sinus tracts and abscess cavities inhibit actinomycosis growth in most cases. (See Schwartz 10th ed., p. 484.)

6. Initial treatment of nonpurulent, complicated cellulitis is
   A. Vancomycin
   B. β-lactam
   C. Linezolid
   D. Clindamycin

Answer: B

Treatment of nonpurulent, complicated cellulitis can begin with a β-lactam, with methicillin-resistant *Staphylococcus aureus* (MRSA) coverage added if no response is observed. Empiric MRSA coverage is warranted in all other complicated skin and subcutaneous infections. Vancomycin is the mainstay of therapy, although it is inferior to β-lactams for methicillin-sensitive *S. aureus* (MSSA) and has a relatively slow onset of efficacy in vitro. Linezolid, daptomycin, tigecycline, and telavancin are other FDA-approved alternatives for MRSA treatment. Clindamycin is also approved for *S. aureus*; however, resistance may develop, and diarrhea can occur in up to 20% (*Clostridium difficile* related). (See Schwartz 10th ed., p. 483.)

7. A 3-mm basal cell carcinoma (BCC) of the skin should be treated with
   A. Biopsy and gross total excision
   B. Dermatologic laser vaporization
   C. Excision with 2- to 4-mm normal margin
   D. Electrodesiccation

Answer: C

Basal cell carcinoma (BCC) arises from the basal layer of non-keratinocytes and represents the most common tumor diagnosed in the United States. Annually it accounts for 25% of all diagnosed cancers and 75% of skin cancers. The primary risk factor for disease development is sun exposure (ultraviolet [UV] B rays more than UVA rays) particularly during adolescence; however, other factors include immune suppression (ie, organ transplant recipients, human immunodeficiency virus [HIV]), chemical exposure, and ionizing radiation exposure. BCC can also be a feature of inherited conditions such as xeroderma pigmentosa, unilateral basal cell nevus syndrome, and nevoid BCC syndrome. The natural behavior of BCC is one of local invasion rather than distant metastasis. Untreated BCC can result in significant morbidity. Thirty percent of cases are found on the nose, and bleeding, ulceration, and itching are often part of the clinical presentation. (See Schwartz 10th ed., p. 486.)

8. Trichilemmal cysts
   A. Are the most common type of cutaneous cysts
   B. Are found between the forehead to nose tip
   C. Are typically found on the scalp of females
   D. Occasionally develop bone, tooth, or nerve tissue

Answer: C

There are three types of cutaneous cysts: epidermal, dermoid, and trichilemmal. All of these benign entities comprise epidermis that grows toward the center of the cyst, resulting in central accumulation of keratin to form a cyst. All clinically appear as a white, creamy substance-containing subcutaneous, thin-walled nodule. Epidermal cysts are the most common cutaneous cyst and histologically characterized by mature epidermis complete with granular layer. Trichilemmal cysts are the second most common lesion; they tend to form on the scalp of females, have a distinct odor after rupture, histologically lack a granular layer, and have an outer layer resembling the root sheath of a hair follicle. Dermoid cysts are congenital, found between the forehead to nose tip, and contain squamous epithelium, eccrine glands, and pilosebaceous units, occasionally developing bone, tooth, or nerve tissue. The eyebrow is the most frequent site of presentation. These cysts are commonly asymptomatic but can become inflamed and infected, thus necessitating incision and drainage. After the acute phase subsides, the entire cyst should be removed to prevent recurrence. (See Schwartz 10th ed., p. 486.)

9. More than half of patients treated for BCC will experience a recurrence within
   A. 6 months
   B. 1 years
   C. 2 years
   D. 3 years

Answer: D

It is critical for each patient to have routine annual follow-up that includes full-body skin examinations. Sixty-six percent of recurrences develop within 3 years, and with a few exceptions occurring decades after initial treatment, the remaining recur within 5 years of initial treatment. A second primary BCC may develop after treatment and, in 40% of cases, presents within the first 3 years after treatment. (See Schwartz 10th ed., p. 487.)

10. The primary risk factor for the development of squamous cell carcinoma (SCC) is
    A. UV exposure
    B. Cigarette smoking
    C. Chemical agents
    D. Chronic, nonhealing wounds

Answer: A

Squamous cell carcinoma (SCC) is the second most common skin cancer, accounting for approximately 100,000 cases each year and generally afflicting individuals of lighter skin color. The primary risk factor and driving force for the development of this common cancer is UV exposure; however, other risks include environmental factors such as chemical agents, physical agents (ionizing radiation), psoralen and UVA (PUVA), HPV-16 and -18 infections (immunosuppression), and smoking. Chronic nonhealing wounds, burn scars, and chronic dermatosis are other risk factors, and many darker skin individuals who develop SCC often have a history of one of these risk factors. Heritable conditions such as xeroderma pigmentosum, epidermolysis bullosa, and oculocutaneous albinism are predisposing risk factors. (See Schwartz 10th ed., p. 487.)

11. In the ABCDE of melanoma, the D stands for *d*iameter greater than
    A. 2 mm
    B. 4 mm
    C. 6 mm
    D. 8 mm

Answer: C

Melanoma most commonly manifests as cutaneous disease, and clinical characteristics include an **A**symmetric outline, changing irregular **B**orders, **C**olor variations, **D**iameter greater than 6 mm, and **E**levation (ABCDE). Other key clinical characteristics include a pigmented lesion that has enlarged, ulcerated, or bled. Amelanotic lesions appear as raised pink, purple, or normal-colored skin papules and are often diagnosed late. (See Schwartz 10th ed., p. 488.)

12. The most common site of distant metastasis for melanoma is
    A. Brain
    B. Lung
    C. Gastrointestinal tract
    D. Distant skin

Answer: B

The most common sites of distant metastasis are the lungs and liver followed by the brain, gastrointestinal tract, distant skin, and subcutaneous tissue. A limited subset of patients with small-volume, limited distant metastases to the brain, gastrointestinal tract, or distant skin will be cured with resection or gamma knife radiation. Liver metastases are better dealt without surgical resection unless they arise from an ocular primary. (See Schwartz 10th ed., p. 491.)

13. The most common subtype of melanoma is
    A. Lentigo maligna
    B. Acral lentiginous
    C. Superficial spreading
    D. Nodular

Answer: C

Melanoma growth most commonly starts as a localized, radial growth phase followed by a vertical growth phase that determines metastatic risk. The subtypes of melanoma include lentigo maligna, superficial spreading, acral lentiginous, mucosal, nodular, polypoid, desmoplastic, amelanotic, and soft tissue. The most common subtype is superficial spreading, accounting for 70% of cases. (See Schwartz 10th ed., p. 488.)

14. Ocular melanoma
    A. Exclusively metastasizes to the lungs
    B. Exclusively metastasizes to the brain
    C. Exclusively metastasizes to regional lymph nodes
    D. Exclusively metastasizes to the liver

Answer: D

Ocular melanoma is the most common noncutaneous disease site, and treatment includes photocoagulation, partial resection, radiation, or enucleation. Ocular melanomas exclusively metastasize to the liver and not regional lymph nodes, and some patients benefit from liver resection. (See Schwartz 10th ed., p. 491.)

15. The following is NOT true in regard to Merkel cell carcinoma
    A. It is commonly found in white men with a median age of 70 years.
    B. It is characterized by a rapidly growing, flesh-colored papule.
    C. Treatment should begin with examination of nodal basins.
    D. Recurrence is uncommon.

Answer: D

This is a rare and aggressive neuroendocrine tumor of the skin most commonly found in white men and diagnosed at a mean age of 70 years. Risk factors include UV radiation, PUVA, and immunosuppression. Approximately one in three cases present on the face, with the remainder occurring on sun-exposed skin. A rapidly growing, flesh-colored papule or plaque characterizes the disease. Regional lymph nodes are involved in 30% of patients, and 50% will develop systemic disease (skin, lymph nodes, liver, lung, bone, brain). There are no standardized diagnostic imaging studies for staging, but computed tomography (CT) of the chest, abdomen, and pelvis and octreotide scans may provide useful information when clinically indicated. After examining the entire skin for other lesions, treatment should begin by evaluating the nodal basins.

Recurrence is common, and one study of 95 patients showed a 47% recurrence, with 80% of recurrences occurring within 2 years and 96% occurring within 5 years. Regional lymph node disease is common, and 70% of patients will have nodal spread within 2 years of disease presentation. Five-year overall survival of head and neck disease in surgically treated patients is between 40 and 68%. (See Schwartz 10th ed., p. 492.)

16. What is the most common melanoma in patients with dark skin?
    A. Nodular
    B. Superficial spreading
    C. Acral lentiginous
    D. Lentigo maligna

Answer: C

Nodular melanoma accounts for 15 to 30% of melanomas, and this variant is unique because it begins with a vertical growth phase that partly accounts for its worse prognosis. Lentigo maligna is typically found in older individuals and primarily located in the head and neck region. The acral lentiginous variant accounts for 29 to 72% of melanomas in dark-skinned individuals, is occasionally seen in Caucasians, and is found on palmar, plantar, and subungual surfaces. (See Schwartz 10th ed., p. 488.)

17. Kaposi sarcoma
    A. Excision is the treatment of choice
    B. Is predominantly found on the skin
    C. Appears as rubbery, blue nodules
    D. Is most often seen in patients in their fifth decade of life

Answer: A

Kaposi sarcoma is diagnosed after the fifth decade of life and predominantly found on the skin but can occur anywhere in the body. In North America, the Kaposi sarcoma herpes virus is transmitted via sexual and nonsexual routes and predominantly affects individuals with compromised immune systems such as those with HIV and transplant recipients on immune-suppressing medications. Clinically, Kaposi sarcoma appears as multifocal, rubbery blue nodules. Treatment of acquired immunodeficiency syndrome (AIDS)-associated Kaposi sarcoma is with antiviral therapy, and many patients experience a dramatic treatment response. Those individuals who do not respond and have limited mucocutaneous disease may benefit from cryotherapy, photodynamic therapy, radiation therapy, intralesional injections, and topical therapy. Surgical biopsy is important for disease diagnosis, but given the high local recurrence and the fact that Kaposi sarcoma represents more of a systemic rather than local disease, the benefit of surgery is limited and generally should not be pursued except for palliation. (See Schwartz 10th ed., p. 492.)

18. The following is NOT a prognostic indicator for patients with a sentinel node containing metastatic melanoma
    A. Patient age
    B. Site of metastasis
    C. Number of positive nodes
    D. Thickness, mitotic rate, and ulceration of primary tumor

Answer: B

Melanoma is characterized according to the American Joint Committee on Cancer (AJCC) as localized disease (stage I and II), regional disease (stage III), or distant metastatic disease (stage IV). Overall tumor thickness, ulceration, and mitotic rate are the most important prognostic indicators of survival. If a sentinel node contains metastatic melanoma, the number of positive nodes; thickness, mitotic rate, and ulceration of the primary tumor; and patient age determine prognosis. With clinically positive nodes, the number of positive nodes, primary tumor ulceration, and patient age determine prognosis. The site of metastasis is strongly associated with prognosis for stage IV disease, and elevated lactate dehydrogenase (LDH) is associated with a worse prognosis. (See Schwartz 10th ed., p. 488.)

19. A patient with a 5-mm deep melanoma of the thigh and no clinically positive nodes should undergo which procedure?
    A. Resection of the primary only
    B. Superficial femoral node resection
    C. Superficial and deep femoral node resection
    D. Resection of femoral and inguinal nodal basins

Answer: A

Nonmetastatic in-transit disease should undergo excision to clear margins when feasible. However, disease not amenable to complete excision derives benefit from isolated limb perfusion (ILP) and isolated limb infusion (ILI) (Fig. 16-1). These two modalities are used to treat regional disease, and their purpose is to administer high doses of chemotherapy, commonly melphalan, to an affected limb while avoiding systemic drug toxicity. ILI was shown to provide a 31% response rate in one study, while hyperthermic ILP provided a 63% complete response rate in an independent study. (See Schwartz 10th ed., Figure 16-15, p. 491.)

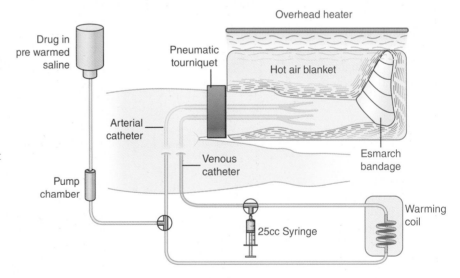

FIG. 16-1. Isolated limb infusion. Schematic of isolated limb infusion of lower extremity. (From Thompson JF, Kam PC. Isolated limb infusion for melanoma: a simple but effective alternative to isolated limb perfusion. *J Surg Onc.* 2004;88:1-3. Copyright 2004 John Wiley and Sons. Reprinted with permission.)

20. A 65-year-old patient who spends winters in Florida presents with a painless, ulcerated lesion on his right cheek. The lesion has been present for 1 year. Physical examination of the patient's neck reveals no lymph node enlargement. The most likely diagnosis is
    A. Melanoma
    B. BCC
    C. SCC
    D. Sebaceous cyst

Answer: B

The most common form of BCC (60%) is the nodular variant, characterized by raised, pearly pink papules and occasionally a depressed tumor center with raised borders giving the classic "rodent ulcer" appearance. This variant tends to develop in sun-exposed areas of individuals older than 60 years. Superficial BCC accounts for 15% of BCC, is diagnosed at a mean age of 57 years, and typically appears on the trunk as a pink or erythematous plaque with a thin pearly border. The infiltrative form appears on the head and neck in the late 60s with similar clinical appearance to the nodular variant. An important variant to keep in mind is the pigmented variant of nodular BCC because this may be difficult to differentiate from nodular melanoma. Other important subtypes include the morpheaform variant, accounting for 3% of cases and characterized by indistinct borders with a yellow hue, and fibroepithelioma of Pinkus. Histologic subtypes of BCC include nodular and micronodular (50%), superficial (15%), and infiltrative. (See Schwartz 10th ed., p. 486.)

21. The chronic inflammatory disease presenting as painful subcutaneous nodules is
    A. Pyoderma gangrenosum
    B. Toxic epidermal necrolysis syndrome
    C. Hidradenitis suppurative
    D. Steven-Johnson syndrome

Answer: C

Hidradenitis suppurativa is a chronic inflammatory disease presenting as painful subcutaneous nodules. Patients experience appreciable physical, psychological, and economical hardship and decreased quality of life when compared with patients who suffer from other chronic dermatologic disease such as psoriasis and alopecia. It is characterized by multiple abscesses, internetworking sinus tracts, foul-smelling exudate from draining sinuses, inflammation in the dermis, both atrophic and hypertrophic scars, ulceration, and infection, which may extend deep into the fascia. The diagnosis is made clinically without the need for imaging or laboratory tests. (See Schwartz 10th ed., p. 467.)

22. Correct statements about toxic epidermal necrolysis (TEN) include all of the following EXCEPT
    A. Toxic epidermal necrolysis is believed to be an immunologic problem.
    B. Lesions are similar in appearance to partial thickness burns.
    C. The process develops at the dermoepidermal junction.
    D. Corticosteroid use is a primary part of therapy.

Answer: D

These inflammatory diseases represent a spectrum of an autoimmune reaction to stimuli such as drugs that result in structural defects in the epidermal-dermal junction. The cutaneous manifestations of toxic epidermal necrolysis syndrome (TENS) follow a prodromal period reminiscent of an upper respiratory tract infection. A symmetrical macular eruption follows starting from the face and trunk and spreading to the extremities. Typically, a Nikolsky sign develops in which lateral pressure causes the epidermis to detach from the basal layer. The macular eruption evolves into blisters, causing an extensive superficial partial-thickness skin injury with exposed dermis. (See Schwartz 10th ed., p. 477.)

23. The rare adenocarcinoma of the apocrine gland that often appears as a nonpigmented plaque is
    A. Angiosarcoma
    B. Extramammary Paget disease
    C. Malignant fibrous histiocytoma
    D. Dermatofibrosarcoma protuberans

Answer: B

This rare adenocarcinoma of apocrine glands arises in perianal and axillary regions and in genitalia of men and women. Clinical presentation is that of erythematous or nonpigmented plaques with an eczema-like appearance that often persist after failed treatment from other therapies. An important characteristic and one that the surgeon must be acutely aware of is the high incidence of concomitant other malignancies with this cutaneous disease. Forty percent of cases are associated with primary gastrointestinal and genitourinary malignancies, and a diligent search should be made after a diagnosis of extramammary Paget disease is made. Treatment is surgical resection with negative microscopic margins, and adjuvant radiation may provide additional locoregional control. (See Schwartz 10th ed., p. 493.)

CHAPTER **17**

Breast

1. Which of the following statements about normal breast anatomy is true?
   A. The breast typically contains 10 lobes.
   B. Cooper ligaments are only found in the upper quadrants of the breast.
   C. The upper inner quadrant of the breast contains the most breast tissue.
   D. The tail of Spence extends across the anterior axillary fold.

Answer: D
The breast is composed of 15 to 20 lobes, which are each composed of several lobules. Fibrous bands of connective tissue travel through the breast (Cooper suspensory ligaments), insert perpendicularly into the dermis, and provide structural support. The mature female breast extends from the level of the second or third rib to the inframammary fold at the sixth or seventh rib. It extends transversely from the lateral border of the sternum to the anterior axillary line. The deep or posterior surface of the breast rests on the fascia of the pectoralis major, serratus anterior, and external oblique abdominal muscles, and the upper extent of the rectus sheath. The retromammary bursa may be identified on the posterior aspect of the breast between the investing fascia of the breast and the fascia of the pectoralis major muscles. The axillary tail of Spence extends laterally across the anterior axillary fold. (See Schwartz 10th ed., p. 500.)

2. Which of the following changes in the breast is NOT associated with pregnancy?
   A. Accumulation of lymphocytes, plasma cells, and eosinophils within the breast.
   B. Enlargement of breast alveoli.
   C. Release of colostrum.
   D. Accumulation of secretory products in minor duct lumina.

Answer: C
With pregnancy, the breast undergoes proliferative and developmental maturation. As the breast enlarges in response to hormonal stimulation, lymphocytes, plasma cells, and eosinophils accumulate within the connective tissues. The minor ducts branch and alveoli develop. Development of the alveoli is asymmetric, and variations in the degree of development may occur within a single lobule. With parturition, enlargement of the breasts occurs via hypertrophy of alveolar epithelium and accumulation of secretory products in the lumina of the minor ducts. Alveolar epithelium contains abundant endoplasmic reticulum, large mitochondria, Golgi complexes, and dense lysosomes. Two distinct substances are produced by the alveolar epithelium: (1) the protein component of milk, which is synthesized in the endoplasmic reticulum (merocrine secretion); and (2) the lipid component of milk (apocrine secretion), which forms as free lipid droplets in the cytoplasm. Milk released in the first few days after parturition is called *colostrum* and has low lipid content but contains considerable quantities of antibodies. (See Schwartz 10th ed., p. 501.)

3. The breast receives its blood supply from all of the following EXCEPT
   A. Branches of the internal mammary artery
   B. Branches of the superior epigastric artery
   C. Branches of the posterior intercostal arteries
   D. Branches of thoracoacromial artery

Answer: B

The breast receives its principal blood supply from: (1) perforating branches of the internal mammary artery; (2) lateral branches of the posterior intercostal arteries; and (3) branches from the axillary artery, including the highest thoracic, lateral thoracic, and pectoral branches of the thoracoacromial artery. The second, third, and fourth anterior intercostal perforators and branches of the internal mammary artery arborize in the breast as the medial mammary arteries. The lateral thoracic artery gives off branches to the serratus anterior, pectoralis major and pectoralis minor, and subscapularis muscles. It also gives rise to lateral mammary branches. (See Schwartz 10th ed., p. 501.)

4. Which of the following statements is INCORRECT?
   A. Level I lymph nodes are those that are lateral to the pectoralis minor muscle.
   B. Level II lymph nodes are located deep to the pectoralis minor muscle.
   C. Level III lymph nodes are located medial to the pectoralis minor muscle.
   D. Level IV lymph nodes are the ipsilateral internal mammary lymph nodes.

Answer: D

Level I includes lymph nodes located lateral to the pectoralis minor muscle; level II includes lymph nodes located deep to the pectoralis minor; and level III includes lymph nodes located medial to the pectoralis minor. (See Schwartz 10th ed., p. 502.)

5. Concerning breast development before and during pregnancy, which hormonal activity pairing is INCORRECT?
   A. Estrogen: Initiates ductal development
   B. Progesterone: Initiates lobular development
   C. Prolactin: Initiates lactogenesis
   D. Follicle stimulating hormone: Cooper ligament relaxation

Answer: D

Estrogen initiates ductal development, whereas progesterone is responsible for differentiation of epithelium and for lobular development. Prolactin is the primary hormonal stimulus for lactogenesis in late pregnancy and the postpartum period. The gonadotropins luteinizing hormone (LH) and follicle-stimulating hormone (FSH) regulate the release of estrogen and progesterone from the ovaries. In turn, the release of LH and FSH from the basophilic cells of the anterior pituitary is regulated by the secretion of gonadotropin-releasing hormone (GnRH) from the hypothalamus. (See Schwartz 10th ed., pp. 503–504.)

6. Concerning gynecomastia, which of the following is true?
   A. During senescence gynecomastia is usually unilateral.
   B. During puberty gynecomastia is usually bilateral.
   C. Is not associated with breast cancer except in Ehlers-Danlos patients.
   D. Is classified as per a three-grade system.

Answer: D

In gynecomastia, the ductal structures of the male breast enlarge, elongate, and branch with a concomitant increase in epithelium. During puberty, the condition often is unilateral and typically occurs between ages 12 and 15. In contrast, senescent gynecomastia is usually bilateral. Gynecomastia generally does not predispose the male breast to cancer. However, the hypoandrogenic state of Klinefelter syndrome (XXY), in which gynecomastia is usually evident, is associated with an increased risk of breast cancer. Gynecomastia is graded based on the degree of breast enlargement, the position of the nipple with reference to the inframammary fold and the degree of breast ptosis and skin redundancy: Grade I: mild breast enlargement without skin redundancy; Grade IIa: moderate breast enlargement without skin redundancy; Grade IIb: moderate breast enlargement with skin redundancy; and Grade 3: marked breast enlargement with skin redundancy and ptosis. (See Schwartz 10th ed., p. 505.)

7. Inflammatory conditions of the breast include all of the following EXCEPT
   A. Necrotizing viral mastitis
   B. Zuska disease (recurrent preductal mastitis)
   C. Mondor disease (superficial breast thrombophlebitis)
   D. Hidradenitis suppurativa

Answer: A

Zuska disease, also called *recurrent periductal mastitis,* is a condition of recurrent retroareolar infections and abscesses. Hidradenitis suppurativa of the nipple-areola complex or axilla is a chronic inflammatory condition that originates within the accessory areolar glands of Montgomery or within the axillary sebaceous glands. Mondor disease is a variant of thrombophlebitis that involves the superficial veins of the anterior chest wall and breast. (See Schwartz 10th ed., pp. 506–507.)

8. Lesions with malignant potential include all of the following EXCEPT
   A. Intraductal papilloma
   B. Atypical ductal hyperplasia
   C. Sclerosing adenosis
   D. Atypical lobular hyperplasia

Answer: C

Sclerosing adenosis is prevalent during the childbearing and perimenopausal years and has no malignant potential. Multiple intraductal papillomas, which occur in younger women and are less frequently associated with nipple discharge, are susceptible to malignant transformation. Individuals with a diagnosis of atypical ductal hyperplasia (ADH) are at increased risk for development of breast cancer and should be counseled appropriately regarding risk reduction strategies. Atypical lobular hyperplasia (ALH) results in minimal distention of lobular units with cells that are similar to those seen in lobular carcinoma in situ (LCIS). (See Schwartz 10th ed., pp. 509–510.)

9. Risk factors for the development of breast cancer include
   A. Early menarche
   B. Nulliparity
   C. Late menopause
   D. Longer lactation period

Answer: D

Increased exposure to estrogen is associated with an increased risk for developing breast cancer, whereas reducing exposure is thought to be protective. Correspondingly, factors that increase the number of menstrual cycles, such as early menarche, nulliparity, and late menopause, are associated with increased risk. Moderate levels of exercise and a longer lactation period, factors that decrease the total number of menstrual cycles, are protective. (See Schwartz 10th ed., p. 511.)

10. Drugs useful in breast cancer prevention include
    A. Raloxifene
    B. Tamoxifen
    C. Aspirin
    D. Aromatase inhibitors

Answer: C

The P-2 trial, the Study of Tamoxifen and Raloxifene (known as the *STAR trial*), randomly assigned 19,747 postmenopausal women at high risk for breast cancer to receive either tamoxifen or raloxifene. The initial report of the P-2 trial showed the two agents were nearly identical in their ability to reduce breast cancer risk, but raloxifene was associated with a more favorable adverse event profile. An updated analysis revealed that raloxifene maintained 76% of the efficacy of tamoxifen in prevention of invasive breast cancer with a more favorable side-effect profile. Aromatase inhibitors (AIs) have been shown to be more effective than tamoxifen in reducing the incidence of contralateral breast cancers in postmenopausal women receiving AIs for adjuvant treatment of invasive breast cancer. (See Schwartz 10th ed., p. 514.)

11. Which of the following is true regarding breast cancer metastasis?
    A. Metastases occur after breast cancers acquire their own blood supply.
    B. Batson plexus facilitates metastasis to the lung.
    C. Natural killer cells have no role in breast cancer immunosurveillance.
    D. Twenty percent of women who develop breast carcinoma metastases will do so within 60 months of treatment.

Answer: A

At approximately the 20th cell doubling, breast cancers acquire their own blood supply (neovascularization). Thereafter, cancer cells may be shed directly into the systemic venous blood to seed the pulmonary circulation via the axillary and intercostal veins or the vertebral column via Batson plexus of veins, which courses the length of the vertebral column. These cells are scavenged by natural killer lymphocytes and macrophages. Sixty percent of the women who develop distant metastases will do so within 60 months of treatment. (See Schwartz 10th ed., p. 518.)

12. All of the following are true concerning breast LCIS EXCEPT
    A. Develops only in the female breast.
    B. Cytoplasmic mucoid globules are a distinctive cellular feature.
    C. Frequency of LCIS cannot be reliably determined.
    D. The average age at diagnosis is 65 to 70 years.

Answer: D

LCIS originates from the terminal duct lobular units and develops only in the female breast. Cytoplasmic mucoid globules are a distinctive cellular feature. The frequency of LCIS in the general population cannot be reliably determined because it usually presents as an incidental finding. The average age at diagnosis is 45 years, which is approximately 15 to 25 years younger than the age at diagnosis for invasive breast cancer. (See Schwartz 10th ed., p. 519.)

13. Which of the following concerning breast cancer staging is correct?
    A. Stage I tumors have no metastases to either lymph nodes or distant sites.
    B. Stage III tumors include some with distant metastases (M1 disease).
    C. Inflammatory carcinoma is considered T4 disease.
    D. N4 disease includes metastases to highest contralateral axillary nodes.

Answer: C

(See Schwartz 10th ed., Tables 17-10 and 17-11, pp. 532 and 534.)

14. Factors that determine the type of therapy offered to patients after diagnosis of breast cancer include all of the following EXCEPT
    A. Whether or not a therapy has been proven effective in clinical trials
    B. Stage of disease
    C. General health of patient
    D. Biologic subtype

Answer: A

Once a diagnosis of breast cancer is made, the type of therapy offered to a breast cancer patient is determined by the stage of the disease, the biologic subtype, and the general health status of the individual. (See Schwartz 10th ed., p. 536.)

15. Which of the following statements about the management of distal carcinoma in situ (DCIS) is true?
    A. DCIS treated by mastectomy has a local recurrence rate of 2%.
    B. Extensive DCIS should be treated with tamoxifen followed by lumpectomy.
    C. Specimen mammography is only useful for patients with small amounts of DCIS.
    D. Postoperative tamoxifen is useful in DCIS patients whose tumors are estrogen-receptor (ER) negative.

Answer: A

Women with DCIS and evidence of extensive disease (>4 cm of disease or disease in more than one quadrant) usually require mastectomy. For women with limited disease, lumpectomy and radiation therapy are generally recommended. For nonpalpable DCIS, needle localization or other image-guided techniques are used to guide the surgical resection. Specimen mammography is performed to ensure that all visible evidence of cancer is excised. Adjuvant tamoxifen therapy is considered for DCIS patients with estrogen-receptor (ER)-positive disease. The gold standard against which breast conservation therapy for DCIS is evaluated is mastectomy. Women treated with mastectomy have local recurrence and mortality rates of <2%. (See Schwartz 10th ed., p. 537.)

16. All of the following are true about accelerated partial breast irradiation (APBI) EXCEPT
    A. APBI is delivered in an abbreviated fashion and a lower total dose than standard course of whole breast radiation.
    B. Suitable patients for APBI include women older than or equal to 60 years.
    C. Suitable patients for APBI include patients whose tumor margins are greater than or equal to 2 mm.
    D. Suitable patients for APBI include those with multifocal disease.

Answer: D
Accelerated partial breast irradiation (APBI) is delivered in an abbreviated fashion (twice daily for 5 days) and at a lower total dose compared with the standard course of 5 to 6 weeks of radiation (50 Gray with or without a boost) in the case of whole breast irradiation. The ASTRO guidelines describe patients "suitable" for APBI to include women older than 60 years with a unifocal, T1, ER-positive tumor with no lymphovascular invasion, and margins of at least 2 mm. Finally, a group felt to be "unsuitable" for APBI includes those with T3 or T4 disease, ER-negative disease, multifocality, multicentricity, extensive lymphovascular invasion (LVI), or positive margins. (See Schwartz 10th ed., p. 539.)

17. Patients not suitable for sentinel lymph node (SLN) biopsy include all of the following EXCEPT
    A. Inflammatory carcinoma of the breast.
    B. Prior axillary surgery.
    C. Biopsy-proven distant metastases.
    D. Lower inner quadrant of breast primary carcinoma.

Answer: D
Clinical situations where sentinel lymph node (SLN) dissection is not recommended include patients with inflammatory breast cancers, those with palpable axillary lymphadenopathy and biopsy-proven metastasis, DCIS without mastectomy, or prior axillary surgery. Although limited data are available, SLN dissection appears to be safe in pregnancy when performed with radioisotope alone. (See Schwartz 10th ed., p. 545.)

18. Which of the following is true concerning breast cancer during pregnancy?
    A. Metastases to lymph nodes occur in approximately 75% of patients.
    B. Approximately 50% of breast nodules developing during pregnancy are malignant.
    C. Mammography is especially useful in localizing small lesions.
    D. There is risk of chemotherapy teratogenicity if used during the second, but not the third, trimester of pregnancy.

Answer: A
Breast cancer occurs in 1 of every 3000 pregnant women, and axillary lymph node metastases are present in up to 75% of these women. Fewer than 25% of the breast nodules developing during pregnancy and lactation will be cancerous. Mammography is rarely indicated because of its decreased sensitivity during pregnancy and lactation; however, the fetus can be shielded if mammography is needed. Chemotherapy administered during the first trimester carries a risk of spontaneous abortion and a 12% risk of birth defects. There is no evidence of teratogenicity resulting from administration of chemotherapeutic agents in the second and third trimesters. (See Schwartz 10th ed., p. 554.)

CHAPTER 18

Disorders of the Head and Neck

1. Which of the following are true about leukoplakia of the vocal cords?
   A. Up to 40% risk of progression to invasive carcinoma.
   B. Ulceration is particularly suggestive of possible malignancy.
   C. Initial therapy includes antihistamines.
   D. Biopsy should be considered only after 6 months of conservative therapy.

Answer: B
Leukoplakia of the vocal fold represents a white patch (which cannot be wiped off) on the mucosal surface, usually on the superior surface of the true vocal cord. Rather than a diagnosis per se, the term *leukoplakia* describes a finding on laryngoscopic examination. The significance of this finding is that it may represent squamous hyperplasia, dysplasia, and/or carcinoma. Lesions exhibiting hyperplasia have a 1 to 3% risk of progression to malignancy. In contrast, that risk is 10 to 30% for those demonstrating dysplasia. Furthermore, leukoplakia may be observed in association with inflammatory and reactive pathologies, including polyps, nodules, cysts, granulomas, and papillomas. Features of ulceration and erythroplasia are particularly suggestive of possible malignancy. A history of smoking and alcohol abuse should also prompt a malignancy workup. In the absence of suspected malignancy, conservative measures are used for 1 month. Any lesions that progress, persist, or recur should be considered for excisional biopsy specimen. (See Schwartz 10th ed., p. 573.)

2. Factors associated with increased incidence of head and neck cancers include all of the following EXCEPT
   A. Human papillomavirus (HPV) exposure
   B. Ultraviolet light exposure
   C. Plummer-Vinson syndrome
   D. Reflux esophagitis

Answer: D
Human papillomavirus (HPV) is an epitheliotropic virus that has been detected to various degrees within samples of oral cavity squamous cell carcinoma. Infection alone is not considered sufficient for malignant conversion; however, results of multiple studies suggest a role of HPV in a subset of head and neck squamous cell carcinoma. Multiple reports reflect that up to 40 to 60% of current diagnoses of tonsillar carcinoma demonstrate evidence of HPV types 16 or 18. Environmental ultraviolet light exposure has been associated with the development of lip cancer. The projection of the lower lip, as it relates to this solar exposure, has been used to explain why the majority of squamous cell carcinomas arise along the vermilion border of the lower lip. In addition, pipe smoking also has been associated with the development of lip carcinoma. Factors such as mechanical irritation, thermal injury, and chemical exposure have been described as an explanation for this finding. Other entities associated with oral malignancy include Plummer-Vinson syndrome (achlorhydria, iron-deficiency anemia, mucosal atrophy of mouth, pharynx, and esophagus), chronic infection with syphilis, and immunocompromised status (30-fold increase with renal transplant). (See Schwartz 10th ed., p. 579.)

3. Features of oral tongue carcinoma include all of the following EXCEPT
   A. Presentation as ulcerated exophytic mass
   B. May involve submandibular and upper cervical lymph nodes
   C. Can result in contralateral paresthesias
   D. CO_2 laser useful for excision of small early tumors

Answer: C

Tumors of the tongue begin in the stratified epithelium of the surface and eventually invade into the deeper muscular structures. The tumors may present as ulcerations or as exophytic masses. The regional lymphatics of the oral cavity are to the submandibular space and the upper cervical lymph nodes. The lingual nerve and the hypoglossal nerve may be directly invaded by locally extensive tumors. Involvement can result in ipsilateral paresthesias and deviation of the tongue on protrusion with fasciculations and eventual atrophy. Tumors on the tongue may occur on any surface, but are most commonly seen on the lateral and ventral surfaces. Primary tumors of the mesenchymal components of the tongue include leiomyomas, leiomyosarcomas, rhabdomyosarcomas, and neurofibromas. Surgical treatment of small (T1–T2) primary tumors is wide local excision with either primary closure or healing by secondary intention. The CO_2 laser may be used for excision. (See Schwartz 10th ed., p. 583.)

4. Branchial cleft cysts, if enlarged, should be removed because of which of the following
   A. Prone to becoming secondarily infected
   B. Prone to cause acute airway obstructions
   C. Possible premalignant concerns
   D. Association with severe halitosis

Answer: A

Congenital branchial cleft remnants are derived from the branchial cleft apparatus that persists after fetal development. There are several types, numbered according to their corresponding embryologic branchial cleft. First branchial cleft cysts and sinuses are associated intimately with the external auditory canal (EAC) and the parotid gland. Second and third branchial cleft cysts are found along the anterior border of the sternocleidomastoid (SCM) muscle and can produce drainage via a sinus tract to the neck skin. Secondary infections can occur, producing enlargement, cellulitis, and neck abscess that requires operative drainage. (See Schwartz 10th ed., p. 598.)

5. All of the following are FALSE about salivary gland neoplasms EXCEPT
   A. Account for less than 2% of all head and neck neoplasms
   B. If in minor salivary glands, less likely to be malignant than if in the parotid gland
   C. Computed tomography (CT) scanning is more accurate than magnetic resonance imaging (MRI) in detecting lesions
   D. Oncocytomas are usually malignant

Answer: A

Tumors of the salivary gland are relatively uncommon and represent less than 2% of all head and neck neoplasms. About 85% of salivary gland neoplasms arise within the parotid gland. The majority of these neoplasms are benign, with the most common histology being pleomorphic adenoma (benign mixed tumor). In contrast, approximately 50% of tumors arising in the submandibular and sublingual glands are malignant. Tumors arising from minor salivary gland tissue carry an even higher risk for malignancy (75%). Diagnostic imaging is standard for the evaluation of salivary gland tumors. Magnetic resonance imaging (MRI) is the most sensitive study to determine soft-tissue extension and involvement of adjacent structures. Benign epithelial tumors include pleomorphic adenoma (80%), monomorphic adenoma, Warthin tumor, oncocytoma, or sebaceous neoplasm. (See Schwartz 10th ed., p. 599.)

6. All of the following are true about tracheostomy EXCEPT
   A. Should be performed in patients anticipated to be intubated more than 2 weeks
   B. Improves patient discomfort as compared to long term oropharyngeal intubation
   C. Usually spontaneously close within 2 months of removal
   D. Does not obligate patient to loss of speech

Answer: C

The avoidance of prolonged orotracheal and nasotracheal intubation decreases the risk of laryngeal and subglottic injury and potential stenosis, facilitates oral and pulmonary suctioning, and decreases patient's discomfort. When the tracheostomy is no longer needed, the tube is removed and closure of the opening usually occurs spontaneously over a 2-week period. Placement of a tracheostomy does not obligate a patient to loss of speech. When a large cuffed tracheostomy tube is in place, expecting a patient to be capable of normal speech is impractical. However, after a patient is downsized to an uncuffed tracheostomy tube, intermittent finger occlusion or Passy-Muir valve placement will allow a patient to communicate while still using the tracheostomy to bypass the upper airway. (See Schwartz 10th ed., p. 602.)

CHAPTER 19

Chest Wall, Pleura, and Mediastinum

1. All of the following increase the risk for tracheal stenosis EXCEPT
   A. Age over 70 years
   B. Radiation
   C. Male gender
   D. Excessive corticosteroid therapy

Answer: C

Intubation-related risk factors include prolonged intubation; high tracheostomy through the first tracheal ring or cricothyroid membrane; transverse rather than vertical incision on the trachea; oversized tracheostomy tube; prior tracheostomy or intubation; and traumatic intubation. Stenosis is also more common in older patients, in females, after radiation, or after excessive corticosteroid therapy, and in the setting of concomitant diseases such as autoimmune disorders, severe reflux disease, or obstructive sleep apnea and the setting of severe respiratory failure. However, even a properly placed tracheostomy can lead to tracheal stenosis because of scarring and local injury. Mild ulceration and stenosis are frequently seen after tracheostomy removal. Use of the smallest tracheostomy tube possible, rapid downsizing, and a vertical tracheal incision minimize the risk for posttracheostomy stenosis. (See Schwartz 10th ed., p. 607.)

2. Adenoid cystic carcinomas
   A. Spread submucosally
   B. Exhibit aggressive growth
   C. Are not radiosensitive
   D. Have a 5-year survival rate of >50%

Answer: A

Squamous cell carcinomas often present with regional lymph node metastases and are frequently unresectable at presentation. Their biologic behavior is similar to that of squamous cell carcinoma of the lung. Adenoid cystic carcinomas, a type of salivary gland tumor, are generally slow-growing, spread submucosally, and tend to infiltrate along nerve sheaths and within the tracheal wall. Although indolent in nature, adenoid cystic carcinomas are malignant and can spread to regional lymph nodes, lung, and bone. Squamous cell carcinoma and adenoid cystic carcinomas represent approximately 65% of all tracheal neoplasms. The remaining 35% comprises small cell carcinomas, mucoepidermoid carcinomas, adenocarcinomas, lymphomas, and others.

Postoperative mortality, which occurs in up to 10% of patients, is associated with the length of tracheal resection, use of laryngeal release, the type of resection, and the histologic type of the cancer. Factors associated with improved long-term survival include complete resection and use of radiation as adjuvant therapy in the setting of incomplete resection. Due to their radiosensitivity, radiotherapy is frequently given postoperatively after resection of both adenoid cystic carcinomas and squamous cell carcinomas. A dose of 50 Gray or greater is usual. Nodal positivity does not seem to be associated with worse survival. Survival at 5 and 10 years is much better for adenoid cystic (73 and 57%, respectively) than for tracheal cancers (47 and 36%, respectively; P <0.05). For patients with unresectable tumors, radiation may be given as the primary therapy to improve local control, but is rarely curative. For recurrent airway compromise, stenting or laser therapies should be considered part of the treatment algorithm. (See Schwartz 10th ed., pp. 610–611.)

3. Which of the following is NOT a non–small-cell tumor of the lung?
   A. Squamous cell carcinoma
   B. Adenocarcinoma
   C. Carcinoid tumor
   D. Large-cell carcinoma

Answer: C

The term non–small-cell lung carcinoma (NSCLC) includes many tumor cell types, including large cell, squamous cell, and adenocarcinoma. Historically, these subtypes were considered to be a uniform group based on limited understanding of the distinct clinical behaviors of the subtypes as well as the fact that there were few treatment options available. With increasing understanding of the molecular biology underlying these tumor subtypes, however, the approach to diagnosis and management and the terminology used in describing these tumors is evolving rapidly. (See Schwartz 10th ed., p. 614.)

4. The most common pattern of benign calcification in hamartomas is
   A. Solid
   B. Diffuse
   C. Central
   D. Popcorn

Answer: D

Computed tomography (CT) findings characteristic of benign lesions include small size, calcification within the nodule, and stability over time. Four patterns of benign calcification are common: diffuse, solid, central, and laminated or "popcorn." Granulomatous infections, such as tuberculosis, can demonstrate the first three patterns, whereas the popcorn pattern is most common in hamartomas. In areas of endemic granulomatous disease, differentiating benign versus malignant can be challenging. Infectious granulomas arising from a variety of organisms account for 70 to 80% of this type of benign solitary nodules; hamartomas are the next most common single cause, accounting for about 10%. (See Schwartz 10th ed., p. 622.)

5. For an adenocarcinoma that has pleural invasion, tumor necrosis, and has lymphovascular invasion the correct subtype is
   A. Minimally invasive adenocarcinoma (MIA)
   B. Lepidic predominant adenocarcinoma (LPA)
   C. Invasive adenocarcinoma
   D. Adenocarcinoma in situ

Answer: B

If lymphovascular invasion, pleural invasion, tumor necrosis, or more than 5 mm of invasion are noted in a lesion that has lepidic growth as its predominant component, minimally invasive adenocarcinoma (MIA) is excluded and the lesion is called *lepidic predominant adenocarcinoma* (LPA), and the size of the invasive component is recorded for the T stage. (See Schwartz 10th ed., p. 615.)

6. The grade of neuroendocrine carcinoma (NEC) that is associated with hemoptysis, pneumonia, and tumor cells arranged in cords and clusters is
   A. Grade VI NEC
   B. Grade IV NEC
   C. Grade II NEC
   D. Grade I NEC

Answer: D

Grade I neuroendocrine carcinoma (NEC) (classic or typical carcinoid) is a low-grade NEC; 80% arise in the epithelium of the central airways. It occurs primarily in younger patients. Because of the central location, it classically presents with hemoptysis, with or without airway obstruction and pneumonia. Histologically, tumor cells are arranged in cords and clusters with a rich vascular stroma. This vascularity can lead to life-threatening hemorrhage with even simple bronchoscopic biopsy maneuvers. Regional lymph node metastases are seen in 15% of patients, but rarely spread systemically or cause death. (See Schwartz 10th ed., p. 617.)

7. Which of the following is NOT a known predictive or prognostic tumor marker for adenocarcinoma?
   A. EGFR
   B. KRAS
   C. AFP
   D. EML4-ALK

Answer: C

Establishing a clear histologic diagnosis early in the evaluation and management of lung cancer is critical to effective treatment. Molecular signatures are also key determinants of treatment algorithms for adenocarcinoma and will likely become important for squamous cell carcinoma as well. Currently, differentiation between adenocarcinoma and squamous cell carcinoma in cytologic specimens or small biopsy specimens is imperative in patients with advanced stage disease, as treatment with pemetrexed or bevacizumab-based chemotherapy is associated with improved progression-free survival in patients with adenocarcinoma but not squamous cell cancer. Furthermore, life-threatening hemorrhage has occurred in patients with squamous cell carcinoma who were treated with bevacizumab. Finally, *EGFR* mutation predicts response to EGFR tumor kinase inhibitors and is now recommended as first-line therapy in advanced adenocarcinoma. Because adequate tissue is required for histologic assessment and molecular testing, each institution should have a clear, multidisciplinary approach to patient evaluation, tissue acquisition, tissue handling/processing, and tissue analysis. In many cases, tumor morphology differentiates adenocarcinoma from the other histologic subtypes. If no clear morphology can be identified, then additional testing for one immunohistochemistry marker for adenocarcinoma and one for squamous cell carcinoma will usually enable differentiation. Immunohistochemistry for neuroendocrine markers is reserved for lesions exhibiting neuroendocrine morphology. Additional molecular testing should be performed on all adenocarcinoma specimens for known predictive and prognostic tumor markers (eg, *EGFR, KRAS*, and *EML4-ALK* fusion gene). Ideally, use of tissue sections and cell block material is limited to the minimum necessary at each decision point. This emphasizes the importance of a multidisciplinary approach; surgeons and radiologists must work in direct cooperation with the cytopathologist to ensure that tissue samples are adequate for morphologic diagnosis as well as providing sufficient cellular material to enable molecular testing. (See Schwartz 10th ed., p. 627.)

8. Desmoid tumors
   A. Arise from the periosteum of the rib
   B. Are treated with wide local excision with a 2- to 4-cm margin
   C. Require radical excision (sacrificing neurovascular structures) to obtain 4-cm margins
   D. Require chemotherapy to treat or prevent metastatic disease

Answer: B

Because the lesions have low cellularity and poor yield with fine needle aspiration (FNA), an open incisional biopsy for lesions over 3 to 4 cm is often necessary. Surgery consists of wide local excision with a 2- to 4-cm margin and intraoperative frozen section assessment of resection margins. Typically, chest wall resection, including the involved rib(s) and one rib above and below the tumor with a 4- to 5-cm margin of rib, is required. A margin of less than 1 cm results in much higher local recurrence rates. If a major neurovascular structure would have to be sacrificed, leading to high morbidity, then a margin of less than 1 cm would have to suffice. Survival after wide local excision with negative margins is 90% at 10 years. (See Schwartz 10th ed., p. 666.)

9. A 57-year-old non–small-cell lung cancer patient with a potentially resectable tumor found on computed tomography (CT) scan who can walk on a flat surface indefinitely without oxygen or stopping to rest, secondary to dyspnea will most likely tolerate
   A. Lobectomy
   B. Pneumonectomy
   C. Single-lung ventilation
   D. Wedge resection

Answer: A

Patients with potentially resectable tumors require careful assessment of their functional status and ability to tolerate either lobectomy or pneumonectomy.

The surgeon should first estimate the likelihood of pneumonectomy, lobectomy, or possibly sleeve resection, based on the CT images. A sequential process of evaluation then unfolds.

A patient's history is the most important tool for gauging risk. Specific questions regarding performance status should be routinely asked. If the patient can walk on a flat surface indefinitely, without oxygen and without having to stop and rest secondary to dyspnea, he will be very likely to tolerate lobectomy. If the patient can walk up two flights of stairs (up two standard levels), without having to stop and rest secondary to dyspnea, he will likely tolerate pneumonectomy. Finally, nearly all patients, except those with carbon dioxide (CO_2) retention on arterial blood gas analysis, will be able to tolerate periods of single-lung ventilation and wedge resection. (See Schwartz 10th ed., pp. 635–636.)

10. An "onion-peel" appearance of a rib on CT is suggestive of
    A. Chondroma
    B. Ewing sarcoma
    C. Plasmacytoma
    D. Osteosarcoma

Answer: B

Primitive neuroectodermal tumors (PNETs) (neuroblastomas, ganglioneuroblastomas, and ganglioneuromas) derive from primordial neural crest cells that migrate from the mantle layer of the developing spinal cord. Histologically, PNETs and Ewing sarcomas are small, round cell tumors; both possess a translocation between the long arms of chromosomes 11 and 22 within their genetic makeup. They also share a consistent pattern of proto-oncogene expression and have been found to express the product of the *MIC2* gene. Ewing sarcoma occurs in adolescents and young adults who present with progressive chest wall pain, but without the presence of a mass. Systemic symptoms of malaise and fever are often present. Laboratory studies reveal an elevated erythrocyte sedimentation rate and mild white blood cell elevation. Radiographically, the characteristic onion peel appearance is produced by multiple layers of periosteum in the bone formation. Evidence of bony destruction is also common. The diagnosis can be made by a percutaneous needle biopsy or an incisional biopsy. (See Schwartz 10th ed., p. 669.)

11. Pancoast tumors are identified as involving all of the following EXCEPT
    A. The chest wall at or below the second rib.
    B. Tumors of the parietal pleura or deeper structures overlying the first rib.
    C. The superior sulcus.
    D. The extreme apex of the chest.

Answer: A

Carcinoma arising in the extreme apex of the chest with associated arm and shoulder pain, atrophy of the muscles of the hand, and Horner syndrome presents a unique challenge to the surgeon. Any tumor of the superior sulcus, including tumors without evidence for involvement of the neurovascular bundle, is now commonly known as *Pancoast tumors*, after Henry Pancoast who described the syndrome in 1932. The designation is reserved for tumors involving the parietal pleura or deeper structures overlying the first rib. Chest wall involvement at or below the second rib is not a Pancoast tumor. Treatment is multidisciplinary; due to the location of the tumor and involvement of the neurovascular bundle that supplies the ipsilateral extremity, preserving postoperative function of the extremity is critical. (See Schwartz 10th ed., p. 642.)

12. The most likely cause of aspiration pneumonia is
    A. A mixture of aerobes and anaerobes
    B. Aerobes only
    C. Anaerobes only
    D. Gram-negative bacteria

Answer: C

Normal oropharyngeal secretions contain many more *Streptococcus* species and more anaerobes (approximately 1×10^8 organisms/mL) than aerobes (approximately 1×10^7 organisms/mL). Pneumonia that follows from aspiration, with or without abscess development, is typically polymicrobial. An average of two to four isolates present in large numbers have been cultured from lung abscesses sampled percutaneously. Overall, at least 50% of these infections are caused by purely anaerobic bacteria, 25% are caused by mixed aerobes and anaerobes, and 25% or fewer are caused by aerobes only. In nosocomial pneumonia, 60 to 70% of the organisms are gram-negative bacteria, including *Klebsiella pneumoniae*, *Haemophilus influenzae*, *Proteus* species, *Pseudomonas aeruginosa*, *Escherichia coli*, *Enterobacter cloacae*, and *Eikenella corrodens*. Immunosuppressed patients may develop abscesses because of the usual pathogens as well as less virulent and opportunistic organisms such as *Salmonella* species, *Legionella* species, *Pneumocystis carinii*, atypical mycobacteria, and fungi. (See Schwartz 10th ed., p. 650.)

13. Laboratory evaluation of a chest wall mass showing elevated erythrocyte sedimentation rates indicates
    A. Osteosarcoma
    B. Plasmacytoma
    C. Ewing sarcoma
    D. Multiple myeloma

Answer: C

Laboratory evaluations are useful in assessing chest wall masses for the following:
1. **Plasmacytoma:** Serum protein electrophoresis demonstrates a single monoclonal spike, which is measuring the overproduction of one immunoglobulin from the malignant plasma cell clone.
2. **Osteosarcoma:** Alkaline phosphatase levels may be elevated.
3. **Ewing sarcoma:** Erythrocyte sedimentation rates may be elevated.
   (See Schwartz 10th ed., Table 19-18, p. 665.)

14. The most common benign chest wall tumor is
    A. Chondromas
    B. Osteochondromas
    C. Desmoid tumors
    D. Fibrous dysplasia

Answer: A

Chondromas, seen primarily in children and young adults, are one of the more common benign tumors of the chest wall. They usually occur at the costochondral junction anteriorly and may be confused with costochondritis, except that a painless mass is present. Radiographically, lesion is lobulated and radiodense; it may have diffuse or focal calcifications; and it may displace the bony cortex without penetration. Chondromas may grow to huge sizes if left untreated. Treatment is surgical resection with a 2-cm margin. Large chondromas may harbor well-differentiated chondrosarcoma and should be managed with a 4-cm margin to prevent local recurrence. (See Schwartz 10th ed., p. 666.)

15. Which of the following is an indication for surgical drainage of a lung abscess?
    A. Abscess >3 cm in diameter.
    B. Hemoptysis.
    C. Failure to decrease in size after 1 week of antibiotic therapy.
    D. Persistent fever.

Answer: B

Surgical drainage of lung abscesses is uncommon since drainage usually occurs spontaneously via the tracheobronchial tree. Indications for intervention are listed in Table 19-1. (See Schwartz 10th ed., Table 19-18, p. 653.)

TABLE 19-1	Indications for surgical drainage procedures for lung abscesses
1. Failure of medical therapy	
2. Abscess under tension	
3. Abscess increasing in size during appropriate treatment	
4. Contralateral lung contamination	
5. Abscess >4–6 cm in diameter	
6. Necrotizing infection with multiple abscesses, hemoptysis, abscess rupture, or pyopneumothorax	
7. Inability to exclude a cavitating carcinoma	

16. What percentages of chest wall masses are malignant?
    A. 10–20%
    B. 20–30%
    C. 50–80%
    D. 40–50%

Answer: C

Patients with chest wall tumors, regardless of etiology, typically complain of a slowly enlarging palpable mass (50–70%), chest wall pain (25–50%), or both. Interestingly, growing masses are often not noticed by the patient until they suffer a trauma to the area. Pain from a chest wall mass is typically localized to the area of the tumor; it occurs more often and more intensely with malignant tumors, but it can also be present in up to one-third of patients with benign tumors. With Ewing sarcoma, fever and malaise may also be present. Benign chest wall tumors tend to occur in younger patients (average age 26 years), whereas malignant tumors tend to be found in older patients (average age 40 years). Overall, between 50 and 80% of chest wall tumors are malignant. (See Schwartz 10th ed., p. 665.)

17. The population most at risk for developing active tuberculosis is
    A. Elderly
    B. Minorities
    C. Urban residents
    D. Human immunodeficiency virus (HIV) infected

Answer: D

Tuberculosis is a widespread problem that affects nearly one-third of the world's population. Between 8.3 and 9 million new cases of tuberculosis and 12 million prevalent cases (range 10–13 million) were estimated worldwide in 2011 according to the World Health Organization. Only 10,521 new cases were reported to the World Health Organization in the United States in 2011. Human immunodeficiency virus (HIV) infection is the strongest risk factor for developing active tuberculosis. The elderly, minorities, and recent immigrants are the most common populations to have clinical manifestations of infection, yet no age group, sex, or race is exempt from infection. In most large urban centers, reported cases of tuberculosis are more numerous among the homeless, prisoners, and drug-addicted populations. Immunocompromised patients additionally contribute to an increased incidence of tuberculosis infection, often developing unusual systemic as well as pulmonary manifestations. (See Schwartz 10th ed., p. 654.)

18. The fungi associated with the highest mortality rate due to invasive mycoses in the United States is
    A. *Aspergillus*
    B. *Cryptococcus*
    C. *Candidia*
    D. *Mucor*

Answer: A

The genus *Aspergillus* comprises over 150 species and is the most common cause of mortality due to invasive mycoses in the United States. It is typically acute in onset and life threatening and occurs in the setting of neutropenia, chronic steroid therapy, or cytotoxic chemotherapy. It can also occur in the general intensive care unit population of critically ill patients, including patients with underlying chronic obstructive pulmonary disease (COPD), postoperative patients, patients with cirrhosis or alcoholism, and postinfluenza patients, without any of these factors present. The species most commonly responsible for clinical disease include *A. fumigatus, A. flavus,*

A. niger, and *A. terreus*. *Aspergillus* is a saprophytic, filamentous fungus with septate hyphae. Spores (2.5–3 μm in diameter) are released and easily inhaled by susceptible patients; because the spores are microns in size, they are able to reach the distal bronchi and alveoli. (See Schwartz 10th ed., p. 655.)

19. A patient presenting with a history and findings of dyspnea, wheezing, hemoptysis, and a mediastinal mass in the visceral compartment yields a diagnosis of
    A. Lymphoma
    B. Thymoma with myasthenia gravis
    C. Mediastinal granuloma
    D. Germ cell tumor

Answer: C
Table 19-2 (See Schwartz 10th ed., Table 19-28, p. 674.)

TABLE 19-2	Signs and symptoms suggestive of various diagnoses in the setting of a mediastinal mass	
Diagnosis	**History and Physical Findings**	**Compartment Location of Mass**
Lymphoma	Night sweats, weight loss, fatigue, extrathoracic adenopathy, elevated erythrocyte sedimentation rate or C-reactive protein level, leukocytosis	Any compartment
Thymoma with myasthenia gravis	Fluctuating weakness, early fatigue, ptosis, diplopia	Anterior
Mediastinal granuloma	Dyspnea, wheezing, hemoptysis	Visceral (middle)
Germ cell tumor	Male gender, young age, testicular mass, elevated levels of human chorionic gonadotropin and/or α-fetoprotein	Anterior

20. A patient with an anterior mediastinal mass and elevated serum α-fetoprotein (AFP) most likely has
    A. A teratoma
    B. A nonseminomatous germ-cell tumor
    C. A seminomatous germ-cell tumor
    D. Metastatic hepatocellular carcinoma

Answer: B
The use of serum markers to evaluate a mediastinal mass can be invaluable in some patients. For example, nonseminomatous and seminomatous germ-cell tumors can frequently be diagnosed and often distinguished from one another by the levels of α-fetoprotein (AFP) and human chorionic gonadotropin (hCG). In over 90% of nonseminomatous germ-cell tumors, either the AFP or the hCG level will be elevated. Results are close to 100% specific if the level of either AFP or hCG is greater than 500 ng/mL. Some centers institute chemotherapy based on this result alone, without biopsy confirmation of the diagnosis. In contrast, the AFP level in patients with mediastinal seminoma is always normal; only 10% will have elevated hCG, which is usually less than 100 ng/mL. Other serum markers, such as intact parathyroid hormone level for ectopic parathyroid adenomas, may be useful for diagnosing and also for intraoperatively confirming complete resection. After successful resection of a parathyroid adenoma, this hormone level should rapidly normalize. (See Schwartz 10th ed., p. 672.)

21. The primary site for male patients with malignant pleural effusions is
    A. Gastrointestinal tract
    B. Lung
    C. Genitourinary tract
    D. Melanoma

Answer: B
Malignant pleural effusions may occur in association with a number of different malignancies, most commonly lung cancer, breast cancer, and lymphomas, depending on the patient's age and gender (Tables 19-3 and 19-4). (See Schwartz 10th ed., Tables 19-35 and 19-36, pp. 682 and 684.)

TABLE 19-3	Primary organ site or neoplasm type in male patients with malignant pleural effusions	
Primary Site or Tumor Type	**No. of Male Patients**	**Percentage of Male Patients**
Lung	140	49.1
Lymphoma/leukemia	60	21.1
Gastrointestinal tract	20	7.0
Genitourinary tract	17	6.0
Melanoma	4	1.4
Miscellaneous less common tumors	10	3.5
Primary site unknown	31	10.9
Total	285	100.0

Source: Reproduced with permission from Johnston WW. The malignant pleural effusion: a review of cytopathologic diagnoses of 584 specimens from 472 consecutive patients. *Cancer.* 1985;56:905. Copyright © 1985 American Cancer Society.

TABLE 19-4	Primary organ site or neoplasm type in female patients with malignant pleural effusions	
Primary Site or Tumor Type	**No. of Female Patients**	**Percentage of Female Patients**
Breast	70	37.4
Female genital tract	38	20.3
Lung	28	15.0
Lymphoma	14	8.0
Gastrointestinal tract	8	4.3
Melanoma	6	3.2
Urinary tract	2	1.1
Miscellaneous less common tumors	3	1.6
Primary site unknown	17	9.1
Total	187	100.0

Source: Reproduced with permission from Johnston WW. The malignant pleural effusion: a review of cytopathologic diagnoses of 584 specimens from 472 consecutive patients. *Cancer.* 1985;56:905. Copyright © 1985 American Cancer Society.

22. Eosinophilic granulomas are associated with
    A. Langerhans cell histiocytosis (LCH)
    B. Parasitic infections
    C. Crohn disease
    D. Gardner syndrome

Answer: A

Eosinophilic granulomas are benign osteolytic lesions. Eosinophilic granulomas of the ribs can occur as solitary lesions or as part of a more generalized disease process of the lymphoreticular system termed Langerhans cell histiocytosis (LCH). In LCH, the involved tissue is infiltrated with large numbers of histiocytes (similar to Langerhans cells seen in skin and other epithelia), which are often organized as granulomas. The cause is unknown. Of all LCH bone lesions, 79% are solitary eosinophilic granulomas, 7% involve multiple eosinophilic granulomas, and 14% belong to other forms of more systemic LCH. Isolated single eosinophilic granulomas can occur in the ribs or skull, pelvis, mandible, humerus, and other sites. They are diagnosed primarily in children between the ages of 5 and 15 years. Because of the associated pain and tenderness, they may be confused with Ewing sarcoma or with an inflammatory process such as osteomyelitis. Healing may occur spontaneously, but the typical treatment is limited surgical resection with a 2-cm margin. (See Schwartz 10th ed., p. 666.)

23. A chylothorax is likely to be present in a patient whose pleural fluid analysis results show a triglyceride level of
    A. 80 mg/100 mL
    B. 100 mg/100 mL
    C. 45 mg/100 mL
    D. 130 mg/100 mL

Answer: D
Laboratory analysis of the pleural fluid shows a high lymphocyte count and high triglyceride levels. If the triglyceride level is greater than 110 mg/100 mL, a chylothorax is almost certainly present (a 99% accuracy rate). If the triglyceride level is less than 50 mg/mL, there is only a 5% chance of chylothorax. (See Schwartz 10th ed., p. 686.)

24. Osteosarcoma of the rib
    A. Is considered nonoperable if pulmonary metastases are present
    B. Is treated with radiation therapy before resection
    C. Is treated with adjuvant chemotherapy before resection
    D. Requires excision with a 6-cm margin

Answer: C
While osteosarcomas are the most common bone malignancy, they represent only 10 to 15% of all malignant chest wall tumors. They primarily occur in young adults as rapidly enlarging, painful masses; however, osteosarcomas can occur in older patients as well, sometimes in association with previous radiation, Paget disease, or chemotherapy. Radiographically, the typical appearance consists of spicules of new periosteal bone formation producing a sunburst appearance. Osteosarcomas have a propensity to spread to the lungs, and up to one-third of patients present with metastatic disease. Osteosarcomas are potentially sensitive to chemotherapy. Currently, preoperative chemotherapy is common. After chemotherapy, complete resection is performed with wide (4-cm) margins, followed by reconstruction. In patients presenting with lung metastases that are potentially amenable to surgical resection, induction chemotherapy may be given, followed by surgical resection of the primary tumor and of the pulmonary metastases. Following surgical treatment of known disease, additional maintenance chemotherapy is usually recommended. (See Schwartz 10th ed., p. 667.)

25. Excisional biopsy of a chest wall mass is allowed if
    A. Needle biopsy was nondiagnostic.
    B. Imaging reveals classic appearance of a chondrosarcoma.
    C. It is >3 cm.
    D. None of the above.

Answer: B
1. **Needle biopsy:** Pathologists experienced with sarcomas can accurately diagnose approximately 90% of patients using FNA cytology. A needle biopsy (FNA or core) has the advantage of avoiding wound and body cavity contamination (a potential complication with an incisional biopsy).
2. **Incisional biopsy:** If a needle biopsy is nondiagnostic, an incisional biopsy may be performed, with caveats. First, the skin incision must be placed directly over the mass and oriented to allow subsequent scar excision; skin flaps and drains should be avoided. However, if the surgeon believes a hematoma is likely to develop, a drain is useful for limiting soft tissue contamination by tumor cells. At the time of definitive surgical resection, the en bloc resection includes the biopsy scar and the drain tract along with the tumor.
3. **Excisional biopsy:** Any lesion less than 2.0 cm can be excised as long as the resulting wound is small enough to close primarily. Otherwise, excisional biopsy is performed only when the initial diagnosis (based on radiographic evaluation) indicates that the lesion is benign or when the lesion has the classic appearance of a chondrosarcoma (in which case, definitive surgical resection can be undertaken). (See Schwartz 10th ed., p. 666.)

CHAPTER 20

Congenital Heart Disease

1. The most common form of atrial septal defect (ASD) is
   A. Sinus venosus defect
   B. Ostium primum defect
   C. Ostium secundum defect
   D. Combined primum and secundum defect

Answer: C
Atrial septal defects (ASDs) can be classified into three different types: (1) sinus venosus defects, comprising approximately 5 to 10% of all ASDs; (2) ostium primum defects, which are more correctly described as partial atrioventricular canal defects; and (3) ostium secundum defects, which are the most prevalent subtype, comprising 80% of all ASDs. (See Schwartz 10th ed., pp. 695–696.)

2. The most common age to close asymptomatic ASDs is
   A. In the immediate newborn period
   B. After the child reaches 10 kg in weight
   C. Age 4–5 years
   D. During puberty

Answer: C
ASDs are closed when patients are between 4 and 5 years of age. Children of this size can usually be operated on without the use of blood transfusion and generally have excellent outcomes. Patients who are symptomatic may require repair earlier, even in infancy. Some surgeons, however, advocate routine repair in infants and children, as even smaller defects are associated with the risk of paradoxical embolism, particularly during pregnancy. Reddy and colleagues, report 116 neonates weighing less than 2500 g who underwent repair of simple and complex cardiac defects with the use of cardiopulmonary bypass and found no intracerebral hemorrhages, no long-term neurologic sequelae, and a low operative-mortality rate (10%). These results correlated with the length of cardiopulmonary bypass and the complexity of repair. These investigators also found an 80% actuarial survival at 1 year and, more importantly, that growth following complete repair was equivalent to weight-matched neonates free from cardiac defects. (See Schwartz 10th ed., p. 697.)

3. Which of the following is NOT an acceptable treatment for aortic valve stenosis with a hypoplastic left ventricle (LV)?
   A. Balloon valvotomy
   B. Intubation and initiation of prostaglandin
   C. Surgical valvotomy
   D. Norwood procedure

Answer: A
In patients with critical aortic stenosis, the degree of left ventricular hypoplasia is assessed and based on this the decision for biventricular and univentricular repair is made. Urgent intervention is needed in these critically ill neonates including intubation, inotropic support, and prostaglandin to maintain ductal patency for systemic blood flow. In the presence of hypoplastic LV, isolated aortic valvotomy should not be performed because studies have demonstrated high mortality in the population following isolated valvotomy. The Norwood procedure is the first part of the staged single ventricle pathway. (See Schwartz 10th ed., p. 699.)

4. The most common location for a coarctation of the aorta (COA) is
   A. Aortic arch
   B. Distal to the left subclavian artery
   C. At the diaphragm
   D. At the level of the renal arteries

Answer: B

Coarctation of the aorta (COA) is defined as a luminal narrowing in the aorta that causes an obstruction to blood flow. This narrowing is most commonly located distal to the left subclavian artery. The embryologic origin of COA is a subject of some controversy. One theory holds that the obstructing shelf, which is largely composed of tissue found within the ductus, forms as the ductus involutes. The other theory holds that a diminished aortic isthmus develops secondary to decreased aortic flow in infants with enhanced ductal circulation. (See Schwartz 10th ed., p. 705.)

5. The treatment of choice for recurrent COA (after surgical repair) in a preschool-aged child
   A. Resection and primary anastomosis
   B. Resection with interposition graft
   C. Balloon dilatation alone
   D. Balloon dilatation with stenting

Answer: C

Children younger than 6 months with native COA should be treated with surgical repair, while those requiring intervention at later ages may be ideal candidates for balloon dilatation or primary stent implantation. Additionally, catheter-based therapy should be employed for those cases of restenosis following either surgical or primary endovascular management. (See Schwartz 10th ed., p. 706.)

6. Which of the following is a true surgical emergency in a newborn?
   A. Tetralogy of Fallot
   B. Truncus arteriosus
   C. Total anomalous pulmonary venous connection (TAPVC)
   D. COA

Answer: C

Total anomalous pulmonary venous connection (TAPVC) occurs in 1 to 2% of all cardiac malformations and is characterized by abnormal drainage of the pulmonary veins into the right heart, whether through connections into the right atrium or into its tributaries. Accordingly, the only mechanism by which oxygenated blood can return to the left heart is through an ASD, which is almost uniformly present with TAPVC.

Unique to this lesion is the absence of a definitive form of palliation. Thus, TAPVC represents one of the only true surgical emergencies across the entire spectrum of congenital heart surgery. (See Schwartz 10th ed., p. 707.)

7. The bidirectional Glenn procedure is used to correct
   A. Tricuspid atresia
   B. Patent ductus arteriosus
   C. Transposition of the great arteries
   D. Total anomalous pulmonary venous connection

Answer: A

Recognizing the inadequacies of the initial repairs for tricuspid atresia, Glenn described the first successful cavopulmonary anastomosis, an end-to-side right pulmonary artery (RPA)-to-superior vena cava (SVC) shunt in 1958, and later modified this to allow flow to both pulmonary arteries. This end-to-side RPA-to-SVC anastomosis was known as the *bidirectional Glenn*, and is the first stage to final Fontan repair in widespread use today. The Fontan repair was a major advancement in the treatment of congenital heart disease, as it essentially bypassed the right heart, and allowed separation of the pulmonary and systemic circulations. (See Schwartz 10th ed., p. 713.)

8. Hypoplastic left heart syndrome is surgically treated with
   A. Bilateral pulmonary artery banding and stent placement in the patent ductus arteriosus.
   B. Norwood procedure with a Blalock-Taussig (B-T) shunt.
   C. Norwood procedure with a right ventricle (RV) to pulmonary artery conduit (Sano shunt).
   D. All of the above.

Answer: D

In 1983, Norwood and colleagues described a two-stage palliative surgical procedure for relief of hypoplastic left heart syndrome that was later modified to the currently used three-stage method of palliation. Stage 1 palliation, also known as the *modified Norwood procedure*, bypasses the LV by creating a single outflow vessel, the neoaorta, which arises from the RV. More recently, Sano introduced a modification that includes arch reconstruction and placement of the shunt between the RV and pulmonary artery (Sano shunt), which diminishes the diastolic flow created by the classical B-T shunt and may augment coronary perfusion, resulting in improved postoperative cardiac function. A newer approach combines surgical and percutaneous techniques (hybrid procedure). The bilateral pulmonary arteries of surgically banded to restrict excess pulmonary blood flow after pulmonary vascular resistance drops and ductal stenting to maintain patency. The hybrid procedure does not require cardiopulmonary bypass. (See Schwartz 10th ed., pp. 717–718.)

9. The arterial switch operation for transposition of the great vessels is best performed
   A. Within 2 weeks of birth
   B. At 1 year of age
   C. At 10 kg of weight
   D. In adolescence

Answer: A

The most important consideration is the timing of surgical repair, because arterial switch should be performed within 2 weeks after birth, before the LV loses its ability to pump against systemic afterload. In patients presenting later than 2 weeks, the LV can be retrained with preliminary pulmonary artery banding and aortopulmonary shunt followed by definitive repair. Alternatively, the unprepared LV can be supported following arterial switch with a mechanical assist device for a few days while it recovers ability to manage systemic pressures. Echocardiography can be used to assess left ventricular performance and guide operative planning in these circumstances. (See Schwartz 10th ed., p. 721.)

10. Which of the following is NOT one of the components of the tetralogy of Fallot (TOF)?
    A. ASD
    B. Ventricular septal defect
    C. Right ventricular hypertrophy
    D. Right ventricular outflow obstruction

Answer: A

The four features of tetralogy of Fallot (TOF) are (1) malalignment ventricular septal defect, (2) dextroposition of the aorta, (3) right ventricular outflow tract obstruction, and (4) right ventricular hypertrophy. This combination of defects arises as a result of underdevelopment and anteroleftward malalignment of the infundibular septum. (See Schwartz 10th ed., p. 724.)

11. The most commonly recommended age for correction of a TOF is
    A. Neonate younger than 3 months
    B. 6 months of age
    C. 1 year of age
    D. 4–5 years of age

Answer: A

However, systemic-to-pulmonary shunts, generally a B-T shunt, may still be preferred with an unstable neonate younger than 3 months, when an extracardiac conduit is required because of an anomalous left anterior descending coronary artery, or when pulmonary atresia, significant branch pulmonary artery hypoplasia, or severe noncardiac anomalies coexist with TOF. (See Schwartz 10th ed., p. 724.)

12. Which of the following is the most common type of ventricular septal defect (VSD) to require surgical correction?
    A. Ostium primum
    B. Ostium secundum
    C. Muscular
    D. Perimembranous

Answer: D

Perimembranous ventricular septal defects (VSDs) are the most common type requiring surgical intervention, comprising approximately 80% of cases. These defects involve the membranous septum and include the malalignment defects seen in TOF. (See Schwartz 10th ed., p. 726.)

13. What is the best predictor of spontaneous closure of a VSD?
    A. Size
    B. Age at diagnosis
    C. Gestational age
    D. Lack of electrocardiogram changes

Answer: B

VSDs may close or narrow spontaneously, and the probability of closure is inversely related to the age at which the defect is observed. Thus, infants at 1 month of age have an 80% incidence of spontaneous closure, whereas a child at 12 months of age has only a 25% chance of closure. This has an important impact on operative decision making, because a small or moderate-size VSD may be observed for a period of time in the absence of symptoms. Large defects and those in severely symptomatic neonates should be repaired during infancy to relieve symptoms because irreversible changes in pulmonary vascular resistance may develop during the first year of life. (See Schwartz 10th ed., p. 727.)

14. Which of the following cardiac abnormalities, all of them well-tolerated during fetal life, becomes a serious problem at birth?
    A. Aortic arch
    B. Ductus arteriosus
    C. Foramen ovale
    D. Tricuspid atresia

Answer: D

In fetal life, blood reaching the right atrium has been oxygenated by the placenta. This blood bypasses the high-resistance pulmonary circulation to enter the systemic circulation through septal defects and the ductus arteriosus. When the child is born, the pulmonary circulation becomes important. Septal defects and the ductus arteriosus can be tolerated by the newborn child, but tricuspid atresia, pulmonic valve stenosis, or other right ventricular outflow obstruction forces a right-to-left shunt, with development of cyanotic heart disease. (See Schwartz 10th ed., p. 712.)

15. Cor triatriatum is
    A. Three atria where the right atrium is divided by a diaphragm with the SVC and inferior vena cava (IVC) drain into separate atria.
    B. Three atria where the SVC and IVC drain into the superior right atrium and the inferior drains through the tricuspid valve in the RV.
    C. Three atria where the left atrium is divided by a diaphragm and the superior and inferior pulmonary veins drain into separate chambers.
    D. Three atria where the left atrium is divided by a diaphragm separating the chamber receiving pulmonary return from the chamber draining through the mitral valve into the LV.

Answer: D

Cor triatriatum results in obstruction of pulmonary venous return to the left atrium with a diaphragm dividing the chamber receiving pulmonary return from the camber in continuity with the mitral valve and LV. The degree of obstruction is variable and depends on the size of fenestrations present in the left atrial membrane, the size of the ASD, and the existence of other associated anomalies. If the communication between the superior and inferior chambers is less than 3 mm, patients are symptomatic during the first year of life. The afflicted infant will present with the stigmata of low cardiac output and pulmonary venous hypertension, as well as congestive heart failure and poor feeding. (See Schwartz 10th ed., p. 710.)

16. Flow across a VSD is dependent upon
    A. Size of defect
    B. Left and right ventricular pressure and size of the defect
    C. Pulmonary and systemic vascular resistance and defect size
    D. Pulmonary and systemic vascular resistance

Answer: C

The size of the VSD determines the initial pathophysiology of the disease. Large VSDs are classified as nonrestrictive and are at least equal in diameter to the aortic annulus. These defects allow free flow of blood from the LV to the RV, elevating right ventricular pressures to the same level as systemic pressure. Consequently, the pulmonary-to-systemic flow ratio (Qp:Qs) is inversely dependent on the ratio of pulmonary vascular resistance to systemic vascular resistance. Nonrestrictive VSDs produce a large increase in pulmonary blood flow, and the afflicted infant will present with symptoms of congestive heart failure. However, if untreated, these defects will cause pulmonary hypertension with a corresponding increase in pulmonary vascular resistance. This will lead to a reversal of flow (a right-to-left shunt), which is known as *Eisenmenger syndrome.*

Small restrictive VSDs offer significant resistance to the passage of blood across the defect, and therefore right ventricular pressure is either normal or only minimally elevated and Qp:Qs rarely exceeds 1.5. These defects are generally asymptomatic because there are few physiologic consequences. However, there is a long-term risk of endocarditis, because endocardial damage from the jet of blood through the defect may serve as a possible nidus for colonization. (See Schwartz 10th ed., p. 727.)

17. A child with a large VSD and no other cardiac lesion can be expected to develop all of the following EXCEPT
    A. Cyanosis
    B. Failure to thrive
    C. Left ventricular hypertrophy greater than left ventricular dilation
    D. Increased susceptibility to lower respiratory tract infection

Answer: C

A VSD produces a left-to-right shunt because systemic vascular resistance is greater than pulmonary vascular resistance. The extra work required by the shunt leads to increased basal energy expenditure and a failure to thrive. The shunt into the pulmonary circulation produces congestion and an associated increased susceptibility to lower respiratory tract infection. Large ventricular defects result in dilation but minimal hypertrophy due to decreased afterload. (See Schwartz 10th ed., p. 727.)

18. Beyond early childhood, high pulmonary blood flow is most apt to produce
    A. Cyanosis on exercise
    B. Diminished exercise tolerance
    C. Periodic episodes of hemoptysis
    D. Right ventricular hypertrophy

Answer: B

High pulmonary blood flow beyond infancy may produce surprisingly little disability for a period of time, and the diminished exercise tolerance may be subtle. Cyanosis, hemoptysis, and pneumonia are not anticipated. With the volume overloading in the RV, ventricular dilatation is more common than ventricular hypertrophy. (See Schwartz 10th ed.)

19. The most important diagnostic assessment modality for evaluating infants and children with congenital heart disease is
    A. Cardiac catheterization
    B. Chest X-ray
    C. Transesophageal echocardiogram
    D. Transthoracic echocardiogram

Answer: D

Although chest X-ray may define heart size and electrocardiograms indicate cardiac rhythm, transthoracic and subcostal echocardiograms provide information on cardiac structure and function. Transesophageal echocardiogram, often very important in adults, is not required in children because children have excellent acoustic windows for the conventional studies. Cardiac catheterization is currently used most frequently for therapeutic reasons such as balloon dilatation of an uncomplicated isolated valvular pulmonic stenosis or coil occlusion of a patent ductus arteriosus. (See Schwartz 10th ed., p. 697.)

20. The major determinant of operability in patients who have a VSD is
    A. The size of the defect.
    B. The location of the defect.
    C. The pulmonary vascular resistance.
    D. The age of the patient.

Answer: C

The specific anatomy of a ventricular defect, its size, and the age of the affected patient are not much hindrance to closure of the defect, and the major determinant of operability is the degree of pulmonary vascular resistance that is present. It is important to differentiate between pulmonary artery pressure and vascular resistance. The pressure may be elevated by a large increase in blood flow, and yet the resistance may be normal; conversely, the pressure may be markedly elevated in the presence of an almost normal blood flow if the resistance is increased. When pulmonary vascular resistance exceeds one-half the systemic resistance, the defect generally is considered inoperable. Those patients who have severe pulmonary vascular resistance increase their cardiac output by right-to-left shunting across the defect because they cannot increase their pulmonary blood flow. If the defect is closed, they have no mechanism to increase cardiac output with exercise. Most cases of VSD are detected today and the affected patient successfully operated on within the first years of life before pulmonary vascular resistance has become severely elevated. (See Schwartz 10th ed., p. 727.)

21. Transplant-free survival after Norwood with B-T shunt (system to pulmonary) versus Sano shunt (RV to pulmonary shunt) in patients with hypoplastic left heart syndrome is
    A. Equal at 12 months, though worse for B-T shunt with longer term follow-up
    B. Worse for B-T shunt at 12 months and at longer term follow-up
    C. Better at 12 months for B-T shunt, but equal at longer term follow-up
    D. Worse at 12 months for B-T shunt, but equal at longer term follow-up

Answer: D

The postoperative management of infants following stage 1 palliation is complex because favorable outcomes depend on establishing a delicate balance between pulmonary and systemic perfusion. Recent literature suggests that these infants require adequate postoperative cardiac output in order to supply both the pulmonary and the systemic circulations and that the use of oximetric catheters to monitor mixed venous oxygen saturation (Svo_2) aids clinicians in both the selection of inotropic agents and in ventilatory management. Recent introduction of a modification that includes arch reconstruction and placement of the shunt between the RV and the pulmonary artery (Sano shunt) diminishes the diastolic flow created by the classical B-T shunt and may augment coronary perfusion, resulting in improved postoperative cardiac function. A recent prospective, randomized, multi-institutional trial sponsored by the National Institutes of Health, the Systemic Ventricle Reconstruction (SVR) trial, compared the outcomes of neonates having either a modified B-T shunt versus a Sano shunt. The SVR trial demonstrated that transplantation-free survival 12 months after randomization was higher with the Sano shunt than with the modified B-T shunt (74 vs 64%, P = 0.01). However, the Sano shunt group had more unintended interventions (P = 0.003) and complications (P = 0.002). Right ventricular size and function at the age of 14 months and the rate of nonfatal serious adverse events at the age of 12 months were similar in the two groups. Data collected over a mean (± standard deviation) follow-up period of 32 ± 11 months showed a nonsignificant difference in transplantation-free survival between the two groups (P = 0.06). (See Schwartz 10th ed., p. 717.)

22. A premature infant is discovered at birth to have a patent ductus arteriosus with moderate respiratory distress. The infant does not improve after 48 hours of medical management with fluid restriction, diuretics, and respiratory support. The next step in management is
    A. Acetylsalicylic acid
    B. Indomethacin
    C. Surgical correction of the ductus
    D. Transvenous occlusion of the ductus

Answer: B
Prostaglandins oppose contraction of the smooth muscle that obliterates the ductus. Indomethacin is a prostaglandin inhibitor and, given intravenously, leads to closure of the ductus in the premature infant. A national cooperative study found that indomethacin effected closure in 79% of 3559 patients studied. Although surgical closure of the ductus is surprisingly well-tolerated in these infants, operation should not be done unless this therapy does not close the ductus and symptoms are poorly controlled. (See Schwartz 10th ed., p. 704.)

23. Which of the following is NOT a type of VSD?
    A. Perimembranous
    B. Atrioventricular canal
    C. Supracristal
    D. Sinus venosal

Answer: D
VSD refers to a hole between the left and RVs. These defects are common, comprising 20 to 30% of all cases of congenital heart disease, and may occur as an isolated lesion or as part of a more complex malformation. VSDs vary in size from 3 to 4 mm to more than 3 cm, and are classified into four types based on their location in the ventricular septum: perimembranous, atrioventricular canal, outlet or supracristal, and muscular. (See Schwartz 10th ed., p. 726.)

24. During left thoracotomy for repair of patent ductus arteriosus the blood pressure is 70/22. Immediately after placement of a clip across the duct the blood pressure is
    A. 70/22
    B. 70/40
    C. 90/22
    D. 90/40

Answer: B
Patent ductus arteriosus results in lower aortic diastolic pressure which increases the potential for myocardial ischemia and underperfusion of other systemic organs, while increased pulmonary blood flow leads to increased work of breathing and decreased gas exchange. Closure of the duct immediately increases diastolic systemic blood pressure, while leaving systolic pressure unchanged. (See Schwartz 10th ed., pp. 706–707.)

25. All of the following are true about truncus arteriosus EXCEPT
    A. Truncal valves most commonly have three leaflets.
    B. Patients usually present with mild to moderate cyanosis and congestive heart failure in the neonatal period.
    C. Patients should undergo repair at 6 months of age.
    D. There is a continuous left to right shunt.

Answer: C
The truncal valve is most commonly trileaflet (60%), but occasionally bicuspid and rarely quadricuspid (25%). Patients present in the neonatal period with signs and symptoms of congestive heart failure and mild to moderate cyanosis. A pansystolic murmur may be noted at the left sternal border and occasionally a diastolic murmur may be heard in the presence of truncal regurgitation. The presence of truncus arteriosus is an indication for surgery. Repair should be undertaken in the neonatal period or as soon as the diagnosis is established to prevent the development of pulmonary hypertension due to pulmonary over circulation. The presence of Eisenmenger physiology, which is found primarily in older children, is the only absolute contraindication to correction. (See Schwartz 10th ed., pp. 706–707)

26. All are true regarding closure of ASDs in adults EXCEPT
    A. Atrial arrhythmias are common postoperatively.
    B. Postoperative mortality is significantly higher with increasing age.
    C. Closure of ASDs in patients older than 60 decreases risk of paradoxical embolism, but has little effect on functional status.
    D. Secundum ASD closure is more commonly performed using transcatheter approach compared with surgical approaches.

Answer: C
After closure, functional capacity as measured by standardized survey instruments was significantly improved in older patients. Atrial arrhythmias are a common complication of ASDs and are not completely mitigated by closure of the defect, though atrial and right ventricular size decrease. Though adults are subject to more complications during the postoperative period, mortality is extremely low, as it is in children who undergo closure. Recent advances in transcatheter technology have resulted in the majority of secundum defects being repaired using these devices. (See Schwartz 10th ed., p. 67.)

CHAPTER 21

Acquired Heart Disease

1. The bypass conduit with the highest patency rate is the
   A. Radial artery
   B. Internal thoracic artery
   C. Greater saphenous vein
   D. Radial artery

2. Which of the following is true about angina pectoris?
   A. Angina is typically substernal and may radiate to the left upper extremity.
   B. "Typical" angina occurs in approximately 50% of patients with coronary disease.
   C. "Atypical" angina occurs more commonly in men.
   D. Angina is a typical symptom for mitral stenosis.

3. A holosystolic murmer that is accompanied by a ventricular septal defect is associated with the following etiology
   A. Ventricular filling that follows atrial contraction
   B. Crescendo-decrescendo; occur as blood is ejected into the left and right ventricular outflow tracts.
   C. Flow between chambers that have widely different pressures throughout systole.
   D. A relative disproportion between valve orifice size and diastolic blood flow volume.

Answer: B
The most important criterion in conduit selection is graft patency. The conduit with the highest patency rate (98% at 5 years and 85–90% at 10 years) is the internal thoracic artery which is most commonly left attached proximally to the subclavian artery (although occasionally used as a free graft) and anastomosed distally to the target coronary artery. The use of both internal thoracic arteries has been shown to increase event-free survival in a number of studies. (See Schwartz 10th ed., pp. 743–744.)

Answer: A
Angina pectoris is the pain or discomfort caused by myocardial ischemia and is typically substernal and may radiate to the left upper extremity, left neck, or epigastrium. The variety of presentations can make myocardial ischemia difficult to diagnose. Characteristics of chest pain that make myocardial ischemia less likely include: pleuritic chest pain, pain reproducible by movement or palpation, or brief episodes lasting only seconds. Typical angina is relieved by rest and/or use of sublingual nitroglycerin. Differential diagnoses to be considered include, but are not limited to, musculoskeletal pain, pulmonary disorders, esophageal spasm, pericarditis, aortic dissection, gastroesophageal reflux, neuropathic pain, and anxiety. (See Schwartz 10th ed., p. 742.)

Answer: C
See Table 21-1. (See Schwartz 10th ed., Table 21-7, p. 748.)

TABLE 21-1	Classification of cardiac murmurs	
Murmur	**Condition**	**Mechanism/Etiology**
		Systolic Murmurs
Holosystolic (pansystolic)	VSD	Flow between chambers that have widely different pressures throughout systole
Mid-systolic (systolic ejection)	High flow rate, MS, MR, TS, TI	Often crescendo-decrescendo in configuration; occur as blood is ejected into the left and right ventricular outflow tracts
Early systolic	Early TI, acute MR	Less common
Mid to late systolic	MR, MVP	Soft to moderate high-pitched murmurs at the LV apex; often due to apical tethering and malcoaptation of MV leaflets; an associated click indicates prolapse of the MV leaflets
		Diastolic Murmurs
Early high-pitched	AI, PR	Generally decrescendo in configuration; occur when the associated ventricular pressure drops sufficiently below that of the outflow tract
Mid-diastolic	MS, TS, PDA*, VSD*, ASD*	Due to a relative disproportion between valve orifice size and diastolic blood flow volume; seen in normal MV and TV with increased diastolic blood flow associated with these conditions*
Presystolic	MS, TS	Occur during the period of ventricular filling that follows atrial contraction (ie, only occur in sinus rhythm)
		Continuous Murmurs
Systolic and diastolic	PDA	Uncommon, due to shunts that persist through the end of systole and the some or all of diastole

AI = aortic insufficiency; ASD = atrial septal defect; MR = mitral regurgitation; MS = mitral stenosis. MVP = mitral valve prolapse; PDA = patent ductus arteriosus; PR = pulmonic regurgitation; TI = tricuspid insufficiency; TS = tricuspid stenosis; VSD = ventricular septal defect.

4. The following is NOT true of left ventricular aneurysms
   A. Rupture is extremely common.
   B. Angina is a common symptom.
   C. Embolic phenomenon is rare.
   D. Ventricular arrhythmias are common.

Answer: A

Symptoms of left ventricle (LV) aneurysms include angina, congestive heart failure (CHF), ventricular arrhythmias, and rarely embolic phenomenon. Rupture is extremely uncommon. Patients generally present for coronary artery bypass or during evaluation of CHF or arrhythmias. While transthoracic echocardiography gives pertinent information regarding LV function, size, mitral valve function, and the presence of thrombus, it is generally accepted that cardiac magnetic resonance imaging (MRI) is the best diagnostic modality to accurately identify areas of scar and viable tissue, and to best define ventricular geometry. (See Schwartz 10th ed., p. 767.)

5. The most common arrhythmia worldwide is
   A. Atrial flutter
   B. Paroxysmal supraventricular tachycardia (PSVT)
   C. Wolff-Parkinson-White (WPW) syndrome
   D. Atrial fibrillation (AF)

Answer: D

Atrial fibrillation (AF) remains the most common arrhythmia in the world with an overall incidence of 0.4 to 1% that increases to 8% in those older than 80 years. The most serious complication of AF is thromboembolism with resultant stroke, but serious morbidity and mortality may also result from hemodynamic compromise due to loss of atrial contraction, exacerbations of CHF from atrioventricular asynchrony and tachycardia-induced cardiomyopathy. (See Schwartz 10th ed., p. 771.)

6. The most common cause of acquired mitral stenosis is
   A. Rheumatic disease
   B. Left atrial myxoma
   C. Ball valve thrombus
   D. Previous chest radiation

Answer: A

Acquired mitral stenosis (MS) is most often caused by rheumatic fever, with approximately 60% of patients with pure MS presenting with a positive clinical history of rheumatic heart disease. Rarely, other conditions can cause obstruction to filling of the LV, mimicking MS. Acquired causes of mitral valve obstruction include left atrial myxoma, ball valve thrombus, mucopolysaccharidosis, previous chest radiation, and severe annular calcification. (See Schwartz 10th ed., p. 751.)

7. What valvular lesion is most commonly found in a patient with Ehlers-Danlos syndrome?
   A. MS
   B. Mitral insufficiency
   C. Aortic stenosis (AS)
   D. Aortic insufficiency (AI)

Answer: D

The most common cause of isolated aortic insufficiency (AI) in patients undergoing aortic valve replacement (AVR) is aortic root disease, and represents over 50% of such patients in some studies. Other common causes of AI include congenital abnormalities of the aortic valve, such as bicuspid aortic valve, calcific degeneration, rheumatic disease, infective endocarditis, systemic hypertension, myxomatous degeneration, dissection of the ascending aorta, and Marfan syndrome. Less common causes of AI include traumatic injuries to the aortic valve, ankylosing spondylitis, syphilitic aortitis, rheumatoid arthritis, osteogenesis imperfecta, giant cell aortitis, Ehlers-Danlos syndrome, Reiter syndrome, discrete subaortic stenosis, and ventricular septal defects with prolapse of an aortic cusp. Although most of these lesions produce chronic aortic insufficiency, rarely acute severe aortic regurgitation can result, often with devastating consequences. (See Schwartz 10th ed., p. 758.)

8. Tricuspid stenosis is
   A. Caused by secondary dilation of the tricuspid annulus due to pulmonary hypertension and/or right heart failure
   B. Commonly the result of organic disease, such as rheumatic heart disease and endocarditis
   C. Commonly caused by mitral valve disease
   D. Commonly associated with Marfan syndrome

Answer: B

Acquired tricuspid valve (TV) disease can be classified as either organic or functional, and affects approximately 0.8% of the general population. Tricuspid stenosis is almost always a result of organic disease, namely rheumatic heart disease and endocarditis. In the case of rheumatic disease, tricuspid stenosis with or without associated insufficiency is invariably associated with mitral valve disease. Other less common causes of obstruction to right atrial emptying include congenital tricuspid atresia, right atrial tumors, and endomyocardial fibrosis. (See Schwartz 10th ed., pp. 762–763.)

9. The most common cardiac tumor is
   A. Papillary fibroelastoma
   B. Lymphangioma
   C. Myxoma
   D. Metastatic tumor

Answer: C

Cardiac myxomas are the most common cardiac tumor and are characterized by several distinguishing features. About 75% of the time, they arise from the interatrial septum near the fossa ovalis in the left atrium. Most others will develop in the right atrium, but, less commonly, they can arise from valvular surfaces and the walls of other cardiac chambers. Macroscopically, these tumors are pedunculated with a gelatinous consistency, and the surface may be smooth (65%), villous, or friable. Size varies greatly with these tumors and ranges from 1 to 15 cm in diameter. Internally, myxomas are heterogeneous and often contain hemorrhage, cysts, necrosis, or calcification. Histologically, these tumors contain cells that arise from a multipotent mesenchyme and are contained within a mucopolysaccharide stroma. (See Schwartz 10th ed., p. 775.)

10. The most common primary cardiac tumor in children is
    A. Fibroelastomas
    B. Hemangiomas
    C. Lipomas
    D. Rhabdomyomas

Answer: D

In children, rhabdomyomas are the most common primary cardiac tumor, whereas fibromas are the most commonly resected cardiac tumor. Rhabdomyomas are myocardial hamartomas that are often multicentric in the ventricles. About 50% of cases are associated with tuberous sclerosis, and while resection is occasionally necessary, most disappear spontaneously. Fibromas are congenital lesions that one-third of the time are found in children younger than 1 year. These tumors, conversely, are ordinarily solitary lesions found in the inner interventricular septum, and they may present with heart failure, cyanosis, arrhythmias, syncopal episodes, chest pain, or sudden cardiac death. (See Schwartz 10th ed., p. 776.)

11. Patients undergoing mechanical mitral valve replacement
    A. Have a target international normalized ratio (INR) of 4 to 5 times normal
    B. Have increased left atrial size
    C. Have AF
    D. Are at lower risk for thromboembolism

Answer: B

Although mechanical valves necessitate systemic anticoagulation, careful monitoring of the international normalized ratio (INR) reduces the risk of thromboembolic events and hemorrhagic complications, and improves overall survival. Patients undergoing mechanical AVR generally have a target INR of 2 to 3 times normal. Patients undergoing mechanical mitral valve replacement frequently have increased left atrial size, concomitant AF, and are at higher risk for thromboembolism than those undergoing mechanical AOR, and are thus recommended to have a target INR 2.5 to 3.5 times normal. When managed appropriately, the yearly thromboembolic and bleeding risks in these patients are 1 to 2%, and 0.5 to 2%, respectively. (See Schwartz 10th ed., p. 749.)

12. An absolute contraindication to a coronary artery bypass operation is
    A. Acute coronary artery insufficiency with persistent or progressive angina despite optimal medical therapy.
    B. Acute subendocardial infarction with multivessel coronary artery disease.
    C. Cardiogenic shock after myocardial infarction.
    D. Chronic CHF and ischemic cardiomyopathy with no signs of angina.

Answer: D

Patients with ischemic cardiomyopathy are a heterogeneous group, and, as with any surgery, appropriate patient selection is central to success. In one retrospective study of 96 patients with ischemic cardiomyopathy (ejection fraction [EF] ≤25%), age, and poor distal vessel quality were predictors of poor outcomes. Mortality in patients with poor vessel quality was 100%, compared with 90% when vessel quality was fair and 10% when it was good. Therefore, poor vessel quality should be considered a contraindication to surgical revascularization even in the presence of angina. (See Schwartz 10th ed., p. 765.)

13. Approximately 50% of benign cardiac tumors are
    A. Figromas
    B. Teratomas
    C. Lipomas
    D. Myxomas

Answer: D

Cardiac neoplasms are rare, with an incidence ranging from 0.001 to 0.3% in autopsy studies and a 0.15% incidence in major echocardiographic series. Benign cardiac tumors are most common and account for 75% of primary neoplasms. Approximately 50% of benign cardiac tumors are myxomas, with the remainder being papillary fibroelastomas, lipomas, rhabdomyomas, fibromas, hemangiomas, teratomas, lymphangiomas, and others, in order of decreasing frequency. Most malignant primary cardiac tumors are sarcomas (angiosarcoma, rhabdomyosarcoma, fibrosarcoma, leiomyosarcoma, and liposarcoma), with a small incidence of malignant lymphomas. Metastatic cardiac tumors, while still infrequent, have been reported to occur 100-fold more often than primary lesions. (See Schwartz 10th ed., p. 774.)

14. The majority of cardiac myxomas arise from
    A. The right atrium
    B. Valvular surfaces
    C. The left atrium
    D. The right ventricle (RV)

Answer: C

Cardiac myxomas are the most common cardiac tumor and are characterized by several distinguishing features. About 75% of the time, they arise from the interatrial septum near the fossa ovalis in the left atrium. Most others will develop in the right atrium, but, less commonly, they can arise from valvular surfaces and the walls of other cardiac chambers. Macroscopically, these tumors are pedunculated with a gelatinous consistency, and the surface may be smooth (65%), villous, or friable. (See Schwartz 10th ed., p. 775.)

15. The following is NOT true of rhabdomyomas.
    A. They often require resection.
    B. They are often multicentric in the ventricles.
    C. They are the most common primary cardiac tumor in children.
    D. They often disappear spontaneously.

Answer: A

In children, rhabdomyomas are the most common primary cardiac tumor, whereas fibromas are the most commonly resected cardiac tumor. Rhabdomyomas are myocardial hamartomas that are often multicentric in the ventricles. About 50% of cases are associated with tuberous sclerosis, and while resection is occasionally necessary, most disappear spontaneously. Fibromas are congenital lesions that one-third of the time are found in children younger than 1 year. These tumors, conversely, are ordinarily solitary lesions found in the inner interventricular septum, and they may present with heart failure, cyanosis, arrhythmias, syncopal episodes, chest pain, or sudden cardiac death. (See Schwartz 10th ed., p. 776.)

16. A patient presents with a history of fatigue and dyspnea. He is found to have hepatomegaly, ascites, and an elevated jugular venous pulse. Heart sounds are normal, no murmurs are present, and the heart is of normal size. The pulse pressure is decreased by palpation. Electrocardiography (ECG) is normal except for low voltage. The most likely diagnosis is
    A. Right atrial myxoma
    B. TV disease
    C. Constrictive pericarditis
    D. Primary pulmonary artery hypertension

Answer: C

Classic physical examination findings include jugular venous distention with Kussmaul sign, diminished cardiac apical impulses, peripheral edema, ascites, pulsatile liver, a pericardial knock, and, in advanced disease, signs of liver dysfunction, such as jaundice or cachexia. The "pericardial knock" is an early diastolic sound that reflects a sudden impediment to ventricular filling, similar to an S_3 but of higher pitch.

Several findings are characteristic on noninvasive and invasive testing. Central venoud pressure (CVP) is often elevated 15 to 20 mm Hg or higher. ECG commonly demonstrates nonspecific low voltage QRS complexes and isolated repolarization abnormalities. Chest X-ray may demonstrate calcification of the pericardium, which is highly suggestive of constrictive pericarditis in patients with heart failure, but this is present in only 25% of cases. Cardiac CT or MRI (cMRI) typically demonstrate increased pericardial thickness (>4 mm) and calcification, dilation of the inferior vena cava, deformed ventricular contours, and flattening or leftward shift of the ventricular septum. Pericardial adhesions may also be seen on tagged cine MRI studies.

As discussed, it is most important to distinguish pericardial constriction from restrictive cardiomyopathy, which is best done with either echocardiography or right heart catheterization. Findings favoring constriction on echocardiography include respiratory variation of ventricular septal motion and mitral inflow velocity, preserved or increased mitral annulus early diastolic filling velocity, and increased hepatic vein flow reversal with expiration. Cardiac catheterization will show increased atrial pressures, equalization of end-diastolic pressure, and early ventricular diastolic filling with a subsequent plateau, called the *square-root sign*. Additional findings upon catheterization that would favor constriction include respiratory variation in ventricular filling and increased ventricular interdependence, manifest as a discordant change in the total area of the LV and RV systolic pressure curve with respiration. (See Schwartz 10th ed., pp. 773–774.)

148

17. Each of the following effects is anticipated after insertion of an intra-aortic balloon pump EXCEPT
    A. Preload decrease
    B. Increased total myocardial oxygen consumption
    C. Improvement in cardiac index
    D. Coronary blood flow increase

Answer: B

The intra-aortic balloon pump (IABP) is the most commonly used device for mechanical circulatory support, and it may be easily deployed in the catheterization laboratory, in the operating room or at the bedside. The device is inserted percutaneously through the femoral artery into the thoracic aorta. It is synchronized so that the balloon is inflated during diastole and deflated during systole, resulting in augmentation of diastolic perfusion of the coronary arteries and decreased afterload. Typically, this improves cardiac index and decreases both preload and myocardial oxygen consumption. (See Schwartz 10th ed., p. 768.)

18. Pericarditis is *usually* treated with
    A. A short course of nonsteroidal anti-inflammatory drugs (NSAIDs).
    B. Use of steroids or intravenous antibiotics.
    C. Surgical exploration and drainage.
    D. Observation.

Answer: A

The preferred treatment depends on the underlying cause of the pericarditis. The disease usually follows a self-limited and benign course and can be successfully treated with a short course of nonsteroidal anti-inflammatory drugs (NSAIDs). Some patients may require judicious use of steroids or IV antibiotics. In cases of purulent pyogenic pericarditis, surgical exploration and drainage are occasionally necessary. Rarely, accumulation of fluid in the pericardium may lead to tamponade, requiring prompt evacuation of the pericardial space. While pericardiocentesis will typically suffice, surgical drainage may be required for thick, viscous, or clotted fluid or in patients with significant scarring from previous surgeries. More commonly, surgical intervention is required to manage recurrent disease. (See Schwartz ed., p. 773.)

19. The most common cause of isolated aortic in AI sufficiency in patients undergoing AVR is
    A. Congenital abnormalities of the aortic valve
    B. Systemic hypertension
    C. Aortic root disease
    D. Calcific degeneration

Answer: C

The most common cause of isolated AI in patients undergoing AVR is aortic root disease, and represents over 50% of such patients in some studies. Other common causes of AI include congenital abnormalities of the aortic valve, such as bicuspid aortic valve, calcific degeneration, rheumatic disease, infective endocarditis, systemic hypertension, myxomatous degeneration, dissection of the ascending aorta, and Marfan syndrome. Less common causes of AI include traumatic injuries to the aortic valve, ankylosing spondylitis, syphilitic aortitis, rheumatoid arthritis, osteogenesis imperfecta, giant cell aortitis, Ehlers-Danlos syndrome, Reiter syndrome, discrete subaortic stenosis, and ventricular septal defects with prolapse of an aortic cusp. Although most of these lesions produce chronic aortic insufficiency, rarely acute severe aortic regurgitation can result, often with devastating consequences. (See Schwartz 10th ed., p. 758.)

20. During cardiopulmonary bypass (CPB) anticoagulation, the range of heparin needed to increase the activated clotting time to greater than 450 seconds is
    A. 200 to 300
    B. 300 to 400
    C. 400 to 500
    D. 450 to 550

Answer: B

The basic cardiopulmonary bypass (CPB) circuit consists of the venous cannulae, a venous reservoir, pump, oxygenator, filter, and the arterial cannula. Anticoagulation is required during CPB, and 300 to 400 units/kg of heparin is given to increase the activated clotting time (ACT) to greater than 450 seconds. Once adequate anticoagulation is achieved, arterial cannulation is performed through a purse-string suture, or through a side graft which is sewn on to the native artery. (See Schwartz 10th ed., p. 740.)

21. Eligibility criteria for mechanical support as destination therapy includes all of the following EXCEPT
    A. Medically refractory NYHA class III
    B. Peak oxygen consumption <12 mL/kg/min
    C. Left ventricular ejection fraction >25%
    D. Age >65

Answer: C

Current eligibility criteria for mechanical support as destination therapy include: (a) medically refractory NYHA class III or IV heart failure for at least 60 days, (b) peak oxygen consumption <12 mL/kg/min or failure to wean from continuous IV inotropes, (c) left ventricular ejection fraction <25%, and (d) presence of a contraindication for heart transplantation (ie, age >65 years, irreversible pulmonary hypertension, chronic renal failure, insulin-dependent diabetes with end organ damage, or other clinically significant comorbidities). Once a patient has a left ventricular assist device inserted as destination therapy, close and intensive follow-up by a multidisciplinary heart failure team is required in order to optimize medical therapy, reduce device-related morbidity, and improve survival. (See Schwartz 10th ed., p. 770.)

22. Angiosarcomas
    A. Are mucous in appearance and are typically found in the posterior wall of the left atrium
    B. Are aggressive and rapidly invade adjacent structures
    C. Are bulky tumors that usually occur in children
    D. Are encapsulated tumors that usually arise from the epicardium

Answer: B

Primary cardiac malignancies are very rare, but when they occur they tend to have a right-sided predominance and frequently demonstrate extracardiac extension and involvement. Malignant cardiac tumors include angiosarcoma, osteosarcoma, leiomyosarcoma, rhabdomyosarcoma, liposarcoma, and primary cardiac lymphomas. Angiosarcomas are aggressive, rapidly invading adjacent structures, and 47 to 89% of patients present with lung, liver, or brain metastases by the time of diagnosis. Leiomyosarcomas are sessile masses with a mucous appearance that are typically found in the posterior wall of the left atrium. Rhabdomyosarcomas are bulky (>10 cm in diameter) tumors that usually occur in children and do not have a predilection for any particular chamber. They frequently invade nearby cardiac structures and are multicentric in 60% of cases. (See Schwartz 10th ed., p. 776.)

23. Age-related calcific AS causes some degree of AI in approximately
    A. 55%
    B. 65%
    C. 75%
    D. 85%

Answer: C

There are also many primary valvular diseases that cause AI, generally in association with AS. One such disorder is age-related calcific AS, which causes some degree of AI in up to 75% of patients. Infective endocarditis may involve the aortic valve apparatus and cause AI through direct destruction of the valve leaflets, perforation of a leaflet, or formation of vegetations that interfere with proper coaptation of the valve cusps. Rheumatic disease causes fibrous infiltration of the valve cusps and subsequent retraction of the valve leaflets, inhibiting apposition of the cusps during diastole and producing a central regurgitant jet. Patients with large ventricular septal defects or membranous subaortic stenosis may develop progressive AI, owing to a Venturi effect that results in prolapse of the aortic valve leaflets. (See Schwartz 10th ed., p. 760.)

CHAPTER 22

Thoracic Aneurysms and Aortic Dissection

1. The type of thoracic aortic aneurysm characterized by an outpouching of the aorta is
   A. Fusiform
   B. Saccular
   C. Pseudoaneurysm
   D. None of the above

Answer: B
Aortic aneurysms can be either "true" or "false." True aneurysms can take two forms: fusiform and saccular. Fusiform aneurysms are more common and can be described as symmetrical dilatations of the aorta. Saccular aneurysms are localized outpouchings of the aorta. False aneurysms, also called *pseudoaneurysms*, are leaks in the aortic wall that are contained by the outer layer of the aorta and/or the periaortic tissue; they are caused by disruption of the aortic wall and lead blood to collect in pouches of fibrotic tissue. (See Schwartz 10th ed., p. 785.)

2. Which of the following is the most common cause of thoracic aortic aneurysms?
   A. Atherosclerosis
   B. Marfan syndrome
   C. Takayasu arteritis
   D. Nonspecific medial degeneration

Answer: D
Nonspecific medial degeneration is the most common cause of thoracic aortic disease. Histologic findings of mild medial degeneration, including fragmentation of elastic fibers and loss of smooth muscle cells, are expected in the aging aorta. However, an advanced, accelerated form of medial degeneration leads to progressive weakening of the aortic wall, aneurysm formation, and eventual dissection, rupture, or both. The underlying causes of medial degenerative disease remain unknown. (See Schwarz 10th ed., p. 787.)

3. The most common complication of extensive repair for distal aortic aneurysms is
   A. Spinal cord ischemia
   B. Renal failure
   C. Pulmonary dysfunction
   D. Left recurrent laryngeal nerve injury

Answer: C
Although spinal cord ischemia and renal failure receive the most attention, several other complications warrant consideration. The most common complication of extensive repairs is pulmonary dysfunction. With aneurysms adjacent to the left subclavian artery, the vagus and left recurrent laryngeal nerves are often adherent to the aortic wall and thus are susceptible to injury. (See Schwartz 10th ed., p. 802.)

4. Marfan syndrome is caused by an abnormality in which of the following proteins?
   A. Elastin
   B. Metalloproteinase
   C. Collagen
   D. Fibrillin

Answer: D

Marfan syndrome is an autosomal-dominant genetic disorder characterized by a specific connective tissue defect that leads to aneurysm formation. The phenotype of patients with Marfan syndrome typically includes a tall stature, high palate, joint hypermobility, eye lens disorders, mitral valve prolapse, and aortic aneurysms. The aortic wall is weakened by fragmentation of elastic fibers and deposition of extensive amounts of mucopolysaccharides (a process previously called *cystic medial degeneration* or *cystic medial necrosis*). Patients with Marfan syndrome have a mutation in the fibrillin gene located on the long arm of chromosome 15. The traditionally held view is that abnormal fibrillin in the extracellular matrix decreases connective tissue strength in the aortic wall and produces abnormal elasticity, which predisposes the aorta to dilatation from wall tension caused by left ventricular ejection impulses. More recent evidence, however, shows that the abnormal fibrillin causes degeneration of the aortic wall matrix by increasing the activity of transforming growth factor-beta (TGF-β). Between 75 and 85% of patients with Marfan syndrome have dilatation of the ascending aorta and annuloaortic ectasia (dilatation of the aortic sinuses and annulus). Such aortic abnormalities are the most common cause of death among patients with Marfan syndrome. Marfan syndrome also is frequently associated with aortic dissection. (See Schwartz 10th ed., p. 787.)

5. The following is NOT true regarding anastomotic pseudoaneurysms
   A. Can arise from deterioration of aortic tissue due to infection
   B. Have increased in incidence with an influx of cardiovascular surgery
   C. Commonly occur in patients with Marfan syndrome
   D. Are associated with high incidence of morbidity and rupture

Answer: B

Anastomotic pseudoaneurysms can be caused by technical problems or by deterioration of the native aortic tissue, graft material, or suture. Commonly, they occur in patients with Marfan syndrome. Tissue deterioration usually is related to either progressive degenerative disease or infection. Improvements in sutures, graft materials, and surgical techniques have decreased the incidence of thoracic aortic pseudoaneurysms. Should thoracic aortic pseudoaneurysms occur, they typically require expeditious surgical or other intervention because they are associated with a high incidence of morbidity and rupture. (See Schwartz 10th ed., p. 788.)

6. The most common cause of death in patients with type IV Ehlers-Danlos syndrome is
   A. Myocardial infarction
   B. Aortic dissection
   C. Ruptured visceral artery
   D. Pulmonary emboli

Answer: C

Ehlers-Danlos syndrome includes a spectrum of inherited connective tissue disorders of collagen synthesis. The subtypes represent differing defective steps of collagen production. Vascular type Ehlers-Danlos syndrome is characterized by an autosomal dominant defect in type III collagen synthesis, which can have life-threatening cardiovascular manifestations. Spontaneous arterial rupture, usually involving the mesenteric vessels, is the most common cause of death in these patients. Thoracic aortic aneurysms and dissections are less commonly associated with Ehlers-Danlos syndrome, but when they do occur, they pose a particularly challenging surgical problem because of the reduced integrity of the aortic tissue. An Ehlers-Danlos variant of periventricular heterotopia associated with joint and skin hyperextensibility and aortic dilation has been described as being caused by mutations in the gene encoding filamin A (*FLNA*), an actin-binding protein that links the smooth muscle cell contractile unit to the cell surface. (See Schwartz 10th ed., p. 787.)

7. The most common presenting symptom in patients with an ascending thoracic aneurysm is
   A. Anterior chest pain
   B. Posterior chest pain
   C. Aortic valve insufficiency
   D. Sudden death

Answer: A

Initially, aneurysmal expansion and impingement on adjacent structures causes mild, chronic pain. The most common symptom in patients with ascending aortic aneurysms is anterior chest discomfort; the pain is frequently precordial in location but may radiate to the neck and jaw, mimicking angina. Aneurysms of the ascending aorta and transverse aortic arch can cause symptoms related to compression of the superior vena cava, the pulmonary artery, the airway, or the sternum. Rarely, these aneurysms erode into the superior vena cava or right atrium, causing acute high-output failure. (See Schwartz 10th ed., p. 789.)

8. Endoleaks
   A. Type I and type IV generally require early and aggressive intervention
   B. Are uncommon
   C. Can occur during the initial procedure or over time
   D. Are benign

Answer: A

Another significant complication of descending thoracic aortic stent grafting is endoleak. An endoleak occurs when there is a persistent flow of blood (visible on radiologic imaging) into the aneurysm sac, and it may occur during the initial procedure or develop over time. Although endoleaks are a relatively common complication, they are not benign, because they lead to continual pressurization of the sac, which can cause expansion or even rupture. These complications are categorized (Table 22-1) according to the site of the leak. Although all endoleaks may progress such that they can be considered life-threatening, type I and type III endoleaks generally necessitate early and aggressive intervention. Recently published reporting guidelines aid standardized reporting. (See Schwartz 10th ed., Table 22-4, p. 806.)

TABLE 22-1	Classification of and common treatment strategies for endoleak

Type I
- Incomplete seal between stent graft and aorta at the proximal landing site (Type Ia), the distal landing site (Type Ib), or branch module, fenestration, or plug (Type Ic)
- Early reintervention to improve seal or conversion to open surgery

Type II
- Retrograde perfusion of sac from excluded collateral arteries
- Surveillance; as-needed occlusion with percutaneous or other interventions

Type III
- Incomplete seal between overlapping stent graft or module (Type IIIa), or tear in graft fabric (Type IIIb)
- Early reintervention to cover gap or tear or conversion to open surgery

Type IV
- Perfusion of sac due to porosity of material
- Surveillance; as-needed reintervention to reline stent graft

Type V
- Expansion of sac with no identifiable source
- Surveillance; as-needed reintervention to reline stent graft

9. The most useful imaging study for thoracic aneurysms is
   A. Echocardiography
   B. Computed tomography (CT) scan
   C. Magnetic resonance angiography
   D. Aortography

Answer: B

Computed tomographic (CT) scanning is widely available, provides visualization of the entire thoracic and abdominal aorta, and permits multiplanar and 3-dimensional aortic reconstructions. Consequently, CT is the most common—and arguably the most useful—imaging modality for evaluating thoracic aortic aneurysms. In addition to establishing the diagnosis, CT provides information about an aneurysm's location, extent, anatomic anomalies, and relationship to major branch vessels. CT is particularly useful in determining the absolute diameter of the aorta, especially in the presence of a laminated clot, and also detects aortic calcification. (See Schwartz 10th ed., pp. 790–791.)

10. A patient with Marfan syndrome who has undergone "aortic surgery" most likely had
    A. Aortic valve annuloplasty (annular plication)
    B. Aortic root replacement (valve and ascending aorta)
    C. Total arch replacement with reattachment of the brachiocephalic branches
    D. Elephant trunk repair of thoracic aneurysm

Answer: B

Mechanical prostheses necessitate following a lifelong anticoagulation regimen. Separate replacement of the aortic valve and ascending aorta is not performed in patients with Marfan syndrome, because progressive dilatation of the remaining sinus segment eventually leads to complications that necessitate reoperation. Therefore, patients with Marfan syndrome or those with annuloaortic ectasia require some form of aortic root replacement. (See Schwartz 10th ed., p. 793.)

11. In the case of aortic dissection
    A. Choice of initial treatment is the dependent on dissection local.
    B. Diagnostic delays are common.
    C. They are categorized as chronic after 14 days.
    D. Contrast-enhanced CT is the diagnostic of choice.

Answer: B

Because of the variations in severity and the wide variety of potential clinical manifestations, the diagnosis of acute aortic dissection can be challenging.[141-143] Only 3 out of every 100,000 patients who present to an emergency department with acute chest, back, or abdominal pain are eventually diagnosed with aortic dissection. Not surprisingly, diagnostic delays are common; delays beyond 24 hours after hospitalization occur in up to 39% of cases (Fig. 22-1.) (See Schwartz 10th ed., Figure 22-20, p. 810.)

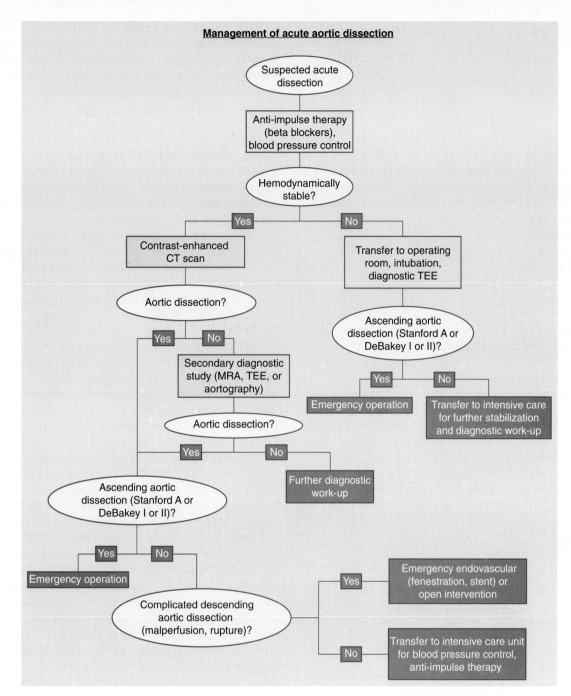

FIG. 22-1. Algorithm used to facilitate decisions regarding treatment of acute aortic dissection. CT = computed tomography; MRA = magnetic resonance angiography; TEE = transesophageal echocardiography.

12. Mortality rates for operative repair of an aortic arch aneurysm have been significantly reduced intraoperatively by
    A. Deep hypothermia to allow circulatory arrest
    B. Innominate and left carotid artery cannulation to permit oxygenation of the brain
    C. Right heart to left subclavian artery bypass to continue brain perfusion
    D. Use of an intraaortic balloon pump to maintain distal circulation

Answer: A
Like the operations themselves, perfusion strategies used during proximal aortic surgery depend on the extent of the repair. Aneurysms that are isolated to the ascending segment can be replaced by using standard cardiopulmonary bypass and distal ascending aortic clamping. This provides constant perfusion of the brain and other vital organs during the repair. Aneurysms involving the transverse aortic arch, however, cannot be clamped during the repair, which necessitates the temporary withdrawal of cardiopulmonary bypass support; this is called *circulatory arrest*. To protect the brain and other vital organs during the circulatory arrest period, hypothermia must be initiated before pump flow is stopped. However, hypothermia is not without risk, and coagulopathy is associated with deep

levels of hypothermia (below 20°C), which have been traditionally used in open arch repair. Recently, more moderate levels of hypothermia (often between 22°C and 24°C) have been introduced that appear to decrease risks associated with deep hypothermia while still providing sufficient brain protection. (See Schwartz 10th ed., p. 797.)

13. According to the Crawford classification scheme, surgical repair of thoracoabdominal aortic aneurysms with repairs beginning near the left subclavian artery but extending distally into the infrarenal abdominal aorta, often reaching the aortic bifurcation is classified as
    A. Extent I
    B. Extent II
    C. Extent III
    D. Extent IV

Answer: B

Extent I thoracoabdominal aortic aneurysm repairs involve most of the descending thoracic aorta, usually beginning near the left subclavian artery, and extend down to the suprarenal abdominal aorta. Extent II repairs also begin near the left subclavian artery but extend distally into the infrarenal abdominal aorta, and they often reach the aortic bifurcation. Extent III repairs extend from the lower descending thoracic aorta (below the sixth rib) and into the abdomen. Extent IV repairs begin at the diaphragmatic hiatus and often involve the entire abdominal aorta. (See Schwartz 10th ed., p. 801.)

14. Treatment of descending aortic dissection by nonoperative, pharmacologic management
    A. Has lower morbidity and mortality rates than traditional surgical treatment.
    B. Most common cause of death during nonoperative treatment is aortic rupture and end-organ malperfusion.
    C. A CT scan obtained on day 2 or 3, compared with the initial scan, is sufficient to rule out significant aortic expansion.
    D. Inadequate blood pressure control has been found to be associated with late aneurysm formation.

Answer: C

Nonoperative, pharmacologic management of acute descending aortic dissection results in lower morbidity and mortality rates than traditional surgical treatment does. The most common causes of death during nonoperative treatment are aortic rupture and end-organ malperfusion. Therefore, patients are continually reassessed for new complications. At least two serial CT scans—usually obtained on day 2 or 3 and on day 8 or 9 of treatment—are compared with the initial scan to rule out significant aortic expansion. Once the patient's condition has been stabilized, pharmacologic management is gradually shifted from intravenous to oral medications. Oral therapy, which usually includes a beta antagonist, is initiated when systolic pressure is consistently between 100 and 110 mm Hg and the neurologic, renal, and cardiovascular systems are stable. Many patients can be discharged after their blood pressure is well controlled with oral agents and after serial CT scans confirm the absence of aortic expansion. Long-term pharmacologic therapy is important for patients with chronic aortic dissection. Beta blockers remain the drugs of choice. In a 20-year follow-up study, DeBakey and colleagues found that inadequate blood pressure control was associated with late aneurysm formation. Aneurysms developed in only 17% of patients with "good" blood pressure control, compared with 45% of patients with "poor" control. (See Schwartz 10th ed., p. 815.)

15. Which of the following is the most typical presenting symptom in a patient with an aortic dissection?
    A. "Tearing" pain
    B. Paraplegia
    C. Abdominal pain
    D. Cold left arm

Answer: A

The onset of dissection often is associated with severe chest or back pain, classically described as *tearing*, that migrates distally as the dissection progresses along the length of the aorta. The location of the pain often indicates which aortic segments are involved. Pain in the anterior chest suggests involvement of the ascending aorta, whereas pain in the back and abdomen generally indicates involvement of the descending and thoracoabdominal aorta. (See Schwartz 10th ed., p. 809.)

16. Delayed treatment for ascending aortic dissection should be considered
    A. In patients who present with severe acute stroke or mesenteric ischemia.
    B. In patients who are elderly and have substantial comorbidity.
    C. In patients who are in stable condition and may benefit from transfer to specialized centers.
    D. In patients who have undergone a cardiac operation in the past 3 weeks.

Answer: D
Because of the risk of aortic rupture, acute ascending aortic dissection is usually considered an absolute indication for emergency surgical repair. However, specific patient groups may benefit from nonoperative management or delayed operation. Delayed repair should be considered for patients who (a) present with severe acute stroke or mesenteric ischemia, (b) are elderly and have substantial comorbidity, (c) are in stable condition and may benefit from transfer to specialized centers, or (d) have undergone a cardiac operation in the remote past. Regarding the last group, it is important that the previous operation not be too recent; dissections that occur during the first 3 weeks after cardiac surgery pose a high risk of rupture and tamponade, and such dissections warrant early operation. (See Schwartz 10th ed., p. 813.)

17. A patient with a subclavian artery malperfusion as a complication of aortic dissection would most likely experience
    A. Paraplegia
    B. Cold, painful extremity
    C. Incontinence
    D. Shock

Answer: B
See Table 22-2. (See Schwartz 10th ed., Table 22-5, p. 811.)

TABLE 22-2	Anatomic complications of aortic dissection and their associated symptoms and signs
Anatomic Manifestation	**Symptoms and Signs**
Aortic valve insufficiency	Dyspnea Murmur Pulmonary rales Shock
Coronary malperfusion	Chest pain with characteristics of angina Nausea/vomiting Shock Ischemic changes on electrocardiogram Elevated cardiac enzymes
Pericardial tamponade	Dyspnea Jugular venous distension Pulsus paradoxus Muffled cardiac tones Shock Low-voltage electrocardiogram
Subclavian or iliofemoral artery malperfusion	Cold, painful extremity Extremity sensory and motor deficits Peripheral pulse deficit
Carotid artery malperfusion	Syncope Focal neurologic deficit (transient or persistent) Carotid pulse deficit Coma
Spinal malperfusion	Paraplegia Incontinence
Mesenteric malperfusion	Nausea/vomiting Abdominal pain
Renal malperfusion	Oliguria or anuria Hematuria

CHAPTER 23

Arterial Disease

1. An ankle-brachial index (ABI) that suggests increased risk of myocardial infarction would be
   A. <0.9
   B. <0.6
   C. >0.9
   D. >0.6

   Answer: A
   There is increasing interest in the use of the ankle-brachial index (ABI) to evaluate patients at risk for cardiovascular events. An ABI less than 0.9 correlates with increased risk of myocardial infarction and indicates significant, although perhaps asymptomatic, underlying peripheral vascular disease. (See Schwartz 10th ed., p. 829.)

2. All of the following are correct regarding abdominal aortic aneurysm (AAA) rupture EXCEPT
   A. It is the 10th leading cause of death for men in the United States.
   B. Risk of rupture is low when below 5.5 cm.
   C. Overall mortality rate of AAA rupture is higher than 70%.
   D. Men have a higher risk of rupture than women.

   Answer: D
   Despite more than 50,000 patients undergoing elective repair of abdominal aortic aneurysm (AAA) each year in the United States, approximately 15,000 patients die annually as a result of ruptured aneurysm, making it the 10th leading cause of death for men. The rupture risk is quite low below 5.5 cm and begins to rise exponentially thereafter. This size can serve as an appropriate threshold for recommending elective repair provided one's surgical mortality is below 5%. For each size strata, however, women appear to be at higher risk for rupture than men, and a lower threshold of 4.5 to 5.0 cm may be reasonable in good-risk patients.

   Overall mortality of AAA rupture is 71 to 77%, which includes all out-of-hospital and in-hospital deaths, as compared with 2 to 6% for elective open surgical repair. Nearly half of all patients with ruptured AAA will die before reaching the hospital. For the remainder, surgical mortality is 45 to 50% and has not substantially changed in the past 30 years. (See Schwartz 10th ed., pp. 850–851.)

3. The compartment most commonly affected in a lower leg compartment syndrome is the
   A. Anterior compartment
   B. Lateral compartment
   C. Deep posterior compartment
   D. Superficial posterior compartment

   Answer: A
   The most commonly affected compartment is the anterior compartment in the leg. Numbness in the web space between the first and second toes is diagnostic due to compression of the deep peroneal nerve. Compartment pressure is measured by inserting an arterial line into the compartment and recording the pressure. Although controversial, pressures greater than 20 mm Hg are an indication for fasciotomy. (See Schwartz 10th ed., p. 888.)

4. Magnetic resonance angiography (MRA) is contraindicated in the following patient groups EXCEPT those with
   A. Pacemakers
   B. Intracerebral shunts
   C. Cochlear implants
   D. Metallic stents

Answer: D

Magnetic resonance angiography (MRA) has the advantage of not requiring iodinated contrast agents to provide vessel opacification (Fig. 23-1). Gadolinium is used as a contrast agent for MRA studies, and because it is generally not nephrotoxic, it can be used in patients with elevated creatinine. MRA is contraindicated in patients with pacemakers, defibrillators, spinal cord stimulators, intracerebral shunts, cochlear implants, and cranial clips. Patients with claustrophobia may require sedation to be able to complete the test. The presence of metallic stents causes artifacts and signal drop-out; however, these can be dealt with using alternations in image acquisition and processing. Nitinol stents produce minimal artifact. Compared to other modalities, MRA is relatively slow and expensive. However, due to its noninvasive nature and decreased nephrotoxicity, MRA is being used more frequently for imaging vasculature in various anatomic distributions. (See Schwartz 10th ed., Figure 23-5, pp. 832–833.)

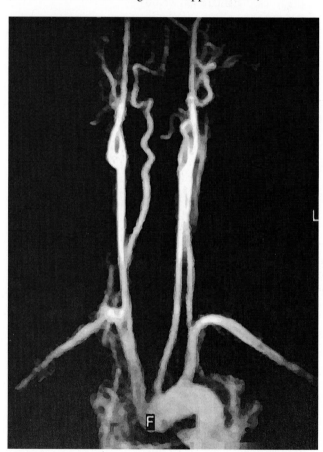

FIG. 23-1. Magnetic resonance angiogram (MRA) of aortic arch and carotid arteries. This study can provide a three-dimensional analysis of vascular structure such as aortic arch branches, carotid and vertebral arteries.

5. The preferred procedure for treatment of typical occlusive disease of the aorta and both iliac arteries is
    A. Endovascular stenting
    B. Extra-anatomic bypass
    C. Aortoiliac endarterectomy
    D. Aortobifemoral bypass

Answer: D

In most cases, aortobifemoral bypass is performed because patients usually have disease in both iliac systems. Although one side may be more severely affected than the other, progression does occur, and bilateral bypass does not complicate the procedure or add to the physiologic stress of the operation. Aortobifemoral bypass reliably relieves symptoms, has excellent long-term patency (approximately 70–80% at 10 years), and can be completed with a tolerable perioperative mortality (2–3%). (See Schwartz 10th ed., p. 876.)

6. The most common cause of ischemic stroke is
    A. Carotid artery disease
    B. Idiopathic
    C. Cardiogenic emboli
    D. Lacunar

Answer: C

Ischemic strokes are due to hypoperfusion from arterial occlusion or, less commonly, to decreased flow resulting from proximal arterial stenosis and poor collateral network. Common causes of ischemic strokes are cardiogenic emboli in 35%, carotid artery disease in 30%, lacunar in 10%, miscellaneous in 10%, and idiopathic in 15%. The term cerebrovascular accident is often used interchangeably to refer to an ischemic stroke. (See Schwartz 10th ed., p. 838.)

7. The treatment of acute embolic mesenteric ischemia is
    A. Observation
    B. Anticoagulation
    C. Thrombolysis
    D. Operative embolectomy

Answer: D

The primary goal of surgical treatment in embolic mesenteric ischemia is to restore arterial perfusion with removal of the embolus from the vessel. The abdomen is explored through a midline incision, which often reveals variable degrees of intestinal ischemia from the mid-jejunum to the ascending or transverse colon. The transverse colon is lifted superiorly, and the small intestine is reflected toward the right upper quadrant. The superior mesenteric artery (SMA) is approached at the root of the small bowel mesentery, usually as it emerges from beneath the pancreas to cross over the junction of the third and fourth portions of the duodenum. Alternatively, the SMA can be approached by incising the retroperitoneum lateral to the fourth portion of the duodenum, which is rotated medially to expose the SMA. Once the proximal SMA is identified and controlled with vascular clamps, a transverse arteriotomy is made to extract the embolus, using standard balloon embolectomy catheters. In the event the embolus has lodged more distally, exposure of the distal SMA may be obtained in the root of the small bowel mesentery by isolating individual jejunal and ileal branches to allow a more comprehensive thromboembolectomy. Following the restoration of SMA flow, an assessment of intestinal viability must be made, and nonviable bowel must be resected. Several methods have been described to evaluate the viability of the intestine, which include intraoperative intravenous fluorescein injection and inspection with a Wood's lamp, and Doppler assessment of antimesenteric intestinal arterial pulsations. A second-look procedure should be considered in many patients and is performed 24 to 48 hours following embolectomy. The goal of the procedure is reassessment of the extent of bowel viability, which may not be obvious immediately following the initial embolectomy. If nonviable intestine is evident in the second-look procedure, additional bowel resections should be performed at that time. (See Schwartz 10th ed., pp. 863–864.)

8. The correct classification for the degree of stenosis in the internal carotid artery of a patient with a luminal diameter of 69% is
   A. Mild
   B. Moderate
   C. Severe
   D. No stenosis

Answer: B

Atherosclerotic plaque formation is complex, beginning with intimal injury, platelet deposition, smooth muscle cell proliferation, and fibroplasia, and leading to subsequent luminal narrowing. With increasing degree of stenosis in the internal carotid artery, flow becomes more turbulent, and the risk of atheroembolization escalates. The severity of stenosis is commonly divided into three categories according to the luminal diameter reduction: mild (<50%), moderate (50–69%), and severe (70–99%). Severe carotid stenosis is a strong predictor for stroke. (See Schwartz 10th ed., p. 838.)

9. The treatment of nonocclusive mesenteric ischemia is
   A. Observation
   B. Catheter infusion of papaverine
   C. Stenting to prevent further spasm
   D. Operative bypass of the SMA

Answer: B

The treatment of nonocclusive mesenteric ischemia is primarily pharmacologic with selective mesenteric arterial catheterization followed by infusion of vasodilatory agents, such as tolazoline or papaverine. Once the diagnosis is made on the mesenteric arteriography (Fig. 23-2), intra-arterial papaverine is given at a dose of 30 to 60 mg/h. This must be coupled with the cessation of other vasoconstricting agents. (See Schwartz 10th ed., Figure 23-42, pp. 863 and 865.)

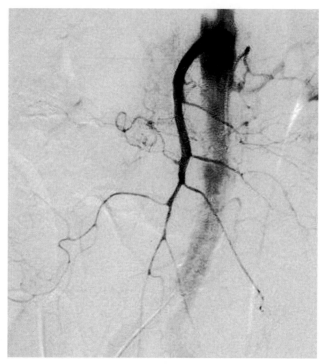

FIG. 23-2. Mesenteric arteriogram showing non-occlusive mesenteric ischemia as evidenced by diffuse spasm of intestinal arcades with poor filling of intramural vessels.

10. Hollenhorst plaque is found within the
    A. Internal carotid artery
    B. Retinal vessels
    C. Peripheral arteries
    D. Renal arteries

Answer: B

Patients who suffer cerebrovascular accidents typically present with three categories of symptoms including ocular symptoms, sensory/motor deficit, and/or higher cortical dysfunction. The common ocular symptoms associated with extracranial carotid artery occlusive disease include amaurosis fugax and presence of Hollenhorst plaques. Amaurosis fugax, commonly referred to as *transient monocular blindness*, is a temporary loss of vision in one eye that patients typically describe as a window shutter coming down or grey shedding of the vision. This partial blindness usually lasts for a few minutes and then resolves. Most of these phenomena (>90%) are due to embolic occlusion of the main artery or the upper or lower divisions. Monocular blindness progressing over a 20-minute period suggests a migrainous etiology. Occasionally, the patient will recall no visual symptoms while the optician notes a yellowish plaque within the retinal vessels, which is also known as *Hollenhorst plaque*. These plaques are frequently derived from cholesterol embolization from the carotid bifurcation and warrant further investigation. (See Schwartz 10th ed., p. 839.)

11. The most accurate diagnostic test with the lowest morbidity in the diagnosis of renal artery stenosis is
    A. Angiography
    B. Computed tomography (CT) scan
    C. MRA
    D. Renal systemic renin index

Answer: C
MRA has the advantage of not requiring iodinated contrast agents to provide vessel opacification (see Fig. 23-1). Gadolinium is used as a contrast agent for MRA studies, and because it is generally not nephrotoxic, it can be used in patients with elevated creatinine. (See Schwartz 10th ed., p. 832.)

12. The risk of a recurrent ipsilateral stroke in patients with severe carotid stenosis is approximately
    A. 20%
    B. 30%
    C. 40%
    D. 50%

Answer: C
Currently, most stroke neurologists prescribe both aspirin and clopidogrel for secondary stroke prevention in patients who have experienced a transient ischemic attack (TIA) or stroke. In patients with symptomatic carotid stenosis, the degree of stenosis appears to be the most important predictor in determining risk for an ipsilateral stroke. The risk of a recurrent ipsilateral stroke in patients with severe carotid stenosis approaches 40%. (See Schwartz 10th ed., p. 841.)

13. Which of the following statements concerning carotid body tumors is true?
    A. Over 50% are hereditary.
    B. Require resection of the underlying carotid artery with reconstruction for cure.
    C. Are associated with catecholamine release.
    D. Are usually benign.

Answer: D
The carotid body originates from the third branchial arch and from neuroectodermal-derived neural crest lineage. The normal carotid body is located in the adventitia or periadventitial tissue at the bifurcation of the common carotid artery (Fig. 23-3). The gland is innervated by the glossopharyngeal nerve. Its blood supply is derived predominantly from the external carotid artery but can also come from the vertebral artery. Carotid body tumor is a rare lesion of the neuroendocrine system. Other glands of neural crest origin are seen in the neck, parapharyngeal spaces, mediastinum, retroperitoneum, and adrenal medulla. Tumors involving these structures have been referred to as *paraganglioma, glomus tumor,* or *chemodectoma*. Approximately 5 to 7% of carotid body tumors are malignant. Although chronic hypoxemia has been invoked as a stimulus for hyperplasia of carotid body, approximately 35% of carotid body tumors are hereditary. The risk of malignancy is greatest in young patients with familial tumors. (See Schwartz 10th ed., Figure 23-27, p. 849.)

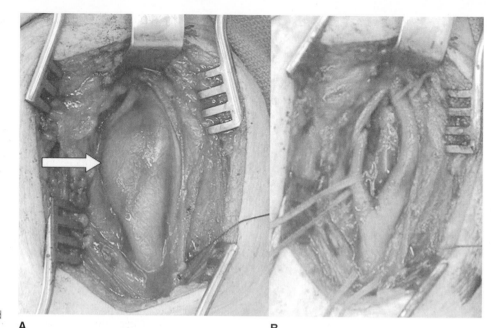

FIG. 23-3A & B. A. Carotid body tumor (arrow) located adjacent to the carotid bulb. **B.** Following periadventitial dissection, the carotid body tumor is removed.

14. The following are major risk factors associated with carotid stenosis disease progression EXCEPT
    A. Diet
    B. Cigarette smoking
    C. Diabetes mellitus
    D. Age

Answer: A

The presence of or progression to a greater than 80% stenosis correlated highly with either the development of a total occlusion of the internal carotid artery or new symptoms. The major risk factors associated with disease progression were cigarette smoking, diabetes mellitus, and age. This study supported the contention that it is prudent to follow a conservative course in the management of asymptomatic patients presenting with a cervical bruit. (See Schwartz 10th ed., p. 842.)

15. Rest pain seen with occlusive peripheral vascular disease in the lower extremity most commonly occurs in
    A. The buttock
    B. The quadriceps
    C. The calf muscles
    D. The metatarsophalangeal joint

Answer: D

Progression of the underlying atherosclerotic process is more likely to occur in patients with diabetes, those who continue to smoke, and those who fail to modify their atherosclerotic risk factors. In comparison, rest pain is constant, and usually occurs in the forefoot across the metatarsophalangeal joint. It is worse at night and requires placing the foot in a dependent position to improve symptoms. (See Schwartz 10th ed., p. 890.)

16. Fibromuscular dysplasia (FMD) is
    A. More common in men than women in the fourth or fifth decade of life.
    B. Commonly present bilaterally in the carotid artery.
    C. Surgical correction is often indicated.
    D. Usually involves short vessels with many branches.

Answer: B

Fibromuscular dysplasia (FMD) usually involves medium-sized arteries that are long and have few branches (Fig. 23-4). Women in the fourth or fifth decade of life are more commonly affected than men. Hormonal effects on the vessel wall are thought to play a role in the pathogenesis of FMD. FMD of the carotid artery is commonly bilateral, and in about 20% of patients, the vertebral artery is also involved. An intracranial saccular aneurysm of the carotid siphon or middle cerebral artery can be identified in up to 50% of the patients with FMD. Four histologic types of FMD have been described in the literature. The most common type is medial fibroplasia, which may present as a focal stenosis or multiple lesions with intervening aneurysmal outpouchings. The disease involves the media with the smooth muscle being replaced by fibrous connective tissue. Commonly, mural dilations and microaneurysms can be seen with this type of FMD. FMD should be suspected when an increased velocity is detected across a stenotic segment without associated atherosclerotic changes on carotid duplex ultrasound. Antiplatelet medication is the generally accepted therapy for asymptomatic lesions. Endovascular treatment is recommended for patients with documented lateralizing symptoms. Surgical correction is rarely indicated. (See Schwartz 10th ed., Figure 23-24, pp. 847–848.)

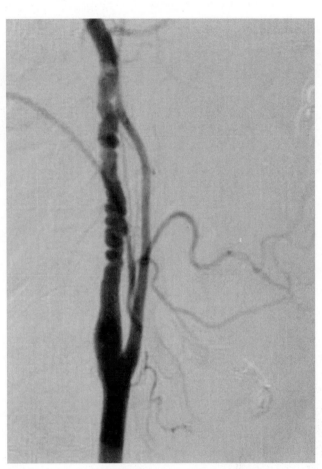

FIG. 23-4. A carotid fibromuscular dysplasia with typical characteristics of multiple stenoses with intervening aneurysmal outpouching dilatations. The disease involves the media with the smooth muscle being replaced by fibrous connective tissue.

17. The best initial treatment for a groin pseudoaneurysm after angiography is
    A. Surgical repair
    B. Ultrasound-guided compression
    C. Ultrasound-guided injection of thrombin
    D. Observation

Answer: C
Percutaneous catheter aspiration should be the initial treatment for calf vessel embolization, but, for larger emboli, such as those that lodge in the profunda femoris or common femoral arteries, surgical embolectomy may be required because the embolic material contains atherosclerotic plaque, which is not amenable to transcatheter aspiration or catheter-directed thrombolysis. The incidence of pseudoaneurysm formation at the puncture site is 0.5%. The treatment of choice for pseudoaneurysms larger than 2 cm in diameter is percutaneous thrombin injection under ultrasound guidance. Arterial rupture may complicate the procedure in 0.3% of cases.

18. The primary cause of renal artery occlusive lesions is
    A. Fibromuscular dysplasia
    B. Atherosclerosis
    C. Renal artery aneurysm
    D. Takayasu arteritis

Tamponade of the ruptured artery with an occlusion balloon should be performed, and a covered stent should be placed. In case of failure, surgical treatment is required. (See Schwartz 10th ed., p. 880.)

Answer: B

Approximately 80% of all renal artery occlusive lesions are caused by atherosclerosis, which typically involves a short segment of the renal artery ostia and represents spillover disease from a severely atheromatous aorta (Fig. 23-5). Atherosclerotic lesions are bilateral in two-thirds of patients. Individuals with this disease commonly present during the sixth decade of life. Men are affected twice as frequently as women. Atherosclerotic lesions in other territories such as the coronary, mesenteric, cerebrovascular, and peripheral arterial circulation are common. When a unilateral lesion is present, the disease process equally affects the right and left renal arteries. The second most common cause of renal artery stenosis is FMD, which accounts for 20% of cases and is most frequently encountered in young, often multiparous women. FMD of the renal artery represents a heterogeneous group of lesions that can produce histopathologic changes in the intima, media, or adventitia. The most common variety consists of medial fibroplasia, in which thickened fibromuscular ridges alternate with attenuated media producing the classic angiographic "string of beads" appearance. The cause of medial fibroplasia remains unclear. Most common theories involve a modification of arterial smooth muscle cells in response to estrogenic stimuli during the reproductive years, unusual traction forces on affected vessels, and mural ischemia from impairment of vasa vasorum blood flow. Fibromuscular hyperplasia usually affects the distal two thirds of the main renal artery, and the right renal artery is affected more frequently than the left. Other less common causes of renal artery stenosis include renal artery aneurysm (compressing the adjacent normal renal artery), arteriovenous malformations, neurofibromatosis, renal artery dissections, renal artery trauma, Takayasu arteritis, and renal arteriovenous fistula. (See Schwartz 10th ed., Figure 23-43, pp. 866–867.)

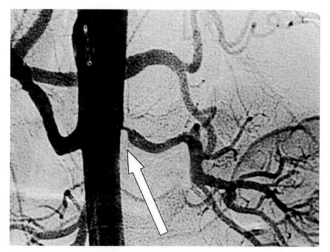

FIG. 23-5. Occlusive disease of the renal artery typically involves the renal ostium (arrow), as a spill over plaque extension from aortic atherosclerosis.

19. Carotid coiling
    A. Is associated with loss of elasticity
    B. Is more common in men than women
    C. Are most often acquired in both children and adults
    D. Are most likely due to embolic episodes

Answer: A

A carotid coil consists of an excessive elongation of the internal carotid artery producing tortuosity of the vessel (Fig. 23-6). Embryologically, the carotid artery is derived from the third aortic arch and dorsal aortic root and is uncoiled as the heart and great vessels descend into the mediastinum. In children, carotid coils appear to be congenital in origin. In contrast, elongation and kinking of the carotid artery in adults are associated with the loss of elasticity and an abrupt angulation of the vessel. Kinking is more common in women than men. Cerebral ischemic symptoms caused by kinks of the carotid artery are similar to those from atherosclerotic carotid lesions but are more likely due to cerebral hypoperfusion than embolic episodes. Classically, sudden head rotation, flexion, or extension can accentuate the kink and provoke ischemic symptoms. Most carotid kinks and coils are found incidentally on carotid duplex scan. However, interpretation of the Doppler frequency shifts and spectral analysis in tortuous carotid arteries can be difficult because of the uncertain angle of insonation. Cerebral angiography, with multiple views taken in neck flexion, extension, and rotation, is useful in the determination of the clinical significance of kinks and coils. (See Schwartz 10th ed., Figure 23-23, p. 847.)

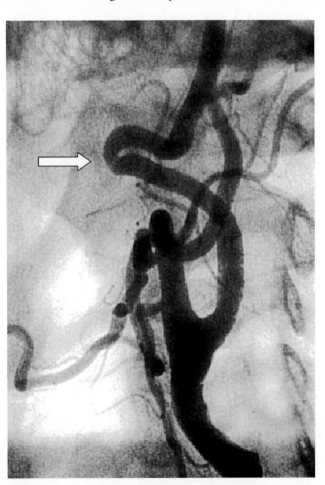

FIG. 23-6. Excessive elongation of the carotid artery can result in carotid kinking (arrow), which can compromise cerebral blood flow and lead to cerebral ischemia.

20. Complications of endovascular treatment for mesenteric ischemia
   A. Often become life threatening.
   B. Can include distal embolization resulting in acute intestinal ischemia.
   C. Can include access-site thrombosis.
   D. Dissections never occur.

Answer: C

Complications are not common and rarely become life threatening. These include access-site thrombosis, hematomas, and infection. Dissection can occur during percutaneous transluminal angioplasty (PTA) and is managed with placement of a stent. Balloon-mounted stents are preferred over the self-expanding ones because of the higher radial force and the more precise placement. Distal embolization has also been reported, but it never resulted in acute intestinal ischemia, likely due to the rich network of collaterals already developed. (See Schwartz 10th ed., p. 865.)

21. The most common location for the development of atherosclerotic disease is
   A. The renal artery.
   B. The coronary arteries.
   C. The abdominal aorta.
   D. The arteries in the circle of Willis.

Answer: A

Obstructive lesions of the renal artery can produce hypertension, resulting in a condition known as *renovascular hypertension,* which is the most common form of hypertension amenable to therapeutic intervention, and affects 5 to 10% of all hypertensive patients in the United States. Patients with renovascular hypertension are at an increased risk for irreversible end-organ dysfunction, including permanent kidney damage, if inadequate pharmacologic therapies are used to control the blood pressure. The majority of patients with renal artery obstructive disease have vascular lesions of either atherosclerotic disease or fibrodysplasia involving the renal arteries. The proximal portion of the renal artery represents the most common location for the development of atherosclerotic disease. It is well established that renal artery intervention, either by surgical or endovascular revascularization, provides an effective treatment for controlling renovascular hypertension as well as preserving renal function. The decision for intervention is complex and needs to consider a variety of anatomic, physiologic, and clinical features, unique for the individual patient. (See Schwartz 10th ed., p. 866.)

22. Angiograph indications for renal artery revascularization include all of the following EXCEPT
   A. Documented renal artery stenosis
   B. FMD lesion
   C. Affected/unaffected kidney renin ration >1.5 to 1
   D. Pressure gradient >10 mm Hg

Answer: D

See Table 23-1. (See Schwartz 10th ed., Table 23-12, p. 869.)

TABLE 23-1	Indications for renal artery revascularization

Angiography Criteria
- Documented renal artery stenosis (>70% diameter reduction)
- Fibromuscular dysplasia lesion
- Pressure gradient >20 mmHg
- Affected/unaffected kidney renin ratio >1.5 to 1

Clinical Criteria
- Refractory or rapidly progressive hypertension
- Hypertension associated with flash pulmonary edema without coronary artery disease
- Rapidly progressive deterioration in renal function
- Intolerance to antihypertensive medications
- Chronic renal insufficiency related to bilateral renal artery occlusive disease or stenosis to a solitary functioning kidney
- Dialysis-dependent renal failure in a patient with renal artery stenosis but without another definite cause of endstage renal disease
- Recurrent congestive heart failure or flash pulmonary edema not attributable to active coronary ischemia

23. Aortoiliac disease represented by diffuse aortoiliac disease above the iliac artery is classified as
    A. Type 1
    B. Type II
    C. Type III
    D. Type IV

Answer: B
See Figure 23-7. (See Schwartz 10th ed., Figure 23-50, p. 873.)

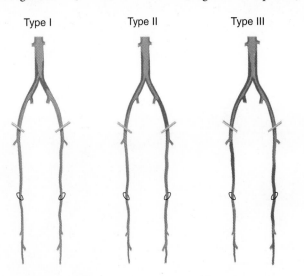

FIG. 23-7. Aortoiliac disease can be classified into three types. Type I represents focal disease affecting the distal aorta and proximal common iliac artery. Type II represents diffuse aortoiliac disease above the inguinal ligament. Type III represents multi-segment occlusive diseases involving aortoiliac and infra-inguinal arterial vessels.

24. The treatment of choice for type B iliac lesions is
    A. Observation
    B. Endovascular therapy
    C. Surgery
    D. Intravenous (IV) antibiotics

Answer: B
The most commonly used classification system of iliac lesions has been set forth by the TransAtlantic Inter-Society Consensus (TASC) group with recommended treatment options. This lesion classification categorizes the extent of atherosclerosis and has suggested a therapeutic approach based on this classification (Table 23-2 and Fig. 23-8). According to this consensus document, endovascular therapy is the treatment of choice for type A lesions, and surgery is the treatment of choice for type D lesions. Endovascular treatment is the preferred treatment for type B lesions, and surgery is the preferred treatment for good-risk patients with type C lesions. In comparison to the 2000 TASC document, the commission has not only made allowances for treatment of more extensive lesions, but also takes into account the continuing evolution of endovascular technology and the skills of individual interventionalists when stating the patient's comorbidities, fully informed patient preference, and the local operator's long-term success rates must be considered when making treatment decisions for type B and type C lesions. (See Schwartz 10th ed., Figure 23-55 and Table 23-14, p. 875.)

TABLE 23-2	TASC classification of aortoiliac occlusive lesions

Type A lesions
- Unilateral or bilateral stenoses of CIA
- Unilateral or bilateral single short (≤3 cm) stenosis of EIA

Type B lesions
- Short (≤3 cm) stenosis of infrarenal aorta
- Unilateral CIA occlusion
- Single or multiple stenosis totaling 3–10 cm involving the EIA not extending into the CFA
- Unilateral EIA occlusion not involving the origins of internal iliac artery or CFA

Type C lesions
- Bilateral CIA occlusions
- Bilateral EIA stenoses 3–10 cm long not extending into the CFA
- Unilateral EIA stenosis extending into the CFA
- Unilateral EIA occlusion that involves the origins of internal iliac artery and/or CFA
- Heavily calcified unilateral EIA occlusion with or without involvement of origins of internal iliac artery and/or CFA

Type D lesions
- Infrarenal aortoiliac occlusion
- Diffuse disease involving the aorta and both iliac arteries requiring treatment
- Diffuse multiple stenoses involving the unilateral CIA, EIA, and CFA
- Unilateral occlusions of both CIA and EIA
- Bilateral occlusions of EIA
- Iliac stenoses in patients with AAA requiring treatment and not amenable to endograft placement or other lesions requiring open aortic or iliac surgery

AAA = abdominal aortic aneurysm; CFA = common femoral artery; CIA = common iliac artery; EIA = external iliac artery.

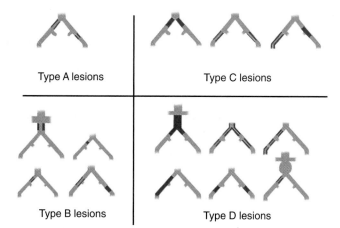

FIG. 23-8. Schematic depiction of TASC classification of aortoiliac occlusive lesions.

25. Carotid bifurcation occlusive disease resulting in stroke is usually caused by
    A. Atheroemboli
    B. Thrombosis
    C. Rupture
    D. Dissection

Answer: A

Stroke due to carotid bifurcation occlusive disease is usually caused by atheroemboli (Fig. 23-9). The carotid bifurcation is an area of low flow velocity and low shear stress. As the blood circulates through the carotid bifurcation, there is separation of flow into the low-resistance internal carotid artery and the high-resistance external carotid artery. (See Schwartz 10th ed., Figure 23-13, p. 838.)

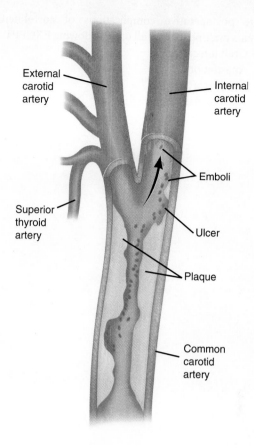

FIG. 23-9. Stroke due to carotid bifurcation occlusive disease is usually caused by atheroemboli arising from the internal carotid artery which provides the majority of blood flow to the cerebral hemisphere. With increasing degree of stenosis in the carotid artery, flow becomes more turbulent, and the risk of atheroembolization escalates.

26. Crescendo TIAs refers to a syndrome comprising repeated TIAs within
   A. A short period of time that is characterized by complete neurologic recovery in between.
   B. A lengthy time period that is characterized by complete neurologic recovery in between.
   C. A short period of time that is characterized by a partial neurologic recovery in between.
   D. A lengthy time period that is characterized by a partial neurologic recovery in between.

Answer: A
TIA is a focal loss of neurologic function, lasting for less than 24 hours. Crescendo TIAs refer to a syndrome comprising repeated TIAs within a short period of time that is characterized by complete neurologic recovery in between. At a minimum, the term should probably be reserved for those with either daily events or multiple resolving attacks within 24 hours. Hemodynamic TIAs represent focal cerebral events that are aggravated by exercise or hemodynamic stress and typically occur after short bursts of physical activity, postprandially, or after getting out of a hot bath. It is implied that these are due to severe extracranial disease and poor intracranial collateral recruitment. Reversible ischemic neurologic deficits refer to ischemic focal neurologic symptoms lasting longer than 24 hours but resolving within 3 weeks. When a neurologic deficit lasts longer than 3 weeks, it is considered a completed stroke. Stroke in evolution refers to progressive worsening of the neurologic deficit, either linearly over a 24-hour period or interspersed with transient periods of stabilization and/or partial clinical improvement. (See Schwartz 10th ed., pp. 838–839.)

27. Late postoperative complications of aortobifemoral bypass grafting include all of the following EXCEPT
    A. Graft infection
    B. Anastomotic fistula
    C. Paraplegia
    D. Aortourinary fistula

Answer: C

See Table 23-3. (See Schwartz 10th ed., Table 23-15, p. 878.)

TABLE 23-3	Perioperative complications of aortobifemoral bypass grafting

Medical Complications
- Perioperative myocardial infarction
- Respiratory failure
- Ischemia-induced renal failure
- Bleeding from intravenous heparinization
- Stroke

Procedure-Related Complications
Early
- Declamping shock
- Graft thrombosis
- Retroperitoneal bleeding
- Groin hematoma
- Bowel ischemia/infarction
- Peripheral embolization
- Erectile dysfunction
- Lymphatic leak
- Chylous ascites
- Paraplegia
Late
- Graft infection
- Anastomotic pseudoaneurysm
- Aortoenteric fistula
- Aortourinary fistula
- Graft thrombosis

28. The best diagnostic imaging modality for identifying lower extremity occlusive disease is
    A. MRA
    B. CT angiography
    C. Ultrasound
    D. Contrast angiography

Answer: D

Contrast angiography remains the gold standard imaging study. Using contrast angiography, interventionists can locate and size the anatomic significant lesions and measure the pressure gradient across the lesion, as well as plan for potential intervention. Angiography is, however, semi-invasive and should be confined to patients for whom surgical or percutaneous intervention is contemplated. Patients with borderline renal function may need to have alternate contrast agents, such as gadolinium or carbon dioxide, to avoid contrast-induced nephrotoxicity. (See Schwartz 10th ed., p. 882.)

29. According to the Fontaine classification system for lower extremity occlusive disease
    A. Patients with tissue loss are classified as stage II.
    B. Patients with rest pain are classified as stage III.
    C. Asymptomatic patients are classified as stage I.
    D. Patients with claudication are classified as stage IV.

Answer: B

The Fontaine classification uses four stages: Fontaine I is the stage when patients are asymptomatic; Fontaine II is when they have mild (IIa) or severe (IIb) claudication; Fontaine III is when they have ischemic rest pain; and Fontaine IV is when patients suffer tissue loss, such as ulceration or gangrene (Table 23-4). (See Schwartz 10th ed., Table 23-17, pp. 883–884.)

TABLE 23-4 Differential diagnosis of intermittent claudication

Condition	Location of pain or Discomfort	Characteristic Discomfort	Onset Relative to Exercise	Effect of Rest	Effect of Body Position	Other Characteristics
Intermittent claudication (calf)	Calf muscles	Cramping pain	After same degree of exercise	Quickly relieved	None	Reproducible
Chronic compartment syndrome	Calf muscles	Tight, bursting pain	After much exercise (e.g., jogging)	Subsides very slowly	Relief speeded by elevation	Typically heavy-muscled athletes
Venous claudication	Entire leg, but usually worse in thigh and groin	Tight, bursting pain	After walking	Subsides slowly	Relief speeded by elevation	History of iliofemoral deep venous thrombosis, signs of venous congestion, edema
Nerve root compression (e.g., herniated disk)	Radiates down leg, usually posteriorly	Sharp lancinating pain	Soon, if not immediately after onset	Not quickly relieved (also often present at rest)	Relief may be aided by adjusting back position	History of back problems
Symptomatic Baker's cyst	Behind knee, down calf	Swelling, soreness, tenderness	With exercise	Present at rest	None	Not intermittent
Intermittent claudication (hip, thigh, buttock)	Hip, thigh, buttocks	Aching discomfort, weakness	After same degree of exercise	Quickly relieved	None	Reproducible
Hip arthritis	Hip, thigh, buttocks	Aching discomfort	After variable degree of exercise	Not quickly relieved (and may be present at rest)	More comfortable sitting, weight taken off legs	Variable, may relate to activity level, weather changes
Spinal cord compression	Hip, thigh, buttocks (follows dermatome)	Weakness more than pain	After walking or standing for same length of time	Relieved by stopping only if position changed	Relief by lumbar spine flexion (sitting or stooping forward) pressure	Frequent history of back problems, provoked by increased intra-abdominal pressure
Intermittent claudication (foot)	Foot, arch	Severe deep pain and numbness	After same degree of exercise	Quickly relieved	None	Reproducible
Arthritic, inflammatory process	Foot, arch	Aching pain	After variable degree of exercise	Not quickly relieved (and may be present at rest)	May be relieved by not bearing weight	Variable, may relate to activity level

30. The most common source of distal emboli is
    A. The heart
    B. Atherosclerotic lesions
    C. Dilated cardiomyopathy
    D. Diseased valves

Answer: A

The heart is the most common source of distal emboli, which accounts for more than 90% of peripheral arterial embolic events. Atrial fibrillation is the most common source. Sudden cardioversion results in the dilated noncontractile atrial appendage regaining contractile activity, which can dislodge the contained thrombus. Other cardiac sources include mural thrombus overlying a myocardial infarction or thrombus forming within a dilated left ventricular aneurysm. Mural thrombi can also develop within a ventricle dilated by cardiomyopathy. Emboli that arise from a ventricular aneurysm or from a dilated cardiomyopathy can be very large and can lodge at the aortic bifurcation (saddle embolus), thus rendering both legs ischemic. Diseased valves are another source of distal embolization. Historically, this occurred as a result of rheumatic heart disease. Currently, subacute endocarditis and acute bacterial endocarditis are the more common causes. Infected emboli can seed the recipient vessel wall, creating mycotic aneurysms. (See Schwartz 10th ed., p. 885.)

31. An absolute contraindication to thrombolytic therapy is
    A. Pregnancy
    B. Intracranial tumor
    C. Intracranial trauma within the past 3 months
    D. Cardiopulmonary resuscitation within the past 10 days

Answer: C

Patients with small-vessel occlusion are poor candidates for surgery because they lack distal target vessels to use for bypass. These patients should be offered a trial of thrombolysis, unless they have contraindications to thrombolysis or their ischemia is so severe that the time needed to achieve adequate lysis is considered too long. The major contraindications of thrombolysis are recent stroke, intracranial primary malignancy, brain metastases, or intracranial surgical intervention. Relative contraindications for performance of thrombolysis include renal insufficiency, allergy to contrast material, cardiac thrombus, diabetic retinopathy, coagulopathy, and recent arterial puncture or surgery (Table 23-5). (See Schwartz 10th ed., Table 23-21, p. 887.)

TABLE 23-5	Contraindications to thrombolytic therapy

Absolute Contraindications
Established cerebrovascular events (including transient ischemic attack) within last 2 months
Active bleeding diathesis
Recent (<10 days) gastrointestinal bleeding
Neurosurgery (intracranial or spinal) within last 3 months
Intracranial trauma within last 3 months
Intracranial malignancy or metastasis

Relative Major Contraindications
Cardiopulmonary resuscitation within last 10 days
Major nonvascular surgery or trauma within last 10 days
Uncontrolled hypertension (>180 mmHg systolic or >110 mmHg diastolic)
Puncture of noncompressible vessel
Intracranial tumor
Recent eye surgery

Minor Contraindications
Hepatic failure, particularly with coagulopathy
Bacterial endocarditis
Pregnancy
Diabetic hemorrhagic retinopathy

32. The term chronic limb ischemia (CLI) is reserved for patients with objectively proven arterial occlusive disease and symptoms lasting for more than
    A. 1 week
    B. 2 weeks
    C. 3 weeks
    D. 4 weeks

Answer: B

The term chronic limb ischemia (CLI) is reserved for patients with objectively proven arterial occlusive disease and symptoms lasting for more than 2 weeks. Symptoms include rest pain and tissue loss, such as ulceration or gangrene (Table 23-6). The diagnosis should be corroborated with noninvasive diagnostic tests, such as the ABI, toe pressures, and transcutaneous oxygen measurements. Ischemic rest pain most commonly occurs below an ankle pressure of 50 mm Hg or a toe pressure less than 30 mm Hg.2 Ulcers are not always of an ischemic etiology (Table 23-7). (See Schwartz 10th ed., Tables 23-24 and 23-25, pp. 889–890.)

TABLE 23-6	Clinical categories of chronic limb ischemia		
Grade	**Category**	**Clinical Description**	**Objective Criteria**
0	0	Asymptomatic—no hemodynamically significant occlusive disease	Normal treadmill or reactive hyperemia test
	1	Mild claudication	Able to complete treadmill exercise[a]; AP after exercise >50 mmHg but at least 20 mmHg lower than resting value
I	2	Moderate claudication	Between categories 1 and 3
	3	Severe claudication	Cannot complete standard treadmill exercise[a] *and* AP after exercise <50 mmHg
II[b]	4	Ischemic rest pain	Resting AP <40 mmHg, flat or barely pulsatile ankle or metatarsal PVR; TP <30 mmHg
III[b]	5	Minor tissue loss—nonhealing ulcer, focal gangrene with diffuse pedal ischemia	Resting AP <60 mmHg, ankle or metatarsal PVR flat or barely pulsatile; TP <40 mmHg
	6	Major tissue loss—extending above TM level, functional foot no longer salvageable	Same as category 5

[a]Five minutes at 2 miles per hour on a 12% incline of treadmill exercise.
[b]Grades II and III, categories 4, 5, and 6, are encompassed by the term chronic *critical* ischemia.
AP = ankle pressure; PVR = pulse volume recording; TM = transmetatarsal; TP = toe pressure.

TABLE 23-7	Symptoms and signs of neuropathic ulcer versus ischemic ulcer
Neuropathic Ulcer	**Ischemic Ulcer**
Painless	Painful
Normal pulses	Absent pulses
Regular margins, typically punched-out appearance	Irregular margin
Often located on plantar surface of foot	Commonly located on toes, glabrous margins
Presence of calluses	Calluses absent or infrequent
Loss of sensation, reflexes, and vibration	Variable sensory findings
Increased in blood flow (arteriovenous shunting)	Decreased in blood flow
Dilated veins	Collapsed veins
Dry, warm foot	Cold foot
Bony deformities	No bony deformities
Red or hyperemic in appearance	Pale and cyanotic in appearance

33. The percentage of patients with vein grafts that will develop intrinsic stenosis within the first 18 months following implantation is
    A. 5%
    B. 10%
    C. 15%
    D. 20%

Answer: C

Fifteen percent of vein grafts will develop intrinsic stenoses within the first 18 months following implantation. Consequently, patients with vein grafts were entered into duplex surveillance protocols (scans every 3 months) to detect elevated (>300 cm/s) or abnormally low (<45 cm/s) graft velocities early. Stenoses greater than 50%, especially if associated with changes in ABI, should be repaired to prevent graft thrombosis. Repair usually entails patch angioplasty or short-segment venous interposition, but PTA/stenting is an option for short, focal lesions. Grafts with stenoses that are identified and repaired prior to thrombosis have assisted primary patency identical to primary patency, whereas a thrombosed autogenous bypass has limited longevity resulting from ischemic injury to the vein wall. (See Schwartz 10th ed., p. 898.)

34. The following are true of cryopreserved grafts EXCEPT
    A. Prone to early thrombosis.
    B. Less expensive than prosthetic grafts.
    C. More prone to failure than prosthetic grafts.
    D. Prone to aneurysmal degeneration.

Answer: B

Cryopreserved grafts are usually cadaveric arteries or veins that have been subjected to rate controlled freezing with dimethyl sulfoxide (DMSO) and other cryopreservants. Cryopreserved vein grafts are more expensive than prosthetic grafts and are more prone to failure. The endothelial lining is lost as part of the freezing process, making these grafts prone to early thrombosis. Cryopreserved grafts are also prone to aneurysmal degeneration. Despite the fact that these grafts have not performed as well as prosthetic bypasses and autogenous vein bypasses in clinical practice, they can still play a role when revascularization is required following removal of infected prosthetic bypass grafts, especially when the autogenous vein is unavailable to create a new bypass through clean tissue planes. (See Schwartz 10th ed., p. 899.)

35. When lower extremity occlusive disease extends to involve the popliteal artery or tibial vessels, the appropriate outflow vessels for performing bypass in order of descending preference are
    A. Below-knee popliteal artery, posterior tibial artery, anterior tibial artery, above-knee popliteal artery
    B. Above-knee popliteal artery, anterior tibial artery, posterior tibial artery, below-knee popliteal artery
    C. Anterior tibial artery, posterior tibial artery, peroneal artery, below-knee popliteal artery, above-knee popliteal artery
    D. Above-knee popliteal artery, below-knee popliteal artery, posterior tibial artery, anterior tibial artery, and peroneal artery

Answer: D

When the disease extends to involve the popliteal artery or the tibial vessels, the surgeon must select an appropriate outflow vessel to perform a bypass. Suitable outflow vessels are defined as uninterrupted flow channels beyond the anastomosis into the foot. Listed in order of descending preference, they are as follows: above-knee popliteal artery, below-knee popliteal artery, posterior tibial artery, anterior tibial artery, and peroneal artery. In patients with diabetes, it is frequently the peroneal artery that is spared. Although it has no direct flow into the foot, collateralization to the posterior tibial and anterior tibial arteries makes it an appropriate outflow vessel. (See Schwartz 10th ed., p. 898.)

36. Giant cell arteritis
    A. Tends to occur in white men older than 50 years
    B. Has low remission rates
    C. Is associated with ischemic optic neuritis in the majority of patients
    D. Is diagnosed by temporal artery biopsy

Answer: D

Giant cell arteritis is also known as *temporal arteritis*, which is a systemic chronic inflammatory vascular disease with many characteristics similar to those of Takayasu disease. The histologic and pathologic changes and laboratory findings are similar. Patients tend to be white women older than 50 years, with a high incidence in Scandinavia and women of Northern European descent. Genetic factors may play a role in disease pathogenesis, with a human leukocyte antigen (HLA) variant having been identified. Differences exist between Takayasu and giant cell arteritis in terms of presentation, disease location, and therapeutic efficacy. The inflammatory process typically involves the aorta and its extracranial branches, of which the superficial temporal artery is specifically affected. The clinical syndrome begins with a prodromal phase of constitutional symptoms, including headache, fever, malaise, and myalgias. The patients may be initially diagnosed with coexisting polymyalgia rheumatica; an HLA-related association may exist between the two diseases. As a result of vascular narrowing and end-organ ischemia, complications may occur such as visual alterations, including blindness and mural weakness, resulting in acute aortic dissection that may be devastating.

Ischemic optic neuritis resulting in partial or complete blindness occurs in up to 40% of patients and is considered a medical emergency. Cerebral symptoms occur when the disease process extends to the carotid arteries. Jaw claudication and temporal artery tenderness may be experienced. Aortic lesions are usually asymptomatic until later stages and consist of thoracic aneurysms and aortic dissections.

The diagnostic gold standard is a temporal artery biopsy, which will show the classic histologic findings of multinucleated giant cells with a dense perivascular inflammatory infiltrate. Treatment regimens are centered on corticosteroids, and giant cell arteritis tends to rapidly respond. Remission rates are high, and treatment tends to have a beneficial and preventative effect on the development of subsequent vascular complications. (See Schwartz 10th ed., p. 901.)

37. The disorder most likely involved in systemic small vessel vasculitis would be
    A. Kawasaki disease
    B. Giant cell arteritis
    C. Hypersensitivity angitis
    D. Buerger disease

Answer: C
See Table 23-8. (See Schwartz 10th ed., Table 23-28, p. 903.)

TABLE 23-8	Classification of vasculitis based on vessel involvement
Large-Vessel Vasculitis	
Takayasu's arteritis	
Giant cell arteritis	
Behçet's disease	
Medium-Vessel Vasculitis	
Polyarteritis nodosa	
Kawasaki's disease	
Buerger's disease	
Small-Vessel Vasculitis	
Hypersensitivity angiitis	

38. The following is true regarding polyarteritis nodosa (PAN) EXCEPT
    A. Is predominantly treated with steroid and cytotoxic agent therapy.
    B. Predominantly affects women over men by a 2:1 ratio.
    C. Presenting symptoms include low-grade fever, malaise, and myalgias.
    D. May be sufficiently diagnosed by skin biopsy.

Answer: B
Polyarteritis nodosa (PAN) is another systemic inflammatory disease process, which is characterized by a necrotizing inflammation of medium-sized or small arteries that spares the smallest blood vessels (ie, arterioles and capillaries). This disease predominantly affects men over women by a 2:1 ratio. PAN develops subacutely, with constitutional symptoms that last for weeks to months. Intermittent, low-grade fevers, malaise, weight loss, and myalgias are common presenting symptoms. As medium-sized vessels lie within the deep dermis, cutaneous manifestations occur in the form of livedo reticularis, nodules, ulcerations, and digital ischemia. Skin biopsies of these lesions may be sufficient for diagnosis. Inflammation may be seen histologically, with pleomorphic cellular infiltrates and segmental transmural necrosis leading to aneurysm formation. Neuritis from nerve infarction occurs in 60% of patients, and gastrointestinal complications occur in

up to 50%. Additionally, renal involvement is found in 40% and manifests as microaneurysms within the kidney or segmental infarctions. Cardiac disease is a rare finding except at autopsy, where thickened, diseased coronary arteries may be seen, as well as patchy myocardial necrosis. Patients may succumb to renal failure, intestinal hemorrhage, or perforation. End-organ ischemia from vascular occlusion or aneurysm rupture can be disastrous complications with high mortality rates. The mainstay of treatment is steroid and cytotoxic agent therapy. Up to 50% of patients with active PAN will experience remission with high dosing. (See Schwartz 10th ed., p. 903.)

CHAPTER 24

Venous and Lymphatic Disease

1. All of the following regarding venous anatomy is true EXCEPT
   A. Veins are thin-walled, collapsible, and highly distensible to a diameter several times greater than that in the supine position.
   B. The venous intima is composed of a nonthrombogenic endothelium that produces endothelium-derived relaxing factors such as nitric oxide and prostacyclin.
   C. Venous valves close in response to caudal-to-cephalad blood flow at a velocity of at least 30 cm/s^2.
   D. The inferior vena cava (IVC), common iliac veins, portal venous system, and cranial sinuses are valveless.

Answer: C

Veins are thin-walled, highly distensible, and collapsible. Their structure specifically supports the primary functions of veins to transport blood toward the heart and serve as a reservoir to prevent intravascular volume overload.

The venous intima is composed of a nonthrombogenic endothelium with an underlying basement membrane and an elastic lamina. The endothelium produces endothelium-derived relaxing factors such as nitric oxide and prostacyclin, which help maintain a nonthrombogenic surface through inhibition of platelet aggregation and promotion of platelet disaggregation.

Circumferential rings of elastic tissue and smooth muscle located in the media of the vein allow for changes in vein caliber with minimal changes in venous pressure. The adventitia is most prominent in large veins and consists of collagen, elastic fibers, and fibroblasts. When a vein is maximally distended, its diameter may be several times greater than that in the supine position.

In the axial veins, unidirectional blood flow is achieved with multiple venous valves. The inferior vena cava (IVC), common iliac veins, portal venous system, and cranial sinuses are valveless. In the axial veins, valves are more numerous distally in the extremities than proximally. Each valve consists of two thin cusps of a fine connective tissue skeleton covered by endothelium. Venous valves close in response to cephalad-to-caudal blood flow at a velocity of at least 30 cm/s^2. (See Schwartz 10th ed., p. 915.)

2. Chronic venous insufficiency (CVI) is characterized by all of the following EXCEPT
   A. Incompetence of venous valves, venous obstruction
   B. Preserved microcirculatory and cutaneous lymphatic anatomy
   C. Eczema and dermatitis
   D. Lipodermatosclerosis

Answer: B

Chronic venous insufficiency (CVI) may lead to characteristic changes in the skin and subcutaneous tissues in the affected limb. CVI results from incompetence of venous valves, venous obstruction, or both. Most CVI involves venous reflux, and severe CVI often reflects a combination of reflux and venous obstruction. It is important to remember that although CVI originates with abnormalities of the veins, the target organ of CVI is the skin, and the underlying physiologic and biochemical mechanisms leading to the cutaneous abnormalities associated with CVI are poorly understood. A typical leg affected by CVI will be edematous, with edema increasing over the course of the day. The leg may also be indurated and pigmented with eczema and dermatitis. These changes are associated with excessive proteinaceous capillary exudate and deposition of a pericapillary fibrin cuff that may limit nutritional exchange. In addition, an increase in white blood cell (WBC) trapping within the skin microcirculation in CVI patients may lead to microvascular congestion and thrombosis. Subsequently, WBCs may migrate into the interstitium and release necrotizing lysosomal enzymes, potentially leading to tissue destruction and eventual ulceration.

Fibrosis can eventually develop from impaired nutrition, chronic inflammation, and fat necrosis (lipodermatosclerosis). Hemosiderin deposition due to the extravasation of red cells and subsequent lysis in the skin contributes to the characteristic pigmentation of chronic venous disease (Fig. 24-1). Ulceration can develop with longstanding venous hypertension and is associated with alterations in microcirculatory and cutaneous lymphatic anatomy and function. The most common location of venous ulceration is approximately 3 cm proximal to the medial malleolus (Fig. 24-2). (See Schwartz 10th ed., Figures 24-2 and 24-3, p. 917.)

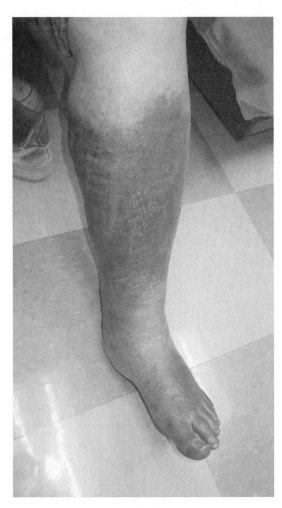

FIG. 24-1. Characteristic hyperpigmentation of chronic venous insufficiency.

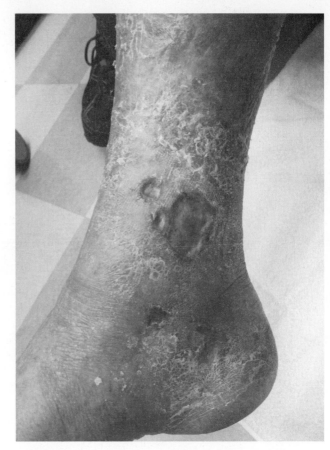

FIG. 24-2. Venous ulceration located proximal to the medial malleolus.

3. Venous thromboembolism (VTE) is associated with all of the following EXCEPT
   A. Increased morbidity and mortality
   B. Pulmonary hypertension
   C. Postthrombotic syndrome
   D. No change in future risk of venous thromboembolism

Answer: D

The incidence of venous thromboembolism (VTE) is approximately 100 per 100,000 people per year in the general population, with 20% of the diagnoses made within 3 months of a surgical procedure. Of the symptomatic patients, one-third will present with pulmonary embolism (PE) and two-thirds with deep vein thrombosis (DVT). The estimated number of cases of VTE may well be over 600,000 per year in the United States, making it a major U.S. health problem. Furthermore, death occurs in 6% of DVT and 12% of PE cases within 1 month of diagnosis. Not only does VTE pose a veritable threat to life, but it also places patients at higher risk for recurrence and post-VTE sequelae such as pulmonary hypertension and postthrombotic syndrome, with 4% and up to 30% incidence, respectively. (See Schwartz 10th ed., p. 918.)

4. Virchow triad is characterized by:
   A. Stasis
   B. Endothelial damage
   C. Hypercoagulability
   D. All of the above

Answer: D

Three conditions, first described by Rudolf Virchow in 1862, contribute to VTE formation: stasis of blood flow, endothelial damage, and hypercoagulability. Of these risk factors, relative hypercoagulability appears most important in most cases of *spontaneous* VTE, or so-called *idiopathic VTE*, whereas stasis and endothelial damage likely play a greater role in *secondary* VTE, or so-called *provoked VTE*, occurring in association with transient risk factors such as immobilization, surgical procedures, and trauma. (See Schwartz 10th ed., p. 918.)

5. Risk factors for inherited VTE include all of the following EXCEPT
   A. Dysfibrinogenemia
   B. Factor V Leiden
   C. Protein C deficiency
   D. von Willebrand disease

Answer: D
Von Willebrand Disease is the most common genetic bleeding disorder and is characterized by a propensity to bleed. All other disorders listed are associated with increased risk of VTE (Table 24-1). (See Schwartz 10th ed., Table 24-2, pp. 918–919)

TABLE 24-1	Risk factors for venous thromboembolism
Acquired	
Advanced age	
Hospitalization/immobilization	
Hormone replacement therapy and oral contraceptive use	
Pregnancy and puerperium	
Prior venous thromboembolism	
Malignancy	
Major surgery	
Obesity	
Nephrotic syndrome	
Trauma or spinal cord injury	
Long-haul travel (>6 hours)	
Varicose veins	
Antiphospholipid antibody syndrome	
Myeloproliferative disease	
Polycythemia	
Inherited	
Factor V Leiden	
Prothrombin 20210A	
Antithrombin deficiency	
Protein C deficiency	
Protein S deficiency	
Factor XI elevation	
Dysfibrinogenemia	
Mixed Etiology	
Homocysteinemia	
Factor VII, VIII, IX, XI elevation	
Hyperfibrinogenemia	
Activated protein C resistance without factor V Leiden	

6. May-Thurner syndrome is an anatomical factor associated with increased DVT formation, and is characterized by which of the following?
   A. Narrowing of the left iliac vein at the site where the right iliac artery crosses over it.
   B. Narrowing of the left renal vein as it traverses beneath the superior mesenteric artery.
   C. Subclavian vein narrowing due to repetitive upper extremity effort.
   D. A rapidly expanding hemangioma.

Answer: A
Anatomic factors may also contribute to development of DVT. At the site where the right iliac artery crosses over the left iliac vein, the left iliac vein may become chronically narrowed predisposing to iliofemoral venous thrombosis, so-called *May-Thurner syndrome*. External compression of major veins by masses of various types can also lead to venous thrombosis. (See Schwartz 10th ed., p. 919.)

7. A Caprini score of ≥5 in a general surgery patient without thromboprophylaxis is associated with what percentage risk of developing a DVT?
   A. 1%
   B. 3%
   C. 6%
   D. 10%

Answer: C
Scoring systems have been developed that take into account the number of VTE risk factors in an individual patient. These risk stratification scores, such as the Rogers score and Caprini score, provide individual patient risk stratification and recommendations for prophylactic anticoagulation. The ninth edition of the American College of Chest Physicians (ACCP) Guidelines for Prevention of VTE in Non-Orthopedic Surgical Patients acknowledges both the Rogers and Caprini scores and provides recommendations for VTE. Orthopedic surgical

patients are generally excluded from risk assessment scores because of the disproportionately increased risk of VTE in orthopedic surgery compared with the general and abdominopelvic surgery population (Table 24-2). (See Schwartz 10th ed., Table 24-3, p. 919.)

TABLE 24-2	Thromboembolism risk and recommended thromboprophylaxis in surgical patients	
Level of Risk	**Approximate Dvt Risk without Thromboprophylaxis (%)**	**Suggested Thromboprophylaxis Options**
Very low risk General or abdominopelvic surgery	<0.5% (Rogers score <7; Caprini score 0)	No specific thromboprophylaxis Early ambulation
Low risk General or abdominopelvic surgery	~1.5% (Rogers score 7–10; Caprini score 1–2)	Mechanical prophylaxis
Moderate risk General or abdominopelvic surgery	~3.0% (Rogers score >10; Caprini score 3–4)	LMWH (at recommended doses), LDUH, or mechanical prophylaxis
High bleeding risk		Mechanical prophylaxis
High risk General or abdominopelvic surgery	~6% (Caprini score ≥5)	LMWH (at recommended doses), fondaparinux and mechanical prophylaxis
High bleeding risk General or abdominopelvic surgery for cancer		Mechanical thromboprophylaxis Extended-duration LMWH (4 weeks)

DVT = deep vein thrombosis; INR = international normalized ratio; LDUH = low-dose unfractionated heparin; LMWH = low molecular weight heparin; VTE = venous thromboembolism.
Source: Summary of recommendations from Gould MK, Garcia DA, Wren SM, et al. Prevention of VTE in nonorthopedic surgical patients: antithrombotic therapy and prevention of thrombosis: American College of Chest Physicians Evidence-Based Clinical Practice Guidelines, 9th ed. *Chest.* 2012;141:227S.

8. *Phlegmasia cerulea dolens* is best described as
   A. Asymptomatic, but extensive DVT.
   B. Isolated popliteal vein thrombosis.
   C. Extensive DVT of the major axial deep venous channels of the lower extremity potentially complicated by venous gangrene and/or the need for amputation.
   D. Painless lower extremity swelling.

Answer: C

Clinical symptoms may worsen as DVT propagates and involves the major proximal deep veins. Extensive DVT of the major axial deep venous channels of the lower extremity with relative sparing of collateral veins causes a condition called *phlegmasia cerulea dolens* (Fig. 24-3). This condition is characterized by pain and pitting edema with associated cyanosis. When the thrombosis extends to the collateral veins, massive fluid sequestration and more significant edema ensue, resulting in a condition known as *phlegmasia alba dolens*. The affected extremity in *phlegmasia alba dolens* is extremely painful and edematous and pale secondary to arterial insufficiency from dramatically elevated below lower knee compartment pressures. Both phlegmasia cerulean dolens and phlegmasia alba dolens can be complicated by venous gangrene and the need for amputation. (See Schwartz 10th ed., Figure 24-4, pp. 919–920.)

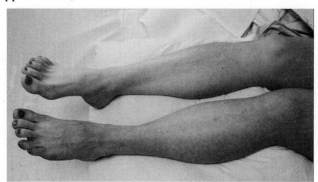

FIG. 24-3. Phlegmasia cerulea dolens of the left leg. Note the bluish discoloration.

9. According to the American College of Chest Physicians, the recommended duration of long-term antithrombotic therapy after provoked DVT is
   A. 2 weeks
   B. 1 month
   C. 3 months
   D. 6 months

Answer: C

The recommended duration of antithrombotic therapy is stratified based on whether the DVT was provoked or unprovoked, whether it was the first or a recurrent episode, where the DVT is located, and whether malignancy or thrombophilia is present. In patients with proximal DVT, several randomized clinical trials have demonstrated that shorter-term antithrombotic therapy (4 to 6 weeks) is associated with a higher rate of VTE recurrence than 3 to 6 months of anticoagulation.[46,47,48] In these trials, most of the patients with transient risk factors had a low rate of recurrent VTE, and most recurrences were in patients with continuing risk factors. The ACCP recommendation, therefore, is that 3 months of anticoagulation are sufficient to prevent recurrent VTE in patients with DVT occurring around the time of a transient risk factor (e.g., hospitalization, orthopedic or major general surgery) (Table 24-3). (See Schwartz 10th ed., Table 24-4, p. 923.)

TABLE 24-3	Summary of American College of Chest Physicians recommendations regarding duration of long-term antithrombotic therapy for deep vein thrombosis (DVT)
Clinical Subgroup	**Antithrombotic Treatment Duration**
First episode DVT/transient risk/ surgery	VKA or LMWH for 3 months
First episode DVT/unprovoked	VKA or LMWH for 3 months Consider for long-term therapy if: • Proximal DVT • Minimal bleeding risk • Stable coagulation monitoring
Distal DVT/unprovoked • Symptomatic • Asymptomatic and no risk factors for progression	VKA for 3 months Serial imaging in 2 weeks, if progression VKA for 3 months
Second episode DVT/ unprovoked DVT and cancer	VKA for extended therapy LMWH for extended therapy over VKA

LMWH = low molecular weight heparin; VKA = vitamin K antagonist.
Source: Summary of recommendations from Kearon C, Akl EA, Comerota AJ, et al. Antithrombotic therapy for VTE disease: antithrombotic therapy and prevention of thrombosis: American College of Chest Physicians Evidence-Based Clinical Practice Guidelines, 9th ed. *Chest.* 2012;141:e419.

10. All of the following are indications for placement of IVC filters EXCEPT
    A. Septic thromboembolism.
    B. Bleeding complication from anticoagulation therapy of acute VTE.
    C. Recurrent DVT or PE despite adequate anticoagulation therapy.
    D. Severe pulmonary hypertension.

Answer: A

Placement of an IVC filter is indicated for patients who have manifestations of lower extremity VTE and absolute contraindications to anticoagulation, those who have a bleeding complication from anticoagulation therapy of acute VTE, or those who develop recurrent DVT or PE despite adequate anticoagulation therapy and for patients with severe pulmonary hypertension. (See Schwartz 10th ed., p. 924.)

11. All of the following are appropriate therapies for suppurative thrombophlebitis EXCEPT
    A. Nonsteroidal anti-inflammatory drugs
    B. Antibiotics
    C. Systemic steroid therapy
    D. Removal of existing indwelling venous catheters

Answer: C

Treatment of superficial vein thrombophlebitis (SVT) is quite variable. A Cochrane Review reported that low-molecular-weight heparins (LMWHs) and nonsteroidal anti-inflammatory drugs both reduce the rate of SVT extension or recurrence. Topical medications appear to improve local symptoms. Surgical treatment, combined with the use of graduated compression stockings, is associated with a lower rate of VTE and SVT progression. The treatment is individualized and depends on the location of the thrombus and the severity of symptoms. In patients with SVT not within 1 cm of the saphenofemoral junction, treatment consists of compression and administration of an anti-inflammatory medication such as indomethacin. In patients with suppurative SVT, antibiotics and removal of any existing indwelling catheters are mandatory. Excision of the vein may be necessary but is usually reserved for patients with systemic symptoms or when excision of the involved vein is straightforward. If the SVT extends proximally to within 1 cm of the saphenofemoral junction, extension into the common femoral vein is more likely to occur. In these patients, anticoagulation therapy for 6 weeks and great saphenous vein (GSV) ligation appear equally effective in preventing thrombus extension into the deep venous system. (See Schwartz 10th ed., p. 928.)

12. Which of following statements regarding injection sclerotherapy for varicose veins is true?
    A. Sclerotherapy can be successful in veins <3 mm in diameter and in telangiectatic vessels. Sclerosing agents include hypertonic saline, sodium tetradecyl sulfate, and polidocanol.
    B. Compressive elastic bandages should be wrapped around the leg after sclerotherapy, and need to be worn for 24 hours.
    C. Elastic stockings should be worn for only 1 week after sclerotherapy.
    D. There are minimal complications associated with sclerotherapy.

Answer: A
Interventional management includes injection sclerotherapy, surgical therapy, or a combination of both techniques. Injection sclerotherapy alone can be successful in varicose veins <3mm in diameter and in telangiectatic vessels. Sclerotherapy acts by destroying the venous endothelium. Sclerosing agents include hypertonic saline, sodium tetradecyl sulfate, and polidocanol. Concentrations of 11.7 to 23.4% hypertonic saline, 0.125 to 0.250% sodium tetradecyl sulfate, and 0.5% polidocanol are used for telangiectasias. Larger varicose veins require higher concentrations: 23.4% hypertonic saline, 0.50 to 1% sodium tetradecyl sulfate, and 0.75 to 1.0% polidocanol. Elastic bandages are wrapped around the leg after injection and worn continuously for 3 to 5 days to produce apposition of the inflamed vein walls and prevent thrombus formation. After the bandages are removed, elastic compression stockings should be worn for a minimum of 2 weeks. Complications from sclerotherapy include allergic reaction, local hyperpigmentation, thrombophlebitis, DVT, and possible skin necrosis. (See Schwartz 10th ed., p. 929.)

13. Heparin-induced thrombocytopenia (HIT) is characterized by which of the following?
    A. Diagnosis based on prior exposure to heparin with platelet count <120,000 and/or platelet decline of 40% following heparin exposure.
    B. Results from heparin-associated antiplatelet antibodies (HAAbs) directed against platelet factor 4 complexed with heparin.
    C. Low incidence in patients with repeat exposure to heparin.
    D. Minimal association with thrombotic complications.

Answer: B
Heparin-induced thrombocytopenia (HIT) results from heparin-associated antiplatelet antibodies (HAAbs) directed against platelet factor 4 complexed with heparin. HIT occurs in 1 to 5% of patients being treated with heparin. In patients with repeat heparin exposure (such as vascular surgery patients), the incidence of HAAbs may be as high as 21%. HIT occurs most frequently in the second week of therapy and may lead to disastrous venous or arterial thrombotic complications. Therefore, platelet counts should be monitored periodically in patients receiving continuous heparin therapy.

HIT is diagnosed based on previous exposure to heparin, platelet count less than 100,000, and/or platelet count decline of 50% following exposure. All heparin must be stopped and alternative anticoagulation initiated immediately to avoid thrombotic complications, which may approach 50% over the subsequent 30 days in affected individuals. (See Schwartz 10th ed., p. 922.)

14. Direct thrombin inhibiting medications include which of the following
    A. Warfarin
    B. Enoxaparin
    C. Argatroban
    D. Fondaparinux

Answer: C

Direct thrombin inhibitors (DTIs) include recombinant hirudin, argatroban, and bivalirudin. These antithrombotic agents bind to thrombin, inhibiting the conversion of fibrinogen to fibrin as well as thrombin-induced platelet activation. These actions are independent of antithrombin. The DTIs should be reserved for (a) patients in whom there is a high clinical suspicion or confirmation of HIT, and (b) patients who have a history of HIT or test positive for heparin-associated antibodies. In patients with established HIT, DTIs should be administered for at least 7 days, or until the platelet count normalizes. Warfarin may then be introduced slowly, overlapping therapy with a DTI for at least 5 days. (See Schwartz 10th ed., p. 922.)

15. Which of the following is a true statement about lymphedema?
    A. Secondary lymphedema is less common than primary lymphedema.
    B. Axillary node dissection leading to lymphedema of the arm is the most common cause of secondary lymphedema in the United States.
    C. Filariasis and other environmental exposures are uncommon causes of lymphedema globally.
    D. Surgery is the mainstay of therapy for lymphedema.

Answer: B

The original classification system, described by Allen, is based on the cause of the lymphedema. Primary lymphedema is further subdivided into congenital lymphedema, lymphedema praecox, and lymphedema tarda. *Congenital lymphedema* may involve a single lower extremity, multiple limbs, the genitalia, or the face. The edema typically develops before 2 years of age and may be associated with specific hereditary syndromes (Turner syndrome, Milroy syndrome, Klippel-Trenaunay-Weber syndrome). *Lymphedema praecox* is the most common form of primary lymphedema, accounting for 94% of cases. Lymphedema praecox is far more common in women, with the gender ratio favoring women 10:1. The onset is during childhood or the teenage years, and the swelling involves the foot and calf. *Lymphedema tarda* is uncommon, accounting for <10% of cases of primary lymphedema. The onset of edema is after 35 years of age.

Secondary lymphedema is far more common than primary lymphedema. Secondary lymphedema develops as a result of lymphatic obstruction or disruption. Axillary node dissection leading to lymphedema of the arm is the most common cause of secondary lymphedema in the United States. Other causes of secondary lymphedema include radiation therapy, trauma, infection, and malignancy. Globally, filariasis (an infection caused by *Wuchereria bancrofti*, *Brugia malayi*, and *Brugia timori*) and environmental exposure to minerals in volcanic soil resulting in podoconiosis in barefoot populations are the most common causes of secondary lymphedema.

Control of chronic limb swelling through compression is the mainstay of therapy for lymphedema. (See Schwartz 10th ed., p. 934.)

16. Mesenteric vein thrombosis (MVT) is associated with all of the following EXCEPT
    A. MVT is less common in patients with hypercoagulable states, malignancy, or cirrhosis.
    B. 5 to 15% of cases of acute mesenteric ischemia occur as a result of MVT.
    C. Patients with MVT are treated with fluid resuscitation, heparin anticoagulation, and bowel rest.
    D. Computed tomography (CT) scan and magnetic resonance imaging (MRI) are 100% sensitive and 98% specific for MVT.

Answer: A

Five to 15% of cases of acute mesenteric ischemia occur as a result of mesenteric vein thrombosis (MVT). Mortality rates in patients with MVT may approach 50%. The usual presenting symptom is nonspecific abdominal pain and distention, often accompanied by nausea, vomiting, and diarrhea. Peritoneal signs, suggesting intestinal infarction, are present in fewer than half of MVT patients. MVT is more common in patients with a hypercoagulable states, malignancy, and cirrhosis. MVT occurs as a rare complication of laparoscopic surgery.

Most cases of MVT are diagnosed with contrast-enhanced computed tomography (CT) scanning or magnetic resonance imaging (MRI) in the course of an evaluation for abdominal pain. The sensitivity and specificity for CT and MRI approach 100% and 98%, respectively. Ultrasound can also be used and has reported sensitivity and specificity of 93% and 99%, respectively.

Patients with MVT are treated with fluid resuscitation, heparin anticoagulation, and bowel rest. (See Schwartz 10th ed., p. 929.)

CHAPTER 25

The Esophagus and Diaphragmatic Hernia

1. Locations of anatomic narrowing of the esophagus seen on an esophagram include all of the following EXCEPT
   A. Lower esophageal sphincter
   B. Crossing of the left mainstem bronchus and aortic arch
   C. Thoracic outlet
   D. Cricopharyngeal muscle

Answer: C
Three normal areas of esophageal narrowing are evident on the barium esophagogram or during esophagoscopy. The uppermost narrowing is located at the entrance into the esophagus and is caused by the cricopharyngeal muscle. Its luminal diameter is 1.5 cm, and it is the narrowest point of the esophagus. The middle narrowing is due to an indentation of the anterior and left lateral esophageal wall caused by the crossing of the left main stem bronchus and aortic arch. The luminal diameter at this point is 1.6 cm. The lowermost narrowing is at the hiatus of the diaphragm and is caused by the gastroesophageal sphincter mechanism. The luminal diameter at this point varies somewhat, depending on the distention of the esophagus by the passage of food, but has been measured at 1.6 to 1.9 cm. These normal constrictions tend to hold up swallowed foreign objects, and the overlying mucosa is subject to injury by swallowed corrosive liquids because of their slow passage through these areas. (See Schwartz 10th ed., p. 942.)

2. The cervical esophagus receives its blood supply primarily from the
   A. Internal carotid artery
   B. Inferior thyroid artery
   C. Superior thyroid artery
   D. Inferior cervical artery
   E. Facial artery

Answer: B
The cervical portion of the esophagus receives its main blood supply from the inferior thyroid artery. The thoracic portion receives its blood supply from the bronchial arteries, with 75% of individuals having one right-sided and two left-sided branches. Two esophageal branches arise directly from the aorta. The abdominal portion of the esophagus receives its blood supply from the ascending branch of the left gastric artery and from inferior phrenic arteries. On entering the wall of the esophagus, the arteries assume a T-shaped division to form a longitudinal plexus, giving rise to an intramural vascular network in the muscular and submucosal layers. As a consequence, the esophagus can be mobilized from the stomach to the level of the aortic arch without fear of devascularization and ischemic necrosis. Caution should be exercised as to the extent of esophageal mobilization in patients who have had a previous thyroidectomy with ligation of the inferior thyroid arteries proximal to the origin of the esophageal branches. (See Schwartz 10th ed., pp. 945–946.)

3. All of the following cranial nerves are involved in the swallowing mechanism EXCEPT
   A. V
   B. VII
   C. VIII
   D. X
   E. XI
   F. XII

Answer: C

Swallowing can be started at will, or it can be reflexively elicited by the stimulation of areas in the mouth and pharynx, among them the anterior and posterior tonsillar pillars or the posterior lateral walls of the hypopharynx. The afferent sensory nerves of the pharynx are the glossopharyngeal nerves and the superior laryngeal branches of the vagus nerves. Once aroused by stimuli entering via these nerves, the swallowing center in the medulla coordinates the complete act of swallowing by discharging impulses through cranial nerves V, VII, X, XI, and XII, as well as the motor neurons of C1 to C3. Discharges through these nerves occur in a rather specific pattern and last for approximately 0.5 second. Little is known about the organization of the swallowing center, except that it can trigger swallowing after a variety of different inputs, but the response is always a rigidly ordered pattern of outflow. Following a cerebrovascular accident, this coordinated outflow may be altered, causing mild to severe abnormalities of swallowing. In more severe injury, swallowing can be grossly disrupted, leading to repetitive aspiration. (See Schwartz 10th ed., p. 948.)

4. All of these are parts of the human antireflux mechanism EXCEPT
   A. Adequate gastric reservoir
   B. Mechanically functioning lower esophageal sphincter (LES)
   C. Mucus secreting cells of the distal esophagus
   D. Efficient esophageal clearance

Answer: C

If the pharyngeal swallow does not initiate a peristaltic contraction, then the coincident relaxation of the lower esophageal sphincter (LES) is unguarded and reflux of gastric juice can occur. This may be an explanation for the observation of spontaneous lower esophageal relaxation, thought by some to be a causative factor in gastroesophageal reflux disease (GERD). The power of the worm-drive pump of the esophageal body is insufficient to force open a valve that does not relax. In dogs, a bilateral cervical parasympathetic blockade abolishes the relaxation of the LES that occurs with pharyngeal swallowing or distention of the esophagus. Consequently, vagal function appears to be important in coordinating the relaxation of the LES with esophageal contraction.

The antireflux mechanism in human beings is composed of three components: a mechanically effective LES, efficient esophageal clearance, and an adequately functioning gastric reservoir. A defect of any one of these three components can lead to increased esophageal exposure to gastric juice and the development of mucosal injury. (See Schwartz 10th ed., p. 949.)

5. Physiologic reflux happens most commonly when a person is
   A. Awake and supine
   B. Awake and upright
   C. Asleep and supine
   D. Asleep and semi-erect

Answer: B

On 24-hour esophageal pH monitoring, healthy individuals have occasional episodes of gastroesophageal reflux. This physiologic reflux is more common when awake and in the upright position than during sleep in the supine position. When reflux of gastric juice occurs, normal subjects rapidly clear the acid gastric juice from the esophagus regardless of their position.

There are several explanations for the observation that physiologic reflux in normal subjects is more common when they are awake and in the upright position than during sleep in the supine position. First, reflux episodes occur in healthy volunteers primarily during transient losses of the gastroesophageal barrier, which may be due to a relaxation of the LES or intragastric pressure overcoming sphincter pressure. Gastric juice can also reflux when a swallow-induced relaxation of the LES is not protected by an oncoming peristaltic wave. The average frequency of these "unguarded moments" or of transient losses of the gastroesophageal barrier is far less while asleep and in the supine position than while awake and in the upright position. Consequently, there are fewer opportunities for reflux to occur in the supine position. Second, in the upright position, there is a 12-mm Hg pressure gradient between the resting, positive intra-abdominal pressure measured in the stomach and the most negative intrathoracic pressure measured in the esophagus at midthoracic level. This gradient favors the flow of gastric juice up into the thoracic esophagus when upright. The gradient diminishes in the supine position. Third, the LES pressure in normal subjects is significantly higher in the supine position than in the upright position. This is due to the apposition of the hydrostatic pressure of the abdomen to the abdominal portion of the sphincter when supine. In the upright position, the abdominal pressure surrounding the sphincter is negative compared with atmospheric pressure, and, as expected, the abdominal pressure gradually increases the more caudally it is measured. This pressure gradient tends to move the gastric contents toward the cardia and encourages the occurrence of reflux into the esophagus when the individual is upright. In contrast, in the supine position, the gastroesophageal pressure gradient diminishes, and the abdominal hydrostatic pressure under the diaphragm increases, causing an increase in sphincter pressure and a more competent cardia. (See Schwartz 10th ed., p. 949.)

6. All of the following hormones decrease LES tone EXCEPT
   A. Gastrin
   B. Estrogen
   C. Somatostatin
   D. CCK
   E. Glucagon

Answer: A

The LES has intrinsic myogenic tone, which is modulated by neural and hormonal mechanisms. Alpha-adrenergic neurotransmitters or beta blockers stimulate the LES, and alpha blockers and beta stimulants decrease its pressure. It is not clear to what extent cholinergic nerve activity controls LES pressure. The vagus nerve carries both excitatory and inhibitory fibers to the esophagus and sphincter. The hormones gastrin and motilin have been shown to increase LES pressure; and cholecystokinin, estrogen, glucagon, somatostatin, and secretin decrease LES pressure. The peptides bombesin, L-enkephalin, and substance P increase LES pressure; and calcitonin gene-related peptide, gastric inhibitory peptide, neuropeptide Y, and vasoactive intestinal polypeptide decrease LES pressure. Some pharmacologic agents such as antacids, cholinergics, agonists, domperidone, metoclopramide, and prostaglandin F2 are known to increase LES pressure; and anticholinergics, barbiturates, calcium channel blockers, caffeine, diazepam, dopamine, meperidine, prostaglandin E1 and E2, and theophylline decrease LES pressure. Peppermint, chocolate, coffee, ethanol, and fat are all associated with decreased LES pressure and may be responsible for esophageal symptoms after a sumptuous meal. (See Schwartz 10th ed., pp. 949–950.)

7. The most common cause of a deficient LES is
   A. Inadequate overall length
   B. Mean resting pressure >6 mm Hg
   C. Inadequate intra-abdominal length
   D. Failure of receptive relaxation

Answer: C

It is important that a portion of the total length of the LES be exposed to the effects of an intra-abdominal pressure. That is, during periods of elevated intra-abdominal pressure, the resistance of the barrier would be overcome if pressure were not applied equally to both the LES and stomach simultaneously. Thus, in the presence of a hiatal hernia, the sphincter resides entirely within the chest cavity and cannot respond to an increase in intra-abdominal pressure because the pinch valve mechanism is lost and gastroesophageal reflux is more liable to occur. Therefore, a permanently defective sphincter is defined by one or more of the following characteristics: An LES with a mean resting pressure of less than 6 mm Hg, an overall sphincter length of <2 cm, and intra-abdominal sphincter length of <1 cm. Compared to normal subjects without GERD these values are below the 2.5 percentile for each parameter. The most common cause of a defective sphincter is an inadequate abdominal length. (See Schwartz 10th ed., p. 966.)

8. Maximal esophageal mucosal damage is caused by exposure to
   A. Acidic fluid alone
   B. Acidic fluid, food contents, and pepsin
   C. Acidic fluid, trypsin, and food contents
   D. Acidic fluid, pepsin, and bile salts
   E. Neutral fluid, pepsin, and trypsin

Answer: D

The potential injurious components that reflux into the esophagus include gastric secretions such as acid and pepsin, as well as biliary and pancreatic secretions that regurgitate from the duodenum into the stomach. There is a considerable body of experimental evidence to indicate that maximal epithelial injury occurs during exposure to bile salts combined with acid and pepsin. These studies have shown that acid alone does minimal damage to the esophageal mucosa, but the combination of acid and pepsin is highly deleterious. Similarly, the reflux of duodenal juice alone does little damage to the mucosa, although the combination of duodenal juice and gastric acid is particularly noxious. (See Schwartz 10th ed., p. 967.)

9. The incidence of metaplastic Barrett esophagus (BE) progressing to adenocarcinoma is
   A. Less than 0.1% per year
   B. 0.2 to 0.5% per year
   C. 1 to 3% per year
   D. 3 to 5% per year
   E. Greater than 5% per year

Answer: B

If reflux of gastric juice is allowed to persist and sustained or repetitive esophageal injury occurs, two sequelae can result. First, a luminal stricture can develop from submucosal and eventually intramural fibrosis. Second, the tubular esophagus may become replaced with columnar epithelium. The columnar epithelium is resistant to acid and is associated with the alleviation of the complaint of heartburn. This columnar epithelium often becomes intestinalized, identified histologically by the presence of goblet cells. This specialized intestinal metaplasia (IM) is currently required for the diagnosis of Barrett esophagus (BE). Endoscopically, BE can be quiescent or associated with complications of esophagitis, stricture, Barrett ulceration, and dysplasia. The complications associated with BE may be due to the continuous irritation from refluxed duodenogastric juice. This continued injury is pH-dependent and may be modified by medical therapy. The incidence of metaplastic Barrett epithelium becoming dysplastic and progressing to adenocarcinoma is approximately 0.2 to 0.5% per year. (See Schwartz 10th ed., pp. 968–969.)

10. The histologic hallmark of BE is
    A. Columnar epithelium
    B. Goblet cells
    C. Parietal cells
    D. Cuboidal epithelium

Answer: B
The definition of BE has evolved considerably over the past decade. Traditionally, BE was identified by the presence of columnar mucosa extending at least 3 cm into the esophagus. It is now recognized that the specialized, intestinal-type epithelium found in the Barrett mucosa is the only tissue predisposed to malignant degeneration. Consequently, the diagnosis of BE is presently made given any length of endoscopically identifiable columnar mucosa that proves, on biopsy, to show IM. Although long segments of columnar mucosa without IM do occur, they are uncommon and might be congenital in origin.

The hallmark of IM is the presence of intestinal goblet cells. There is a high prevalence of biopsy-demonstrated IM at the cardia, on the gastric side of the squamocolumnar junction, in the absence of endoscopic evidence of a columnar-lined esophagus (CLE). Evidence is accumulating that these patches of what appears to be Barrett in the cardia have a similar malignant potential as in the longer segments, and are precursors for carcinoma of the cardia. (See Schwartz 10th ed., p. 969.)

11. Relief from respiratory symptoms can be expected in approximately what percent of patients with reflux associated asthma with medical therapy
    A. <10%
    B. 25%
    C. 50%
    D. 75%

Answer: C
Once the diagnosis is established, treatment may be initiated with either proton pump inhibitor (PPI) therapy or antireflux surgery. A trial of high-dose PPI therapy may help establish the facts that reflux is partly or completely responsible for the respiratory symptoms. It is important to note that the persistence of symptoms in the face of aggressive PPI treatment does not necessarily rule out reflux as a possible cofactor or sole etiology.

Although there is probably some elements of a placebo effect, relief of respiratory symptoms can be anticipated in up to 50% of patients with reflux-induced asthma treated with antisecretory medications. However, when examined objectively, <15% of patients can be expected to have improvement in their pulmonary function with medical therapy. In properly selected patients, antireflux surgery improves respiratory symptoms in nearly 90% of children and 70% of adults with asthma and reflux disease. Improvements in pulmonary function can be demonstrated in around 30% of patients. Uncontrolled studies of the two forms of therapy (PPI and surgery) and the evidence from the two randomized controlled trials of medical versus surgical therapy indicate that surgical valve reconstruction is the most effective therapy for reflux-induced asthma. The superiority of the surgery over PPI is most noticeable in the supine position, which corresponds with the nadir of PPI blood levels and resultant acid breakthrough and is the time in the circadian cycle when asthma symptoms are at their worst. (See Schwartz 10th ed., p. 971.)

12. All of the following patients are good candidates for anti-reflux surgery EXCEPT
    A. A 31-year-old man with typical GERD with disease becoming resistant to medical therapy.
    B. A 55-year-old woman with disease well controlled with PPIs who wishes to discontinue medical therapy.
    C. A 75-year-old man with new onset heartburn which is not relieved by PPIs.
    D. A 52-year-old man with volume reflux and a large paraesophageal hernia.

Answer: C
Studies of the natural history of GERD indicate that most patients have a relatively benign form of the disease that is responsive to lifestyle changes and dietary and medical therapy, and do not need surgical treatment. Approximately 25 to 50% of the patients with GERD have persistent or progressive disease, and it is this patient population that is best suited to surgical therapy. In the past, the presence of esophagitis and a structurally defective LES were the primary indications for surgical treatment, and many internists and surgeons

were reluctant to recommend operative procedures in their absence. However, one should not be deterred from considering antireflux surgery in a symptomatic patient with or without esophagitis or a defective sphincter, provided the disease process has been objectively documented by 24-hour pH monitoring. This is particularly true in patients who have become dependent upon therapy with PPIs, or require increasing doses to control their symptoms. It is important to note that a good response to medical therapy in this group of patients predicts an excellent outcome following antireflux surgery.

In general, the key indications for antireflux surgery are (a) objectively proven gastroesophageal reflux disease, and (b) typical symptoms of gastroesophageal reflux disease (heartburn and/or regurgitation) despite adequate medical management, or (c) a younger patient unwilling to take lifelong medication. In addition, a structurally defective LES can also predict which patients are more likely to fail with medical therapy. Patients with normal sphincter pressures tend to remain well controlled with medical therapy, whereas patients with a structurally defective LES may not respond as well to medical therapy, and often develop recurrent symptoms within 1 to 2 years of beginning therapy. Such patients should be considered for an antireflux operation, regardless of the presence or absence of endoscopic esophagitis. (See Schwartz 10th ed., p. 972.)

13. Preoperative testing for antireflux surgery typically includes all of the following EXCEPT
   A. Computed tomography (CT) scan of the chest and abdomen
   B. Contrast esophagram
   C. 24 hour pH probe
   D. Esophageal manometry
   E. Esophagogastroduodenostomy

Answer: A

Before proceeding with an antireflux operation, several factors should be evaluated. The clinical symptoms should be consistent with the diagnosis of gastroesophageal reflux. Patients presenting with the typical symptoms of heartburn and/or regurgitation who have responded, at least partly, to PPI therapy, will generally do well following surgery, whereas patients with atypical symptoms have a less predictable response. Reflux should also be objectively confirmed by either the presence of ulcerative esophagitis or an abnormal 24-hour pH study.

The propulsive force of the body of the esophagus should be evaluated by esophageal manometry to determine if it has sufficient power to propel a bolus of food through a newly reconstructed valve. Patients with normal peristaltic contractions can be considered for a 360° Nissen fundoplication or a partial fundoplication, depending on patient and surgeon preferences. When peristalsis is absent a partial fundoplication is probably the procedure of choice, but only if achalasia has been ruled out.

Hiatal anatomy should also be assessed. In patients with smaller hiatal hernias endoscopy evaluation usually provides sufficient information. However, when patients present with a very large hiatus hernia or for revision surgery after previous antireflux surgery, contrast radiology provides better anatomical information. The concept of anatomic shortening of the esophagus is controversial, with divergent opinions held about how common this problem is. Believers claim that anatomic shortening of the esophagus compromises the ability of the surgeon to perform an adequate repair without tension, and that this can lead to an increased incidence of breakdown or thoracic displacement of the repair. Some of those who hold this view claim that esophageal shortening is present when a barium swallow X-ray identifies a sliding hiatal hernia that will not reduce in the upright position, or that measures more than 5 cm in length at endoscopy. When identified these surgeons usually undertake add a gastroplasty to the antireflux procedure. Others claim that esophageal shortening is overdiagnosed and rarely seen, and that the morbidity of adding a gastroplasty outweighs any benefits. These surgeons would recommend a standard antireflux procedure in all patients undergoing primary surgery. (See Schwartz 10th ed., pp. 972–973.)

14. The valve created during an antireflux procedure should be at least
    A. 1 cm
    B. 2 cm
    C. 3 cm
    D. 4 cm
    E. 5 cm

Answer: C
The primary goal of antireflux surgery is to safely create a new antireflux valve at the gastroesophageal junction (GEJ), while preserving the patient's ability to swallow normally and to belch to relieve gaseous distention. Regardless of the choice of the procedure, this goal can be achieved if attention is paid to some basic principles when reconstructing the antireflux mechanism. First, the operation should create a flap valve which prevents regurgitation of gastric contents into the esophagus. This will result in an increase in the pressure of the distal esophageal sphincter region. Following a Nissen fundoplication, the expected increase is to a level twice the resting gastric pressure (ie, 12 mm Hg for a gastric pressure of 6 mm Hg). The extent of the pressure rise is often less following a partial fundoplication, although with all types of fundoplication the length of the reconstructed valve should be at least 3 cm. This not only augments sphincter characteristics in patients in whom they are reduced before surgery, but prevents unfolding of a normal sphincter in response to gastric distention. Preoperative and postoperative esophageal manometry measurements have shown that the resting sphincter pressure and the overall sphincter length can be surgically augmented over preoperative values, and that the change in the former is a function of the degree of gastric wrap around the esophagus. However, the aim of any fundoplication is to create a loose wrap, and to maintain the position of the gastric fundus close to the distal intra-abdominal esophagus, in a flap valve arrangement. The efficacy of this relies on the close relationship between the fundus and the esophagus, not the "tightness" of the wrap. (See Schwartz 10th ed., p. 973.)

15. A Toupet fundoplication involves
    A. A 180° anterior wrap
    B. A 90° posterior wrap
    C. A 180° posterior wrap
    D. A 270° posterior wrap

Answer: D
Partial fundoplications were developed as an alternative to the Nissen procedure in an attempt to minimize the risk of postfundoplication side effects, such as dysphagia, inability to belch, and flatulence. The commonest approach has been a posterior partial or Toupet fundoplication. Some surgeons use this type of procedure for all patients presenting for antireflux surgery, whereas others apply a tailored approach in which a partial fundoplication is constructed in patients with impaired esophageal motility, in which the propulsive force of the esophagus is thought to be insufficient to overcome the outflow obstruction of a complete fundoplication. The Toupet posterior partial fundoplication consists of a 270° gastric fundoplication around the distal 4 cm of esophagus. It is usually stabilized by anchoring the wrap posteriorly to the hiatal rim. (See Schwartz 10th ed., pp. 975–976.)

16. What percentage of patients should be expected to have relief of symptoms at 5 years out from antireflux surgery?
    A. <50%
    B. 50–60%
    C. 60–80%
    D. 80–90%
    E. >90%

Answer: D

Studies of long-term outcome following both open and laparoscopic fundoplication document the ability of laparoscopic fundoplication to relieve typical reflux symptoms (heartburn, regurgitation, and dysphagia) in more than 90% of patients at follow-up intervals averaging 2 to 3 years and 80 to 90% of patients 5 years or more following surgery. This includes evidence-based reviews of antireflux surgery, prospective randomized trials comparing antireflux surgery to PPI therapy and open to laparoscopic fundoplication and analysis of U.S. national trends in use and outcomes. (See Schwartz 10th ed., p. 977.)

17. An upward dislocation of both the cardia and gastric fundus is which type of hiatal hernia?
    A. I
    B. II
    C. III
    D. IV

Answer: C

With the advent of clinical radiology, it became evident that a diaphragmatic hernia was a relatively common abnormality and was not always accompanied by symptoms. Three types of esophageal hiatal hernia were identified: (a) the sliding hernia, type I, characterized by an upward dislocation of the cardia in the posterior mediastinum; (b) the rolling or paraesophageal hernia (PEH), type II, characterized by an upward dislocation of the gastric fundus alongside a normally positioned cardia; and (c) the combined sliding-rolling or mixed hernia, type III, characterized by an upward dislocation of both the cardia and the gastric fundus. The end stage of type I and type II hernias occurs when the whole stomach migrates up into the chest by rotating 180° around its longitudinal axis, with the cardia and pylorus as fixed points. In this situation the abnormality is usually referred to as an *intrathoracic stomach* (Fig. 25-1). In some taxonomies, a type IV hiatal hernia is declared when an additional organ, usually the colon, herniates as well. Type II-IV hiatal hernias are also referred to as *paraesophageal hernia* (PEH), as a portion of the stomach is situated adjacent to the esophagus, above the GEJ. (See Schwartz 10th ed., Figure 25-39D, pp. 980–981.)

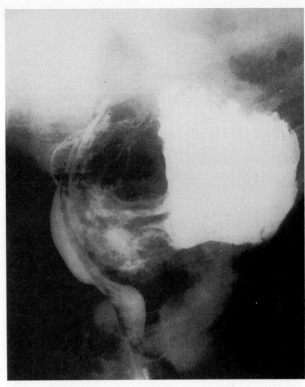

FIG. 25-1. Radiogram of an intrathoracic stomach. This is the end stage of a large hiatal hernia regardless of its initial classification. Note that the stomach has rotated 180° around its longitudinal axis, with the cardia and pylorus as fixed points. (Reproduced with permission from DeMeester TR, Bonavina L. Paraesophageal hiatal hernia, in: Nyhus LM, Condon RE eds. *Hernia*, 3rd ed. Philadelphia: Lippincott; 1989, p 684.)

18. The most common form of esophageal cancer diagnosed in the United States is
    A. Adenocarcinoma
    B. Squamous carcinoma
    C. Anaplastic carcinoma
    D. Leiomyosarcoma

Answer: A

Adenocarcinoma of the esophagus, once an unusual malignancy, is diagnosed with increasing frequency and now accounts for more than 50% of esophageal cancer in most Western countries. The shift in the epidemiology of esophageal cancer from predominantly squamous carcinoma seen in association with smoking and alcohol, to adenocarcinoma in the setting of BE, is one of the most dramatic changes that have occurred in the history of human neoplasia. Although esophageal carcinoma is a relatively uncommon malignancy, its prevalence is exploding, largely secondary to the well-established association between gastroesophageal reflux, BE, and esophageal adenocarcinoma. Once a nearly uniformly lethal disease, survival has improved slightly because of advances in the understanding of its molecular biology, screening and surveillance practices, improved staging, minimally invasive surgical techniques, and neoadjuvant therapy. (See Schwartz 10th ed., p. 1003.)

19. Squamous cell carcinomas of the esophagus most commonly occur
    A. At the GEJ
    B. In the cervical and upper thoracic esophagus
    C. In the lower thoracic esophagus
    D. Evenly distributed throughout the esophagus

Answer: B

It is estimated that 8% of the primary malignant tumors of the esophagus occur in the cervical portion. They are almost always squamous cell cancer, with a rare adenocarcinoma arising from a congenital inlet patch of columnar lining. These tumors, particularly those in the postcricoid area, represent a separate pathologic entity for two reasons: (a) They are more common in women and appear to be a unique entity in this regard; and (b) the efferent lymphatics from the cervical

20. The preoperative test most heavily correlated with the ability to tolerate an esophagectomy is
    A. DLCO
    B. FEV1
    C. Ability to climb a flight of stairs
    D. FVC

21. Which test most accurately assess the T stage of esophageal cancer?
    A. High-resolution CT scan
    B. Magnetic resonance imaging (MRI)
    C. Echocardiography
    D. Endoscopic ultrasonography (EUS)
    E. Esophagogastroduodenoscopy (EGD)

22. Which of the following patients would not be considered a candidate for esophagectomy?
    A. A 55-year-old man with GEJ adenocarcinoma confined to the muscularis mucosa.
    B. A 47-year-old woman with mid-esophageal cancer and an involved cervical LN.
    C. A 60-year-old man with a large GEJ carcinoma with invasion into the pleura without a malignant effusion.
    D. A 70-year-old woman with a small GEJ cancer and three pathologic LNs nearby on EUS.

esophagus drain completely differently from those of the thoracic esophagus. The latter drain directly into the paratracheal and deep cervical or internal jugular lymph nodes (LNs) with minimal flow in a longitudinal direction. Except in advanced disease, it is unusual for intrathoracic LNs to be involved. (See Schwartz 10th ed., p. 1005.)

Answer: B
Patients undergoing esophageal resection should have sufficient cardiopulmonary reserve to tolerate the proposed procedure. The respiratory function is best assessed with the forced expiratory volume in 1 second, which ideally should be 2 L or more. Any patient with a forced expiratory volume in 1 second of <1.25 L is a poor candidate for thoracotomy, because he or she has a 40% risk of dying from respiratory insufficiency within 4 years. In patients with poor pulmonary reserve, the transhiatal esophagectomy should be considered, as the pulmonary morbidity of this operation is less than is seen following thoracotomy. Clinical evaluation and electrocardiogram are not sufficient indicators of cardiac reserve. Echocardiography and dipyridamole-thallium imaging provide accurate information on wall motion, ejection fraction, and myocardial blood flow. A defect on thallium imaging may require further evaluation with preoperative coronary angiography. A resting ejection fraction of <40%, particularly if there is no increase with exercise, is an ominous sign. In the absence of invasive testing, observed stair-climbing is an economical (albeit not quantitative) method of assessing cardiopulmonary reserve. Most individuals who can climb three flights of stairs without stopping will do well with two-field open esophagectomy, especially if an epidural catheter is used for postoperative pain relief. (See Schwartz 10th ed., p. 1007.)

Answer: D
For years, clinical staging, contrast radiography, endoscopy, and CT scanning formed the backbone of esophageal cancer staging. More recently, preoperative decision making is guided by endoscopic ultrasonography (EUS) and positron emission tomography (PET) scanning.

EUS provides the most reliable method of determining depth of cancer invasion. In the absence of enlarged LNs, the degree of wall invasion dictates surgical therapy. (See Schwartz 10th ed., p. 1008.)

Answer: B
If the tumor invades into the submucosa, without visible LN involvement, most individuals would suggest esophagectomy with LN dissection, as positive nodes can be found in 20 to 25% of those with cancer limited to the mucosa and submucosa. If EUS demonstrates spread through the wall of the esophagus, especially if LNs are enlarged, then induction chemoradiation therapy (neoadjuvant therapy) should be strongly considered. Lastly, when the EUS demonstrates invasion of the trachea, bronchus, aorta, or spine, then surgical resection is

rarely indicated. If there is invasion into the pleura (T4a), then surgical resection can be considered in the absence of a malignant effusion. Thus, it can be seen that the therapy of esophageal cancer is largely driven by the findings of an endoscopic ultrasonography. It is difficult to provide modern treatment of esophageal cancer without access to this modality. (See Schwartz 10th ed., p. 1008.)

23. The technique of resecting an esophageal cancer which remains symptomatic after definitive chemoradiotherapy is referred to as
    A. Palliative esophagectomy
    B. Salvage esophagectomy
    C. Rescue esophagectomy
    D. None of the above, the procedure is not performed

Answer: B

Salvage esophagectomy is the nomenclature applied to esophagectomy performed after failure of definitive radiation and chemotherapy. The most frequent scenario is one in which distant disease (bone, lung, brain, or wide LN metastases) renders the patient nonoperable at initial presentation. Then, systemic chemotherapy, usually with radiation of the primary tumor, destroys all foci of metastasis, as demonstrated by CT and CT-PET, but the primary remains present and symptomatic. Following a period of observation, to make sure no new disease will become evident, salvage esophagectomy is performed, usually with an open two-field approach. Surprisingly, the cure rate of salvage esophagectomy is not inconsequential. One in four patients undergoing this operation will be disease free 5 years later, despite the presence of residual cancer in the operative specimen. Because of the dense scarring created by radiation treatment, this procedure is the most technically challenging of all esophagectomy techniques. (See Schwartz 10th ed., p. 1011.)

24. Patients with dysphagia secondary to esophageal cancer treated with radiation can expect the benefit to last
    A. <1 month
    B. 2–3 months
    C. 6–12 months
    D. >12 months

Answer: B

Primary treatment with radiation therapy does not produce results comparable with those obtained with surgery. Currently, the use of radiotherapy is restricted to patients who are not candidates for surgery, and is usually combined with chemotherapy. Radiation alone is used for palliation of dysphagia but the benefit is short-lived, lasting only 2 to 3 months. Furthermore, the length and course of treatment are difficult to justify in patients with a limited life expectancy. Radiation is effective in patients who have hemorrhage from the primary tumor. (See Schwartz 10th ed., p. 1012.)

25. How long after completion of neoadjuvant chemoradiotherapy should esophagectomy be performed?
    A. 2 weeks
    B. 4–6 weeks
    C. 6–8 weeks
    D. 8–10 weeks
    E. >10 weeks

Answer: C

The timing of surgery after chemoradiation induction is generally felt to be optimal between 6 and 8 weeks following the completion of induction therapy. Earlier than this time, active inflammation may make the resection hazardous, and the patients have not had time to recover fully from the chemoradiation. After 8 weeks, edema in the periesophageal tissue starts to turn to scar tissue, making dissection more difficult.

With chemoradiation, the complete response rates for adenocarcinoma range from 17 to 24%. No tumor is detected in the specimen after esophagectomy. Patients demonstrating a complete response to chemoradiation have a better survival rate than those without complete response, but distant failure remains common. (See Schwartz 10th ed., pp. 1012–1013.)

26. The optimal treatment of an incidentally discovered 3 cm leiomyoma of the upper esophagus in a 45-year-old otherwise healthy man is?
    A. Observation
    B. Esophagectomy
    C. Enucleation
    D. Endoscopic resection

Answer: C

Despite their slow growth and limited potential for malignant degeneration, leiomyomas should be removed unless there are specific contraindications. The majority can be removed by simple enucleation. If, during removal, the mucosa is inadvertently entered, the defect can be repaired primarily. After tumor removal, the outer esophageal wall should be reconstructed by closure of the muscle layer. The location of the lesion and the extent of surgery required will dictate the approach. Lesions of the proximal and middle esophagus require a right thoracotomy, whereas distal esophageal lesions require a left thoracotomy. Videothoracoscopic and laparoscopic approaches are now frequently used. The mortality rate associated with enucleation is low, and success in relieving the dysphagia is near 100%. Large lesions or those involving the GEJ may require esophageal resection. (See Schwartz 10th ed., pp. 1017–1018.)

27. Following a night of heavy drinking, a 43-year-old otherwise healthy man has sudden onset of severe chest pain after vomiting. Esophagram confirms esophageal rupture just proximal to the GEJ. What is the preferred operative exposure?
    A. Right thoracotomy
    B. Right thoracotomy with laparotomy
    C. Left thoracotomy
    D. Left thoracotomy with laparotomy
    E. Midline laparotomy

Answer: C

The key to optimum management is early diagnosis. The most favorable outcome is obtained following primary closure of the perforation within 24 hours, resulting in 80 to 90% survival. The most common location for the injury is the left lateral wall of the esophagus, just above the GEJ. To get adequate exposure of the injury, a dissection similar to that described for esophageal myotomy is performed. A flap of stomach is pulled up and the soiled fat pad at the GEJ is removed. The edges of the injury are trimmed and closed primarily. The closure is reinforced with the use of a pleural patch or construction of a Nissen fundoplication. (See Schwartz 10th ed., pp. 1018–1019.)

28. A 34-year-old man presents to the emergency department (ED) after an episode of hematemesis. EGD confirms a Mallory-Weiss tear with no residual bleeding. Treatment should consist of
    A. Esophagectomy
    B. Observation
    C. Proximal gastrectomy with esophago-jejunostomy
    D. Injection of botulinum toxin

Answer: B

Mallory-Weiss tears are characterized by arterial bleeding, which may be massive. Vomiting is not an obligatory factor, as there may be other causes of an acute increase in intra-abdominal pressure, such as paroxysmal coughing, seizures, and retching. The diagnosis requires a high index of suspicion, particularly in the patient who develops upper gastrointestinal (GI) bleeding following prolonged vomiting or retching. Upper endoscopy confirms the suspicion by identifying one or more longitudinal fissures in the mucosa of the herniated stomach as the source of bleeding.

In the majority of patients, the bleeding will stop spontaneously with nonoperative management. In addition to blood replacement, the stomach should be decompressed and antiemetics administered, as a distended stomach and continued vomiting aggravate further bleeding. A Sengstaken-Blakemore tube will not stop the bleeding, as the pressure in the balloon is not sufficient to overcome arterial pressure. Endoscopic injection of epinephrine may be therapeutic if bleeding does not stop spontaneously. Only occasionally will surgery be required to stop blood loss. The procedure consists of laparotomy and high gastrotomy with oversewing of the linear tear. Mortality is uncommon, and recurrence is rare. (See Schwartz 10th ed., p. 1020.)

29. Successful treatment of a Zenker diverticulum involves
    A. Diverticulopexy
    B. Resection of the diverticulum
    C. Observation
    D. Either diverticulopexy or resection with cricopharyngeal myotomy

Answer: D

When a pharyngoesophageal diverticulum is present, localization of the pharyngoesophageal segment is easy. The diverticulum is carefully freed from the overlying areolar tissue to expose its neck, just below the inferior pharyngeal constrictor and above the cricopharyngeus muscle. It can be difficult to identify the cricopharyngeus muscle in the absence of a diverticulum. A benefit of local anesthesia is that the patient can swallow and demonstrate an area of persistent narrowing at the pharyngoesophageal junction. Furthermore, before closing the incision, gelatin can be fed to the patient to ascertain whether the symptoms have been relieved, and to inspect the opening of the previously narrowed pharyngoesophageal segment. Under general anesthesia, and in the absence of a diverticulum, the placement of a nasogastric tube to the level of the manometrically determined cricopharyngeal sphincter helps in localization of the structures. The myotomy is extended cephalad by dividing 1 to 2 cm of inferior constrictor muscle of the pharynx, and caudad by dividing the cricopharyngeal muscle and the cervical esophagus for a length of 4 to 5 cm. If a diverticulum is present and is large enough to persist after a myotomy, it may be sutured in the inverted position to the prevertebral fascia using a permanent suture (ie, diverticulopexy). If the diverticulum is excessively large so that it would be redundant if suspended, or if its walls are thickened, then a diverticulectomy should be performed. This is best performed under general anesthesia by placing a Maloney dilator (48F) in the esophagus, after controlling the neck of the diverticulum and after myotomy. A linear stapler is placed across the neck of the diverticulum and the diverticulum is excised distal to the staple line. The security of this staple line and effectiveness of the myotomy may be tested before hospital discharge with a water soluble contrast esophagogram. Postoperative complications include fistula formation, abscess, hematoma, recurrent nerve paralysis, difficulties in phonation, and Horner syndrome. The incidence of the first two can be reduced by performing a diverticulopexy rather than diverticulectomy. (See Schwartz 10th ed., p. 989.)

30. Which of the following disorders involves simultaneous nonperistaltic contractions of the esophagus?
    A. Achalasia
    B. Diffuse esophageal spasm (DES)
    C. Hypertensive lower esophageal sphincter
    D. Nutcracker esophagus

Answer: B

The classic manometric findings in these patients are characterized by the frequent occurrence of simultaneous waveforms and multipeaked esophageal contractions, which may be of abnormally high amplitude or long duration (Table 25-1). Key to the diagnosis of diffuse esophageal spasm (DES) is that there remain some peristaltic waveforms in excess of those seen in achalasia. A criterion of 30% or more peristaltic waveforms out of 10 wet swallows has been used to differentiate DES from vigorous achalasia. However, this figure is arbitrary and often debated.

The LES in patients with DES usually shows a normal resting pressure and relaxation on swallowing. A hypertensive sphincter with poor relaxation may also be present. In patients with advanced disease, the radiographic appearance of tertiary contractions appears helical, and has been termed corkscrew esophagus or pseudodiverticulosis. Patients with segmental or DES can compartmentalize the esophagus and develop an epiphrenic or midesophageal diverticulum between two areas of high pressure occurring simultaneously. (See Schwartz 10th ed., Table 25-9, pp. 991–992.)

TABLE 25-1	Manometric characteristics of the primary esophageal motility disorders

Achalasia

Incomplete lower esophageal sphincter (LES) relaxation (<75% relaxation)

Aperistalsis in the esophageal body

Elevated LES pressure ≤26 mmHg

Increased intraesophageal baseline pressures relative to gastric baseline

Diffuse Esophageal Spasm (DES)

Simultaneous (nonperistaltic contractions) (>20% of wet swallows)

Repetitive and multipeaked contractions

Spontaneous contractions

Intermittent normal peristalsis

Contractions may be of increased amplitude and duration

Nutcracker Esophagus

Mean peristaltic amplitude (10 wet swallows) in distal esophagus ≥180 mmHg

Increased mean duration of contractions (>7.0 s)

Normal peristaltic sequence

Hypertensive Lower Esophageal Sphincter

Elevated LES pressure (≥26 mmHg)

Normal LES relaxation

Normal peristalsis in the esophageal body

Ineffective Esophageal Motility Disorders

Decreased or absent amplitude of esophageal peristalsis (<30 mmHg)

Increased number of nontransmitted contractions

Source: Reproduced with permission from DeMeester TR, et al.: Physiologic diagnostic studies, in Zuidema GD, Orringer MB, (eds): *Shackelford's Surgery of the Alimentary Tract*, 3rd ed, Vol. I. Philadelphia: W.B. Saunders, 1991, p. 115. Copyright Elsevier.

CHAPTER 26

Stomach

1. The consistently largest artery to the stomach is the
   A. Right gastric
   B. Left gastric
   C. Right gastroepiploic
   D. Left gastroepiploic

Answer: B

The consistently largest artery to the stomach is the left gastric artery, which usually arises directly from the celiac trunk and divides into an ascending and descending branch along the lesser gastric curvature. Approximately 20% of the time, the left gastric artery supplies an aberrant vessel that travels in the gastrohepatic ligament (lesser omentum) to the left side of the liver. Rarely, this is the only arterial blood supply to this part of the liver, and inadvertent ligation may lead to clinically significant hepatic ischemia in this unusual circumstance. (See Schwartz 10th ed., p. 1037.)

2. Which of the following inhibits gastrin secretion?
   A. Histamine
   B. Acetylcholine
   C. Amino acids
   D. Acid

Answer: D

Luminal peptides and amino acids are the most potent stimulants of gastrin release, and luminal acid is the most potent inhibitor of gastrin secretion. The latter effect is predominantly mediated in a paracrine fashion by somatostatin released from antral D cells. Gastrin-stimulated acid secretion is significantly blocked by H_2 antagonists, suggesting that the principal mediator of gastrin-stimulated acid production is histamine from mucosal enterochromaffin-like (ECL) cells. Acetylcholine released by the vagus nerve leads to stimulation of ECL cells, which in turn produce histamine. (See Schwartz 10th ed., p. 1045.)

3. *Helicobacter pylori* infection primarily mediates duodenal ulcer pathogenesis via
   A. Antral alkalinization leading to inhibition of somatostatin release
   B. Direct stimulation of gastrin release
   C. Local inflammation with autoimmune response
   D. Upregulation of parietal cell acid production

Answer: A

Helicobacter pylori possess the enzyme urease, which converts urea into ammonia and bicarbonate, thus creating an environment around the bacteria that buffers the acid secreted by the stomach. *H. pylori* infection is associated with decreased levels of somatostatin, decreased somatostatin messenger RNA production, and fewer somatostatin-producing D cells. These effects are probably mediated by *H. pylori*-induced local alkalinization of the antrum (antral acidification is the most potent antagonist to antral gastrin secretion), and *H. pylori*-mediated increases in other local mediators and cytokines. The result is hypergastrinemia and acid hypersecretion, presumably leading to the parietal cell hyperplasia seen in many patients with duodenal ulcer. Other mechanisms whereby *H. pylori* can induce gastroduodenal mucosal injury include the production of toxins (vacA and cagA), local elaboration of cytokines (particularly interleukin-8) by infected mucosa, recruitment of inflammatory cells and release of inflammatory mediators, recruitment and activation of local immune factors, and increased apoptosis. (See Schwartz 10th ed., pp. 1054–1055.)

4. The effect of erythromycin on gastric emptying is through its function as a
   A. Dopamine antagonist
   B. Cholinergic agonist
   C. Motilin agonist
   D. Cholinergic antagonist

Answer: C
Erythromycin is a common prokinetic agent used to treat delayed gastric empting, and works as a motilin agonist. Domperidone and metoclopramide, two other commonly used medications, function as dopamine antagonists (Table 26-1). (See Schwartz 10th ed., Table 26-4, p. 1050.)

TABLE 26-1	Drugs that accelerate gastric emptying	
Agent	**Typical Adult Dose**	**Mechanism of Action**
Metoclopramide	10 mg PO qid	Dopamine antagonist
Erythromycin	250 mg PO qid	Motilin agonist
Domperidone	10 mg PO qid	Dopamine antagonist

5. Which of the following is secreted by gastric parietal cells?
   A. Pepsinogen
   B. Intrinsic factor
   C. Gastrin-releasing peptide
   D. Ghrelin
   E. Histamine

Answer: B
Activated parietal cells secrete intrinsic factor in addition to hydrochloric acid. Presumably the stimulants are similar, but acid secretion and intrinsic factor secretion may not be linked. Intrinsic factor binds to luminal vitamin B_{12}, and the complex is absorbed in the terminal ileum via mucosal receptors. Vitamin B_{12} deficiency can be life-threatening, and patients with total gastrectomy or pernicious anemia require B_{12} supplementation by a nonenteric route. (See Schwartz 10th ed., p. 1044.)

6. The most accurate diagnostic test for Zollinger-Ellison syndrome (ZES) is
   A. Fasting serum gastrin
   B. Computed tomography (CT) scan
   C. Endoscopy
   D. Secretin stimulation test

Answer: D
All patients with gastrinoma have an elevated gastrin level, and hypergastrinemia in the presence of elevated basal acid output (BAO) strongly suggests gastrinoma. Patients with gastrinoma usually have a BAO >15 mEq/h or >5 mEq/h if they have had a previous procedure for peptic ulcer. Acid secretory medications should be held for several days before gastrin measurement, because acid suppression may falsely elevate gastrin levels. Causes of hypergastrinemia can be divided into those associated with hyperacidity and those associated with hypoacidity (Fig. 26-1). The diagnosis of Zollinger-Ellison syndrome (ZES) is confirmed by the secretin stimulation test. An intravenous (IV) bolus of secretin (2 U/kg) is given and gastrin levels are checked before and after injection. An increase in serum gastrin of 200 pg/mL or greater suggests the presence of gastrinoma. Patients with gastrinoma should have serum calcium and parathyroid hormone levels determined to rule out multiple endocrine neoplasia type 1 (MEN1) and, if present, parathyroidectomy should be considered before resection of gastrinoma. (See Schwartz 10th ed., Figure 26-46, p. 1072.)

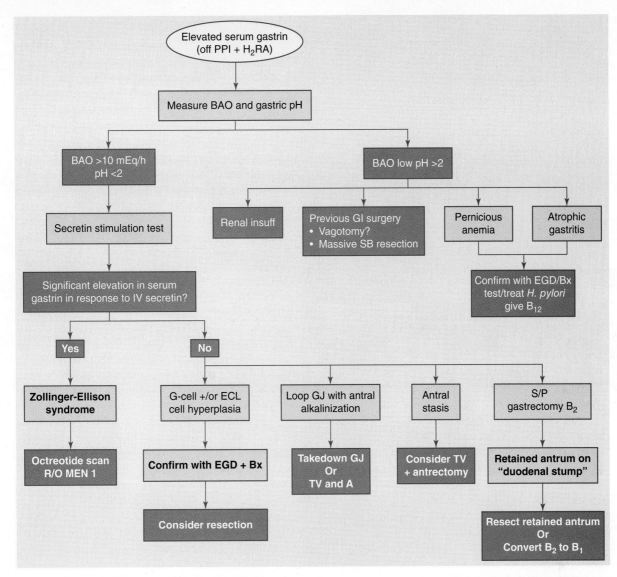

FIG. 26-1. Algorithm for diagnosis and management of hypergastrinemia. B_1 = Billroth I; B_2 = Billroth II; BAO = basal acid output; Bx = biopsy; ECL = enterochromaffin-like; EGD = esophagogastroduodenoscopy; GJ = gastrojejunostomy; H_2RA = histamine 2 receptor antagonist; insuff = insufficiency; MEN1 = multiple endocrine neoplasia type 1; PPI = proton pump inhibitor; R/O = rule out; SB = small bowel; S/P = status post; TV = truncal vagotomy; TV and A = truncal vagotomy and antrectomy.

7. Which of the following is the preoperative imaging study of choice for gastrinoma?
   A. CT scan
   B. Magnetic resonance imaging (MRI)
   C. Endoscopic ultrasound (EUS)
   D. Angiographic localization
   E. Somatostatin receptor scintigraphy

Answer: E

CT will detect most lesions >1cm in size and magnetic resonance imaging (MRI) is comparable. Endoscopic ultrasound (EUS) is more sensitive than these other noninvasive imaging tests, but it still misses many of the smaller lesions, and may confuse normal lymph nodes for gastrinomas. Currently, the preoperative imaging study of choice for gastrinoma is somatostatin-receptor scintigraphy (the octreotide scan). When the pretest probability of gastrinoma is high, the sensitivity and specificity of this modality approach 100%. Gastrinoma cells contain type II somatostatin receptors that bind the indium-labeled somatostatin analogue (octreotide) with high affinity, making imaging with a gamma camera possible. Currently, angiographic localization studies are infrequently performed for gastrinoma. (See Schwartz 10th ed., pp.1072–1073.)

8. Patients taking nonsteroidal anti-inflammatory drugs (NSAIDs) or aspirin need concomitant acid suppressing medication if which of the following is present?
   A. Age over 50
   B. Heavy smoking history
   C. Concurrent steroid intake
   D. Heavy alcohol consumption

Answer: C

The overall risk of significant serious adverse gastrointestinal (GI) events in patients taking nonsteroidal anti-inflammatory drugs (NSAIDs) is more than three times that of controls (Table 26-2). This risk increases to five times in patients older than 60 years. Factors that clearly put patients at increased risk for NSAID-induced GI complications include age >60, prior GI event, high NSAID dose, concurrent steroid intake, and concurrent anticoagulant intake. Alcohol is commonly mentioned as a risk factor for peptic ulcer disease (PUD), but confirmatory data are lacking. High doses of H_2 blockers have been shown to be less effective than proton pump inhibitors (PPIs) in preventing GI complications in these high risk patients on antiplatelet therapy, but clearly they are better than no acid suppression. (See Schwartz 10th ed., Table 26-6, p. 1058.)

TABLE 26-2   Hospitalization rates for GI events with and without NSAID use in selected large populations

Study[a]	Therapies Used		Clinical Upper GI Events[c]		Complicated Upper GI Events[d]	
	NSAID Control	Study Drugs	Control	Study Drug	Control	Study Drug
MUCOSA	NSAIDs (n = 4439)	Misoprostol 200 μg qid + NSAID (n = 4404)	3.1%	1.6%	1.5%	0.7%
CLASS	Ibuprofen 800 mg tid, diclofenac 75 mg bid (n = 3987)	Celecoxib 400 mg bid (n = 3995)	3.5%	2.1%	1.5%	0.8%
			(No aspirin[e]: 2.9%)	1.4%	1.3%	0.4%
VIGOR	Naproxen 500 mg bid (n = 4047)	Rofecoxib 50 mg qd (n = 4029)	4.5%	2.1%	1.4%	0.6%

[a]MUCOSA and VIGOR trials included only rheumatoid arthritis patients; CLASS trial included osteoarthritis (73%) and rheumatoid arthritis (27%).
[b]Incidence for MUCOSA trial represents doubling of results provided at 6 months (although median follow-up was <6 months). Incidences for VIGOR and CLASS trials represent rates per 100 patient-years, although VIGOR median follow-up was 9 months and CLASS data include only the first 6 months of the study.
[c]Includes perforations, obstructions, bleeding, and uncomplicated ulcers discovered on clinically indicated work-up.
[d]Includes perforation, obstruction, bleeding (documented due to ulcer or erosions in MUCOSA and CLASS; major bleeding in VIGOR).
[e]21% of patients in CLASS study were taking low-dose aspirin.
Note: All differences between controls and study drugs were significant except clinical upper GI events in overall CLASS study (P = .09).
Source: Reproduced with permission from Laine L. Approaches to nonsteroidal anti-inflammatory drug use in the high-risk patient. *Gastroenterology* 120:594, 2001. Copyright Elsevier.

9. The optimal initial management of a patient hospitalized for a bleeding peptic ulcer is
   A. Ulcer oversew
   B. Vagotomy and pyloroplasty
   C. Distal gastrectomy
   D. Intravenous PPIs

Answer: D

The management of bleeding peptic ulcer is summarized in the algorithm in Fig. 26-2. All patients admitted to hospital with bleeding peptic ulcer should be adequately resuscitated and started on continuous IV PPI. Seventy-five percent of patients will stop bleeding with these measures alone, but 25% will continue to bleed or will rebleed in hospital. Among the high risk group, endoscopic hemostatic therapy is indicated and usually successful. Only then should surgical intervention be considered, with indications including massive hemorrhage unresponsive to endoscopic control and transfusion requirement of more than four to six units of blood, despite attempts at endoscopic control. Long-term maintenance PPI therapy should be considered in all patients admitted to hospital with ulcer complications. (See Schwartz 10th ed., Figure 26-42, pp. 1061, 1064–1065, and 1069.)

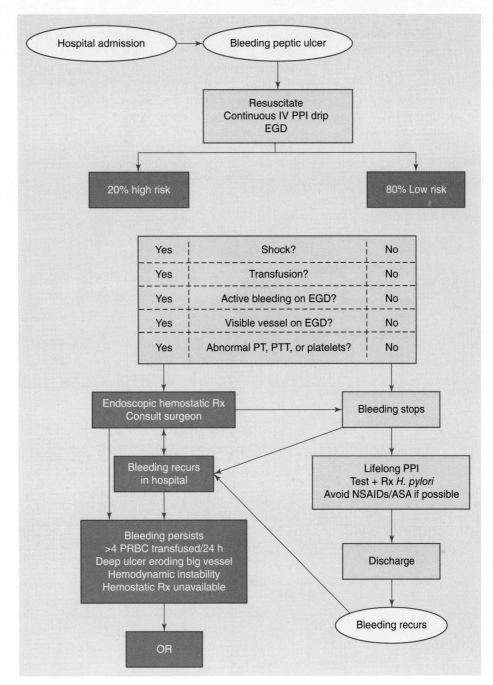

FIG. 26-2. Algorithm for the treatment of bleeding peptic ulcer. ASA = acetylsalicylic acid; EGD = esophagogastroduodenoscopy; IV = intravenous; OR = operating room; PPI = proton pump inhibitor; PRBC = unit of packed red blood cells; PT = prothrombin time; PTT = partial thromboplastin time; Rx = treatment.

10. Which of the following options is the least preferable reconstruction for patients undergoing antrectomy for PUD?
    A. Billroth I.
    B. Billroth II.
    C. Roux-en-Y gastrojejunostomy.
    D. All are equally preferable.

Answer: C
Following antrectomy, GI continuity may be reestablished with a Billroth I gastroduodenostomy or a Billroth II loop gastrojejunostomy. Since antrectomy routinely leaves a 60 to 70% gastric remnant, routine reconstruction as a Roux-en-Y gastrojejunostomy should be avoided. Although the Roux-en-Y operation is an excellent procedure for keeping duodenal contents out of the stomach and esophagus, in the presence of a large gastric remnant, this reconstruction will predispose to marginal ulceration and/or gastric stasis. (See Schwartz 10th ed., p. 1063.)

11. A 55-year-old executive who is seen because of severe epigastric pain is found on esophagogastroduodenoscopy to have a large ulcer in the duodenal bulb and tests positive for *H. pylori*. He is treated for *H. pylori* and instructed to quit smoking, but his symptoms persist and he is referred to you for further management. At this time, it would be most appropriate to recommend
    A. NSAID cessation and urea breath test
    B. Highly selective vagotomy
    C. Truncal vagotomy and antrectomy
    D. Truncal vagotomy and pyloroplasty

Answer: A

The indications for surgery in PUD are bleeding, perforation, obstruction, and intractability or nonhealing. Intractability should be an unusual indication for peptic ulcer operation nowadays. The patient referred for surgical evaluation because of intractable PUD should raise red flags for the surgeon: maybe the patient has a missed cancer, is noncompliant, or has *Helicobacter* despite the presence of a negative test or previous treatment (differential for intractability, Table 26-3). In this setting, the patient with persistent symptoms despite appropriate treatment requires further evaluation before any consideration of operative treatment. If surgery is necessary, a lesser operation may be preferable. (See Schwartz 10th ed., Table 26-13, pp. 1059 and 1069–1071.)

TABLE 26-3	Differential diagnosis of intractability or nonhealing peptic ulcer disease
Cancer	
Gastric	
Pancreatic	
Duodenal	
Persistent *H. pylori* infection	
Tests may be false-negative	
Consider empiric treatment	
Noncompliant patient	
Failure to take prescribed medication	
Surreptitious use of NSAIDs	
Motility disorder	
Zollinger-Ellison syndrome	

12. Which blood group is associated with an increased risk of gastric cancer?
    A. A
    B. B
    C. AB
    D. O

Answer: A

Gastric cancer is more common in patients with pernicious anemia, blood group A, or a family history of gastric cancer. When patients migrate from a high-incidence region to a low-incidence region, the risk of gastric cancer decreases in the subsequent generations born in the new region. This strongly suggests an environmental influence on the development of gastric cancer. Environmental factors appear to be more related etiologically to the intestinal form of gastric cancer than the more aggressive diffuse form. The commonly accepted risk factors for gastric cancer are listed in Table 26-4. (See Schwartz 10th ed., Table 26-15, pp. 1074–1075.)

TABLE 26-4	Factors increasing or decreasing the risk of gastric cancer
Increase risk	
Family history	
Diet (high in nitrates, salt, fat)	
Familial polyposis	
Gastric adenomas	
Hereditary nonpolyposis colorectal cancer	
H. pylori infection	
Atrophic gastritis, intestinal metaplasia, dysplasia	
Previous gastrectomy or gastrojejunostomy (>10 years ago)	
Tobacco use	
Ménétrier's disease	
Decrease risk	
Aspirin	
Diet (high fresh fruit and vegetable intake)	
Vitamin C	

13. A subtotal gastrectomy with D2 dissection performed for Stage 3 gastric adenocarcinoma in the antrum includes
    A. Grossly negative margins of 2 cm
    B. More than 15 lymph nodes removed
    C. Billroth II reconstruction
    D. Splenectomy

Answer: B

Surgical resection is the only curative treatment for gastric cancer and most patients with clinically resectable locoregional disease should have gastric resection. The standard operation for gastric cancer is radical subtotal gastrectomy, which entails ligation of the left and right gastric and gastroepiploic arteries at the origin, as well as the en bloc removal of the distal 75% of the stomach, including the pylorus and 2 cm of duodenum, the greater and lesser omentum, and all associated lymphatic tissue. Generally, the surgeon strives for a grossly negative margin of at least 5 cm. More than 15 resected lymph nodes are required for adequate staging, even in the low-risk patient. The operation is deemed an adequate cancer operation provided that tumor-free margins are obtained, >15 lymph nodes are removed, and all gross tumor is resected. In the absence of involvement by direct extension, the spleen and pancreatic tail are not removed. Reconstruction is usually by Billroth I gastrojejunostomy or Roux-en-Y reconstruction. (See Schwartz 10th ed., p. 1081.)

14. The standard treatment for an isolated 3 cm gastrointestinal stromal tumor (GIST) in the body of the stomach is
    A. Imatinib
    B. Endoscopic ablation
    C. Wedge resection
    D. Subtotal gastrectomy

Answer: C

Gastrointestinal stromal tumors (GISTs) are submucosal tumors that are slow growing, and arise from interstitial cells of Cajal (ICC). Prognosis in patients with GISTs depends mostly on tumor size and mitotic count, and metastasis, when it occurs, is typically by the hematogenous route. Any lesion >1cm can behave in a malignant fashion and may recur. Thus, all GISTs are best resected along with a margin of normal tissue—wedge resection with clear margins is adequate surgical treatment. True invasion of adjacent structures by the primary tumor is evidence of malignancy. If safe, en bloc resection of involved surrounding organs is appropriate to remove all tumor when the primary is large and invasive. Five-year survival following resection for GIST is about 50%. Most patients with low-grade lesions are cured (80% 5-year survival), but most patients with high-grade lesions are not (30% 5-year survival). Imatinib, a chemotherapeutic agent that blocks the activity of the tyrosine kinase product of c-kit, yields excellent results in many patients with metastatic or unresectable GIST, and is also recommended in high risk groups as an adjuvant therapy. Fig. 26-3 shows an algorithm for treatment of patients with GIST (See Schwartz 10th ed., Figure 26-59, pp. 1085–1086.)

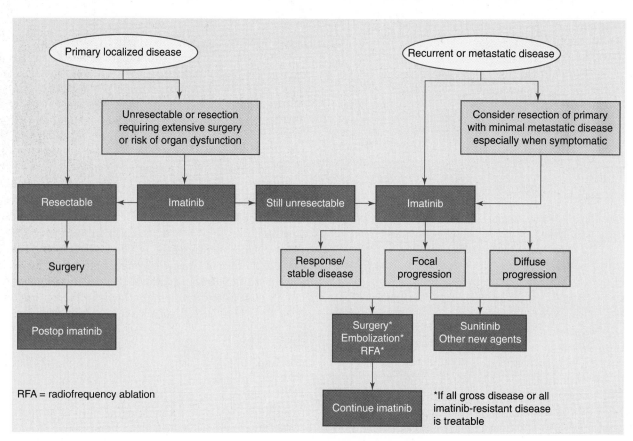

FIG. 26-3. Algorithm for the treatment of gastrointestinal stromal tumor. (Reproduced with permission from Gold JS, DeMatteo RP, Combined surgical and molecular therapy: *The gastrointestinal stromal tumor model*. Ann Surg 244:176, 2006.)

15. Which of the following options is the best management of a low-grade gastric lymphoma of the gastric antrum?
    A. *H. pylori* eradication
    B. Chemotherapy ± radiation therapy
    C. Wedge resection
    D. Antrectomy

Answer: A

Low-grade mucosa-associated lymphoid tissue (MALT) lymphoma, essentially a monoclonal proliferation of B cells, presumably arises from a background of chronic gastritis associated with *H. pylori*. These relatively innocuous tumors then undergo degeneration to high-grade lymphoma, which is the usual variety seen by the surgeon. Remarkably, when the *H. pylori* are eradicated and the gastritis improves, the low-grade MALT lymphoma often disappears. Thus, low-grade MALT lymphoma is not a surgical lesion. An algorithm for gastric lymphoma treatment is found in Fig. 26-4. (See Schwartz 10th ed., Figure 26-58, pp. 1084–1085.)

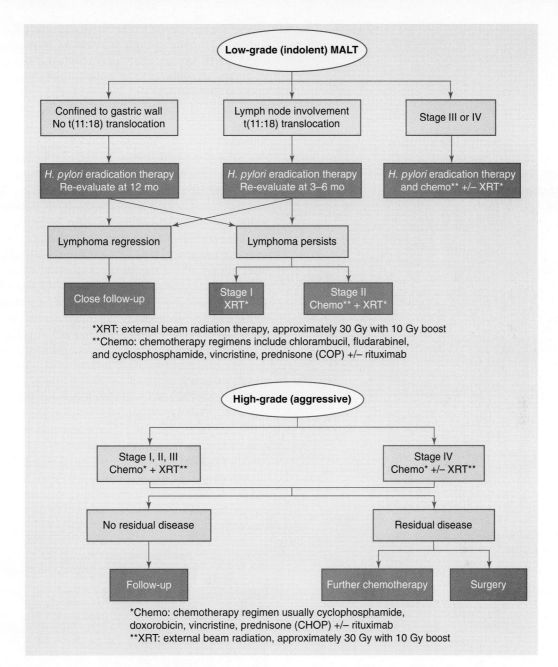

FIG. 26-4. Algorithm for the treatment of gastric lymphoma. MALT = mucosa-associated lymphoid tissue. (Reproduced with permission from Yoon SS, Coit DG, Portlock CS, et al, *The diminishing role of surgery in the treatment of gastric lymphoma.* Ann Surg 240:28, 2004.)

16. Type III gastric carcinoid tumors
    A. Often do not require resection
    B. Are associated with hypergastrinemia
    C. Are sporadic lesions
    D. Have better outcomes than type I and II tumors

Answer: C

Type III gastric carcinoids are sporadic tumors, most often solitary (usually >2 cm), occur more commonly in men, and behave more aggressively than types I and II. Unlike types 1 and II, they are not associated with hypergastrinemia. Type I gastric carcinoids are the most common type of gastric carcinoid, and occur in patients with chronic hypergastrinemia secondary to pernicious anemia or chronic atrophic gastritis. Type II is rare, and is associated with MEN1 and ZES. Gastric carcinoids should all be resected, and small lesions (<2 cm) confined to the mucosa may be treated endoscopically with endoscopic mucosal resection (EMR) if there are only a few lesions (<5) and if margins are histologically negative. Locally invasive lesions, or those >2 cm, should be removed by radical gastric resection and lymphadenectomy. Survival is excellent for node-negative patients (>90% 5-year survival); node-positive patients have

17. Watermelon stomach is best treated by
   A. Acid-reducing agents
   B. Beta blockers
   C. Antrectomy
   D. Total gastrectomy

a 50% 5-year survival. The 5-year survival for patients with type I gastric carcinoid is close to 100%; for patients with type III lesions, the 5-year survival is less than 50%. Most type III patients have nodal or distant metastases at the time of diagnosis, and some present with symptoms of carcinoid syndrome. (See Schwartz 10th ed., p. 1086.)

Answer: C
The parallel red stripes atop the mucosal folds of the distal stomach give this rare entity its name. Histologically, gastric antral vascular ectasia (GAVE) is characterized by dilated mucosal blood vessels that often contain thrombi, in the lamina propria. Mucosal fibromuscular hyperplasia and hyalinization often are present (Fig. 26-5). The histologic appearance can resemble portal hypertensive gastropathy, but the latter usually affects the proximal stomach, whereas watermelon stomach predominantly affects the distal stomach.

Beta blockers and nitrates, useful in the treatment of portal hypertensive gastropathy, are ineffective in patients with gastric antral vascular ectasia. Patients with GAVE are usually elderly women with chronic GI blood loss requiring transfusion. Most have an associated autoimmune connective tissue disorder, and at least 25% have chronic liver disease. Nonsurgical treatment options include estrogen and progesterone, and endoscopic treatment with the neodymium yttrium-aluminum garnet (Nd:YAG) laser or argon plasma coagulator. Antrectomy may be required to control blood loss, and this operation is quite effective but carries increased morbidity in this elderly patient group. Patients with portal hypertension and antral vascular ectasia should be considered for transjugular intrahepatic portosystemic shunt (TIPSS). (See Schwartz 10th ed., Figure 26-61, pp. 1088–1089.)

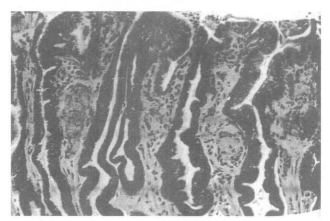

FIG. 26-5. Gastric antral vascular ectasia (watermelon stomach). (Reproduced with permission from Goldman H. Mucosal hypertrophy and hyperplasia of the stomach, in Ming S-C, Goldman H, eds. *Pathology of the Gastrointestinal Tract,* 2nd ed. Baltimore: Williams & Wilkins; 1998, p. 548.)

18. Treatment for severe early dumping after gastrectomy that is persistent despite an antidumping diet and fiber is
    A. Expectant management
    B. Oral glucose for symptoms
    C. Octreotide
    D. Surgical conversion to a Roux-en-Y drainage

Answer: C

Dumping is a phenomenon consisting of a constellation of postprandial symptoms thought to be the result of the abrupt delivery of a hyperosmolar load into the small bowel due to ablation of the pylorus or decreased gastric compliance. Early dumping occurs 15 to 30 minutes after a meal, with patients becoming diaphoretic, weak, light-headed, and tachycardic. Late dumping occurs hours later, and is due to a reactive hypoglycemia. Late dumping is relieved by the administration of sugar. The medical therapy for the dumping syndrome consists of dietary management and somatostatin analogue (octreotide). Often, symptoms improve if the patient avoids liquids during meals. Hyperosmolar liquids (eg, milk shakes) may be particularly troublesome. There is some evidence that adding dietary fiber compounds at mealtime may improve the syndrome. If dietary manipulation fails, the patient is started on octreotide, 100 µg subcutaneously twice daily. This can be increased up to 500 µg twice daily if necessary. The long-acting depot octreotide preparation is useful. Octreotide not only ameliorates the abnormal hormonal pattern seen in patients with dumping symptoms, but also promotes restoration of a fasting motility pattern in the small intestine (ie, restoration of the migrating motor complex [MMC]). Only a very small percentage of patients with dumping symptoms ultimately require surgery. Therefore, the surgeon should not rush to re-operate on the patient with dumping syndromes. (See Schwartz 10th ed., p. 1091.)

19. Ménétrier disease is characterized by
    A. Hypertrophic gastric folds and hypoproteinemia
    B. A tortuous submucosal congenital arteriovenous malformation
    C. Gastric antral vascular ectasia
    D. Epithelial hyperplasia and hypergastrinemia

Answer: A

There are two clinical syndromes characterized by epithelial hyperplasia and giant gastric folds: ZES and Ménétrier disease. The latter is characteristically associated with protein-losing gastropathy and hypochlorhydria. A few patients with these unusual diseases have been successfully treated with the epidermal growth factor receptor blocking monoclonal antibody cetuximab. There may be an increased risk of gastric cancer with this disease, and gastric resection may be indicated for bleeding, severe hypoproteinemia, or cancer. The other options describe Dieulafoy lesions, watermelon stomach, and ZES, respectively. (See Schwartz 10th ed., p. 1088.)

CHAPTER 27

The Surgical Management of Obesity

1. What body mass index (BMI or weight(kg)/height [m²]) definition of obesity serves as the standard indication for bariatric surgery when medical therapy has failed and comorbid conditions exist?
   A. Overweight (BMI 25.0–29.9)
   B. Class I obesity (BMI 30.0–34.9)
   C. Class II obesity (BMI 35.0–39.9)
   D. Class III obesity (BMI 40.0 and greater)

2. Which of the following bariatric procedures is primarily intended to induce weight loss through malabsorption of ingested nutrients?
   A. Adjustable gastric band
   B. Sleeve gastrectomy
   C. Roux-en-Y gastric bypass (RYGB)
   D. Duodenal switch

3. Complications of adjustable gastric banding which have diminished its popularity as a bariatric procedure include all of the following EXCEPT
   A. Mortality risk
   B. Slippage of the band
   C. Failure to lose weight
   D. Port and tubing complications

4. Early postoperative complications after a RYGB procedure include all of the following EXCEPT
   A. Anastomotic leak from a staple line
   B. Dilation of the distal gastric remnant
   C. Pulmonary embolus
   D. Hyperglycemia

Answer: C
A 1991 NIH Consensus Conference recommended that bariatric surgery was indicated for a body mass index (BMI) of 35.0–39.9 when medical therapy has failed and comorbid conditions exist. When no comorbid conditions exist, a BMI of 40 or greater is required. This standard continues to be used by insurers, although recent studies have shown benefit in lower BMI groups. (See Schwartz 10th ed., p. 1100.)

Answer: D
Bariatric procedures are classified as restrictive, malabsorptive, or a combination of restrictive and malabsorptive in the mechanism of weight loss that they induce. Restrictive operations include adjustable gastric band and gastric sleeve, malabsorptive operations include duodenal switch and biliopancreatic diversion, and combined restrictive and malabsorptive procedures include the Roux-en-Y gastric bypass (RYGB). (See Schwartz 10th ed., p. 1103.)

Answer: A
The adjustable gastric band procedure, usually performed laparoscopically, has the lowest cost and mortality risk of all the bariatric procedures, but is the least effective for weight loss. In addition, slippage and erosion of the band and complications related to the maintenance and use of the port for adjusting the size of the band contribute to its loss of popularity. (See Schwartz 10th ed., p. 1112.)

Answer: D
Early postoperative complications after RYGB include anastomotic leak from a staple line, gastric remnant dilation due to downstream obstruction, intra-abdominal bleeding, and pulmonary complications such as atelectasis and pulmonary embolus. Diabetes, if present, usually improves promptly after RYGB and hyperglycemia is unlikely to be problematic. (See Schwartz 10th ed., pp. 1116–1117.)

5. Small bowel obstruction after RYGB should be treated as an urgent surgical emergency because
   A. It is frequently due to an incarcerated internal hernia which can progress to bowel necrosis and perforation.
   B. Abdominal distension risks disruption of suture lines.
   C. Signs and symptoms of peritonitis, such as pain, fever, and leukocytosis, are usually masked in the obese.
   D. Nasogastric intubation will not decompress the distal gastric remnant.

Answer: A
Small bowel obstruction after RYGB is frequently due to an incarcerated internal hernia at the location of the closure, or lack thereof, of the mesenteric defect. This can progress rapidly to strangulation and necrosis of the bowel with subsequent perforation. Adverse outcomes with this complication have resulted in the uniform recommendation that small bowel obstruction in this setting should be regarded as a surgical emergency. Abdominal distention and difficulties with nasogastric intubation are not relevant concerns. (See Schwartz 10th ed., p. 1117.)

6. In addition to weight loss, the benefits of RYGB include all of the following EXCEPT
   A. Reduced long-term mortality.
   B. Resolution of type 2 diabetes mellitus.
   C. Resolution of sleep apnea.
   D. Resolution of craving for sweets.

Answer: D
The long-term benefits of RYGB include a high incidence of resolution of the comorbidities of obesity, such as type 2 diabetes and sleep apnea, and a reduced mortality risk due to these and other illnesses. The success of the operation is dependent upon the patient's success in adopting a healthy eating habit, despite continued cravings for snacks and sweets. (See Schwartz 10th ed., p. 1116.)

7. The gastric sleeve procedure originated as part of what operation?
   A. Esophageal resection
   B. Billroth I gastrectomy
   C. Duodenal switch
   D. Resection of the gastric cardia

Answer: C
The first stage of the duodenal switch procedure is creation of a gastric sleeve. This is intended to promote weight loss in morbidly obese candidates whose massive obesity creates an unacceptable risk of perioperative complications of a prolonged procedure. The gastric sleeve portion of the procedure was seen to be so effective that the second stage of the duodenal switch was sometimes postponed indefinitely, and the gastric sleeve became a treatment option alone. (See Schwartz 10th ed., p. 1121.)

8. In addition to the effects of weight loss, the resolution of type 2 diabetes mellitus after the gastric sleeve procedure and RYGB is thought to be contributed to by
   A. Reduced ghrelin production
   B. Increased secretion of glucagon-like peptide-1 (GLP-1)
   C. Appetite suppression
   D. All of the above

Answer: D
Gastrectomy removes much of the ghrelin-producing portion of the stomach, and is thought to contribute to weight loss after both gastric sleeve and RYGB procedures. GLP-1, the enteric hormone which augments insulin release, is dramatically increased after RYGB, and is increased after gastric sleeve as well. A profound suppression of appetite and food craving has been found to follow these procedures, presumably due to the altered hormonal status of peptides which affect the satiety centers of the central nervous system. (See Schwartz 10th ed., p. 1125.)

9. Adolescent patients with morbid obesity are increasingly being referred for consideration of bariatric procedures due to failure of medical management and the risks associated with a lifetime of obesity. What nutritional deficiencies require life-long treatment after RYGB, the most common procedure performed in this age group?
   A. Pernicious anemia due to vitamin B$_{12}$ deficiency
   B. Iron deficiency anemia
   C. Deficiencies of vitamins A, E, D, and K
   D. All of the above

Answer: D
Loss of intrinsic factor produced in the gastric fundus, impaired iron absorption, and a deficiency of the fat-soluble vitamins present life-long risks after RYGB and other malabsorptive bariatric procedures. Vitamin replacement and nutritional monitoring are therefore mandatory in bariatric patients. (See Schwartz 10th ed., p. 1120.)

10. The gastric sleeve procedure and RYGB result in similar degrees of resolution of all of the following EXCEPT
    A. Gastroesophageal reflux disease (GERD)
    B. Hypertension
    C. Type 2 diabetes mellitus
    D. Obstructive sleep apnea

Answer: A

The resolution of obesity-related comorbidities after gastric sleeve procedures is nearly equivalent to that seen after RYGB, with the exception of the resolution of gastroesophageal reflux disease (GERD). Whereas more than 90% of RYGB patients report relief of GERD, some studies show an increase in GERD symptoms after gastric sleeve surgery. (See Schwartz 10th ed., p. 1128.)

CHAPTER 28

Small Intestine

1. Where is the largest number of hormone-producing cells found in the body?
   A. The pituitary
   B. The small intestine
   C. The pancreas
   D. The liver

Answer: B
The small intestine is the body's largest reservoir of hormone-producing cells. Multiple specialized cells within the intestinal mucosa respond to luminal stimuli and secrete over 30 peptide hormones which regulate the functions of the intestine, other organs in the gastro-entero-pancreato-biliary system, the heart, and the brain (See Schwartz 10th ed., p. 1145.)

2. Which of the following features is characteristic of the ileum, as opposed to the jejunum?
   A. The presence of valvulae conniventes
   B. The presence of Peyer patches
   C. Larger vasa recta
   D. Less fatty mesentery

Answer: B
The entire small intestine contains valvulae conniventes, also known as *plicae circularis*. The jejunum has larger vasa recta, a larger diameter, and a less fatty mesentery. The ileum contains prominent lymphoid follicles called *Peyer patches*. (See Schwartz 10th ed., p. 1138.)

3. Within the intestine, epithelial cells originate from stem cells, proliferate in the crypts, and migrate up the villus in 2 to 5 days. This process replaces cells that are removed due to apoptosis or exfoliation. This rapid turnover makes the small intestine susceptible to
   A. Radiation damage
   B. Starvation
   C. Exogenous steroids
   D. Hypothermia

Answer: A
The high cellular turnover rate of enterocytes makes the small intestine susceptible to damage by inhibitors of proliferation such as radiation and cytotoxic chemotherapy. (See Schwartz 10th ed., p. 1138.)

4. A pocket- or sock-like outpouching on the anti-mesenteric side of the distal ileum, called a *Meckel diverticulum*, is caused by
   A. Excessive traction on the intestine during childbirth.
   B. Increased intraluminal pressure.
   C. A persistent vitelline duct.
   D. A mutation of the *c-Mec* gene.

Answer: C
The embryonic gut communicates with the yolk sac by mean of the vitelline duct. Failure of this structure to obliterate by the end of gestation can result in a Meckel diverticulum. (See Schwartz 10th ed., p. 1139.)

5. How much fluid normally enters the adult small intestine each day?
   A. 2 L
   B. 4 L
   C. 6 L
   D. 8 L

Answer: D
Eight to nine liters of fluid enters the small intestine daily, of which over 80% is absorbed. This includes 2 L from oral intake, 1.5 L of saliva, 2.5 L of gastric juice, 1.5 L of biliopancreatic secretions, and 1 L of fluid secreted by the small intestine. (See Schwartz 10th ed., p. 1140.)

6. How are the digestion products of carbohydrates, such as glucose, galactose, and fructose, absorbed through the intestine?
   A. By passive diffusion across enterocyte plasma membranes.
   B. By facilitated diffusion via specific transporters such as sodium-glucose cotransporter 1 (SGLT1), glucose transporter 2 (GLUT2), and glucose transporter 5 (GLUT5).
   C. By endocytosis of enterocytes on the villus.
   D. By facilitated diffusion through tight junctions between enterocytes.

Answer: B
The three terminal products of carbohydrate digestion are transported through the enterocyte brush border membrane via facilitative transporter proteins such as the sodium-glucose cotransporter 1 (SGLT1), glucose transporter 2 (GLUT2), and glucose transporter 5 (GLUT5). There is evidence of overexpression of these transporters, particularly SGLT1, in diabetes and obesity, and new therapeutic approaches for these conditions are designed to inhibit these transporters. (See Schwartz 10th ed., p. 1141.)

7. What does the "enterohepatic circulation" refer to?
   A. The superior mesenteric-portal venous circuit.
   B. The secretion of cholesterol in the bile and its reabsorption in the distal ileum.
   C. The secretion of bile acids by the liver and their reabsorption in the distal ileum.
   D. The secretion of cholecystokinin by the jejunum and its stimulation of bile flow.

Answer: C
Bile acids act as detergents which increase the solubility of lipid micelles which are taken up by the brush border membrane of the jejunum, where over 90% of fat is absorbed. The bile acids themselves remain in the intestinal lumen and are reabsorbed in the distal ileum where they enter the portal venous circulation and are re-secreted in the bile. (See Schwartz 10th ed., p. 1143.)

8. The secretin-glucagon family of gut hormones includes all of the following structurally related peptides EXCEPT
   A. Somatostatin (SST)
   B. Glucose-dependent insulinotropic polypeptide (GIP)
   C. Glucagon-like peptide-1 (GLP-1)
   D. Vasoactive intestinal polypeptide (VIP)

Answer: A
Peptide hormones produced by enteroendocrine cells of the intestine are grouped into families based on their amino acid structural similarity. The secretin-glucagon family of hormones includes glucose-dependent insulinotropic polypeptide (GIP), glucagon-like peptide-1 (GLP-1), vasoactive intestinal polypeptide (VIP), peptide histidine isoleucine (PHI), growth hormone-releasing hormone (GHRH), and pituitary adenylyl cyclase-activating peptide (PACAP). (See Schwartz 10th ed., p. 1145.)

9. The most common cause of small bowel obstruction is
   A. Incarcerated hernia
   B. Crohn's disease
   C. Malignancy
   D. Postoperative adhesions

Answer: D
Intra-abdominal adhesions related to prior abdominal surgery accounts for 75% of cases of small bowel obstruction. Cancer-related small bowel obstruction is almost always due to extrinsic compression or entrapment of the bowel by a primary or metastatic tumor; primary small bowel malignancies are rare. (See Schwartz 10th ed., p. 1146.)

10. A closed-loop obstruction is particularly dangerous because
    A. Intraluminal pressure rises high enough to cause ischemia and necrosis.
    B. The obstruction is painless.
    C. Bacterial overgrowth results in sepsis.
    D. The obstructive segment is not apparent on imaging studies.

Answer: A
A closed-loop obstruction, in which an intestinal segment is obstructed both proximally and distally, as in a volvulus, is particularly dangerous because intraluminal pressure rises quickly and can cause venous congestion and arterial obstruction which leads to necrosis of the intestinal wall and perforation. It classically presents with "pain out of proportion to the physical exam," and is usually apparent on CT scan which frequently shows a U-shaped or C-shaped dilated bowel loop associated with a radial distribution of mesenteric vessels converging toward a torsion point. (See Schwartz 10th ed., p. 1147.)

11. Therapy of a small bowel obstruction usually consists of prompt surgical correction. In patients with no evidence of closed-loop obstruction, and in whom there is no fever or leukocytosis or tachycardia, a period of careful observation with nasogastric decompression may be successful in all of the following conditions EXCEPT
A. Partial small bowel obstruction.
B. Obstruction in the early postoperative period.
C. Obstruction due to Crohn disease.
D. Obstruction due to an internal hernia.

Answer: D

Partial small bowel obstruction and early postoperative obstruction can mimic ileus, and may respond to nonoperative therapy. Crohn disease usually responds to medical therapy, although recurrent obstruction is an indication for surgical correction. Obstruction due to an internal hernia requires prompt surgical intervention to avoid strangulation and necrosis. (See Schwartz 10th ed., p. 1149.)

12. Interventions which may reduce the incidence and duration of postoperative ileus include all of the following EXCEPT
A. Epidural analgesia
B. A μ-opioid receptor antagonist
C. Intravenous erythromycin
D. Avoiding excess intra- and postoperative fluid administration

Answer: C

Epidural analgesia (with reduced systemic narcotic administration), avoiding excess intra- and postoperative fluid administration, and administration of alvimopan, a mu-opioid receptor antagonist, have all been associated with reduced incidence and/or duration of postoperative ileus. Prokinetic agents such as metoclopramide and erythromycin are rarely useful. (See Schwartz 10th ed., p. 1153.)

13. Risk factors for the development of Crohn's disease include all of the following EXCEPT
A. Having a family member with Crohn's disease
B. Smoking
C. Having Chinese ancestry
D. Having Ashkenazi Jewish ancestry

Answer: C

The risk of having Crohn's disease is two- to fourfold higher in Ashkenazi Jewish families, 15 times higher in family members of a patient with Crohn's disease, and is increased in higher socioeconomic groups, and among smokers. The incidence in China is 1% of the incidence in the United States, although this number is increasing. (See Schwartz 10th ed., p. 1153.)

14. The primary genetic defect associated with Crohn's disease is a mutation of the *NOD2* gene on chromosome 16. This gene encodes for a protein product which
A. Mediates the innate immune response to microbial pathogens
B. Activates stellate cells to produce collagen
C. Regulates the rate of crypt-to-villus enterocyte migration
D. Mediates the production of enterocyte alkaline phosphatase

Answer: A

The protein product of the *NOD2* gene mediates the innate immune response to microbial pathogens. A variety of defects in immune regulatory mechanisms such as overresponsiveness of mucosal T cells to enteric flora-derived antigens can lead to defective immune tolerance and sustained inflammation. (See Schwartz 10th ed., p. 1153.)

15. In the resection of a stenotic area of intestine in a patient with Crohn's disease, the best approach is
A. A resection margin of 2 cm from gross disease.
B. A resection margin of 12 cm from gross disease.
C. A resection margin 2 cm from microscopic disease on frozen section.
D. A resection margin 12 cm from microscopic disease on frozen section.

Answer: A

There are no differences in the recurrence rates for resection with a 2-cm margin or a 12-cm margin from gross disease. The additional bowel lost may contribute to eventual short gut syndrome in a patient who requires multiple resections, so minimizing bowel loss is a priority. There is no benefit to achieving frozen section negative margins in the resection of Crohn's strictures; positive margin resections have the same recurrence rate as negative margin resections. The effort to obtain a frozen section negative margin carries the risk of removing more intestine than is necessary. (See Schwartz 10th ed., p. 1157.)

16. The failure of an enterocutaneous fistula to heal on a regimen of total parenteral nutrition and antisecretory therapy may be due to which of the following?
A. A foreign body in the fistula tract.
B. Epithelialization of the fistula tract.
C. Downstream obstruction of the fistulized segment of intestine.
D. All of the above.

Answer: D

Factors which prevent healing of an enterocutaneous fistula include foreign body, epithelialization of the fistula tract, downstream obstruction, radiation enteritis, associated infection (abscess or sepsis), malignancy, and a short (<2 cm) fistula tract. (See Schwartz 10th ed., p. 1158.)

17. Which primary malignancy of the small intestine is most common?
    A. Adenocarcinoma of the duodenum
    B. Carcinoid tumor of the ileum
    C. Lymphoma of the jejunum
    D. Gastrointestinal stromal tumor (GIST) of the duodenum

Answer: A

Adenocarcinomas of the duodenum are the most common primary small bowel malignancy and account for 35 to 50% of the total. Lymphoma and gastrointestinal stromal tumors (GISTs) of the small bowel are the least common and each accounts for 10 to 15% of the total. (See Schwartz 10th ed., p. 1159.)

18. Adenocarcinoma of the duodenum is associated with what hereditary oncologic syndrome?
    A. Hereditary nonpolyposis colorectal cancer (HNPCC)
    B. Familial adenomatous polyposis (FAP)
    C. Peutz-Jeghers syndrome
    D. Von Hippel-Lindau (VHL) syndrome

Answer: B

Duodenal carcinoma is a late manifestation of the familial adenomatous polyposis (FAP) syndrome. After resolution of the colonic disease by total colectomy, patients with FAP must be followed with periodic upper gastrointestinal (GI) endoscopy to maintain surveillance for duodenal tumors. Duodenal cancer is the leading cause of death among patients with FAP. (See Schwartz 10th ed., p. 1158.)

19. Which of the following statements is true regarding GISTs?
    A. Most occur in the small intestine.
    B. GISTs are usually metastatic when first diagnosed.
    C. GISTs typically present with GI hemorrhage.
    D. GISTs are usually responsive to cytotoxic chemotherapy.

Answer: C

GISTs are a form of sarcoma which occur most commonly (70%) in the stomach. They more frequently present with GI hemorrhage than other small bowel malignancies. They are usually refractory to conventional cytotoxic chemotherapy, but are not usually metastatic on initial diagnosis. A radical lymphadenectomy is not usually required; a segmental resection of the involved portion of the small intestine is usually sufficient surgical treatment. (See Schwartz 10th ed., p. 1162.)

20. Methods to prevent radiation enteritis of the small bowel during pelvic irradiation for gynecologic or rectal malignancy include which of the following?
    A. Tilt table positioning in Trendelenburg position during radiation therapy treatments.
    B. Closure (reapproximation) of the pelvic peritoneum after primary resection.
    C. Placement of an absorbable mesh sling to suspend small intestine out of the pelvis during postoperative radiation therapy.
    D. All of the above.

Answer: D

In addition to limiting radiation exposure to less than 5000 cGy, avoiding radiation to the small intestine after pelvic surgery can involve steep Trendelenburg positioning during radiation therapy sessions, closure of the pelvic peritoneum at the level of the sacral promontory to prevent small bowel filling the pelvis, and creating of an absorbable mesh sling to prevent the small intestine from filling the pelvic cavity. (See Schwartz 10th ed., p. 1163.)

21. What ectopic tissue is commonly found in a Meckel diverticulum?
    A. Gastric mucosa
    B. Ectopic pancreas
    C. Splenic follicles
    D. Ovarian follicles

Answer: A

Approximately 60% of Meckel diverticula contain ectopic tissue, of which over 60% consists of gastric mucosa. Pancreatic acini are next most common, followed by pancreatic islets, endometriosis, and hepatobiliary tissues. Gastric mucosa can ulcerate and bleed, the etiology of which can be hard to determine unless the Meckel diverticulum is known. (See Schwartz 10th ed., pp. 1163–1164).

22. A patient with recent onset of ascites after an episode of acute pancreatitis undergoes paracentesis, which reveals cloudy white fluid. What therapy is indicated?
    A. Surgical exploration
    B. Low-fat diet
    C. Total parenteral nutrition (TPN) and octreotide
    D. Octreotide and weekly paracentesis

Answer: C

Chylous ascites can develop as a complication of operative procedures or inflammatory conditions such as acute pancreatitis. Lymphatic drainage from damaged lymphatics can heal when the patient is made NPO, and maintained on TPN and octreotide. Medium-chain triglycerides have been advocated as an oral diet, but temporary cessation of oral feeding and octreotide comprise the most successful therapy. (See Schwartz 10th ed., pp. 1169–1170.)

23. Short bowel syndrome has been arbitrarily defined in adults as having a small intestine of less than what length?
    A. 300 cm
    B. 200 cm
    C. 100 cm
    D. 50 cm

Answer: B
A functional definition, in which insufficient absorptive capacity results in diarrhea, dehydration, and malnutrition is more appropriate, but a standard definition of short bowel syndrome of 200 cm has been used widely. (See Schwartz 10th ed., p. 1171.)

24. Common causes of short bowel syndrome include all of the following EXCEPT
    A. Mesenteric ischemia
    B. Malignancy
    C. Crohn's disease
    D. Radiation enteritis

Answer: D
In adults, the common etiologies of short bowel syndrome include mesenteric ischemia, malignancy, and Crohn's disease. In pediatric patients, common causes include intestinal atresias, volvulus, and necrotizing enterocolitis. Radiation enteritis usually involves isolated segments of small bowel of less than 50% of total small intestinal length. (See Schwartz 10th ed., p. 1171.)

25. After an emergency operation for bowel infarction in which more than half of the small intestine was removed and a jejunostomy created, high volume ostomy losses cause recurrent dehydration. Management of this condition includes which of the following?
    A. Proton pump inhibitors or histamine-2 receptor antagonists
    B. Octreotide
    C. Loperamide
    D. All of the above

Answer: D
Reducing gastric secretion with proton pump inhibitors or histamine-2 receptor antagonist, reducing gastroenteropancreatic secretions with octreotide, and inhibiting motility with agents such as loperamide or diphenoxylate, are useful approaches to prevent dehydration as the short gut adapts to its new length. Total parenteral nutrition is also often required. (See Schwartz 10th ed., p. 1171.)

Colon, Rectum, and Anus

1. A 74-year-old man with biopsy-proven rectal adenocarcinoma is undergoing a low anterior resection. Which layers must be stapled through when resecting the distal portion of resection specimen?
   A. Mucosa, submucosa, circular muscle layer, longitudinal muscle layer, and serosa
   B. Mucosa, submucosa, longitudinal muscle layer, circular muscle layer, and serosa
   C. Mucosa, submucosa, longitudinal muscle layer, and circular muscle layer
   D. Mucosa, submucosa, circular muscle layer, and serosa

   Answer: C
   The wall of the colon and rectum are made of five separate layers: mucosa, submucosa, circular muscle layer, longitudinal muscle layer, and serosa. The mid and lower rectum lack serosa so this layer would not be stapled through if the surgeon were stapling through the mid or lower rectum. (See Schwartz 10th ed., p. 1176.)

2. Which layer of muscle joins together to form the internal anal sphincter?
   A. Circumferential muscle layer
   B. Longitudinal muscle layer
   C. Puborectalis muscle
   D. Circular muscle layer

   Answer: A
   The inner circular muscle joins to form the internal anal sphincter. The subcutaneous, superficial, and deep external sphincter surrounds it. The deep external anal sphincter is an extension of the puborectalis muscle. (See Schwartz 10th ed., p. 1176.)

3. A 24-year-old woman with medically refractory ulcerative colitis decides to undergo a total colectomy. During this procedure, where would it be most appropriate to look for the inferior mesenteric vein in order to ligate it?
   A. Look for the inferior mesenteric artery; the veins of the colon usually parallel with the corresponding arteries.
   B. The inferior mesenteric artery can be ligated within the peritoneum, where it joins with the superior mesenteric artery.
   C. The inferior mesenteric vein is often ligated at the inferior edge of the pancreas, just below where it joins with the splenic vein.
   D. The inferior mesenteric vein will not be ligated for this procedure.

   Answer: C
   The inferior mesenteric vein does not run with the inferior mesenteric artery. Instead, it travels cranially in the retroperitoneum over the psoas and then posterior to the pancreas to join the splenic vein. The vein is often ligated at the inferior edge of the pancreas during a colectomy. (See Schwartz 10th ed., p. 1177.)

4. An anatomy class is dissecting out the rectum. What are the correct fascial arrangements that they will encounter during this dissection?
    A. The presacral fascia separates the rectum from the presacral venous plexus and the pelvic nerves; Waldeyer fascia extends forward and downward and attaches to the fascia propria at the anorectal junction. Denonvilliers fascia separates the rectum from the prostate and seminal vesicles in men and from the vagina in women.
    B. The presacral fascia extends forward and downward and attaches to the fascia propria at the anorectal junction; Waldeyer fascia separates the rectum from the prostate and seminal vesicles in men and from the vagina in women; Denonvilliers fascia separates the rectum from the presacral venous plexus and the pelvic nerves.
    C. The presacral fascia separates the rectum from the prostate and seminal vesicles in men and from the vagina in women; Waldeyer fascia extends forward and downward and attaches to the fascia propria at the anorectal junction; Denonvilliers fascia separates the rectum from the presacral venous plexus and the pelvic nerves.
    D. The presacral fascia separates the rectum from the prostate and seminal vesicles in men and from the vagina in women; Waldeyer fascia extends backward and downward and attaches to the fascia propria at the anorectal junction; Denonvilliers fascia separates the rectum from the presacral venous plexus and the pelvic nerves.

Answer: A

The *presacral fascia* separates the rectum from the presacral venous plexus and the pelvic nerves. The rectosacral fascia (*Waldeyer fascia*) extends forward and downward and attaches to the fascia propria at the anorectal junction. Anteriorly, *Denonvilliers fascia* separates the rectum from the prostate and seminal vesicles in men and from the vagina in women. (See Schwartz 10th ed., p. 1177.)

5. Choose the correct definition of intestinal malrotation
    A. At the 4th week of gestation the midgut herniates through the abdominal cavity, rotates 270° clockwise around the superior mesenteric artery and then travels to its resting place in the abdomen during the 10th week.
    B. At the 4th week of gestation the midgut herniates through the abdominal cavity, rotates 270° counterclockwise around the superior mesenteric artery and then travels to its resting place in the abdomen during the 12th week.
    C. At the 6th week of gestation the midgut herniates through the abdominal cavity, rotates 270° clockwise around the superior mesenteric artery and then travels to its resting place in the abdomen during the 12th week.
    D. At the 6th week of gestation the midgut herniates through the abdominal cavity, rotates 270° counterclockwise around the superior mesenteric artery and then travels to its resting place in the abdomen during the 10th week.

Answer: D

During the 6th week of gestation, the midgut herniates out of the abdominal cavity and rotates 270° counterclockwise around the superior mesenteric artery and travels to its resting position in the 10th week of gestation. Failure of the midgut to rotate and return to the abdominal cavity during the 10th week of gestation results in intestinal malrotation. (See Schwartz 10th ed., pp. 1175, 1179.)

6. A 62-year-old man has perforated diverticulitis and undergoes an emergent left hemicolectomy with a diverting loop ileostomy. If he has a high output ileostomy and is at risk of diversion colitis, which fatty acids are not being absorbed?
   A. Butyric acid and propionic acid
   B. Propionic acid and palmitic acid
   C. Tricosic acid and butyric acid
   D. Lauric acid and palmitic acid

Answer: A
Short-chain fatty acids (acetic acid, butyric acid, and propionic acid) are produced by bacterial fermentation of dietary carbohydrates and are an important source of energy for the colonic mucosa, and metabolism by colonocytes provides energy for processes such as active transport of sodium. Diversion of feces by an ileostomy or colostomy can result in "diversion colitis" which is associated with mucosal atrophy and inflammation. (See Schwartz 10th ed., p. 1179.)

7. A 58-year-old mother of 10 suffers from fecal incontinence. Usually, defecation occurs by increased intra-abdominal pressure via the Valsalva maneuver, increased rectal contraction, and relaxation of the puborectalis muscle, which forms a "sling" around the distal rectum, forming a relatively acute angle that distributes intra-abdominal forces onto the pelvic floor. With defecation, this angle straightens, allowing downward force to be applied along the axis of the rectum and anal, and opening of the anal canal. A dysfunction at which point of this pathway can lead to fecal incontinence?
   A. Injury to the puborectalis.
   B. Decreased rectal contraction.
   C. Repair of the internal or external sphincter during delivery.
   D. Hypertrophic internal and external anal sphincters.

Answer: A
Defecation proceeds by coordination of increasing intra-abdominal pressure via the Valsalva maneuver, increased rectal contraction, relaxation of the puborectalis muscle, and opening of the anal canal. Impaired continence may result from poor rectal compliance, injury to the internal and/or external sphincter or puborectalis, or nerve damage or neuropathy. (See Schwartz 10th ed., p. 1180.)

8. A healthy 48-year-old physician with no family history of cancer and who strictly adheres to a high protein, high fiber diet, exercises five times per week for 50 minutes, and takes vitamin C supplements daily performs a fecal occult blood test (FOBT) on herself and tests positive. Should she have any further colon screening?
   A. No, vitamin C can produce a false-positive result.
   B. Yes, all positive FOBT requires further investigation with a colonoscopy.
   C. Yes, all positive FOBT requires further investigation with FOBT in 1 year.
   D. No, she has no risk factors for colon cancer and should follow the USPSTF screening guidelines for colorectal cancer.

Answer: B
Fecal occult blood test (FOBT) has been a nonspecific test for peroxidase contained in hemoglobin; consequently, occult bleeding from any gastrointestinal source will produce a positive result. Similarly, many foods (red meat, some fruits and vegetables, and vitamin C) will produce a false-positive result. Any positive FOBT mandates further investigation, usually by colonoscopy. (See Schwartz 10th ed., p. 1182.)

9. A 22-year-old college student presents to clinic with a history of intermittent diarrhea for the past 5 days after returning from Mexico. On further questioning, she has had previous episodes of diarrhea for the past 2 years, unrelated to travel. After a physical examination, what are appropriate tests that should be ordered to appropriately work up this patient?
   A. Stool wet-mount and stool culture.
   B. Sigmoidoscopy and colonoscopy, but only if no peritoneal signs on physical examination.
   C. Add Sudan red to stool sample.
   D. All of the above.

Answer: D
Stool wet-mount and culture can often diagnose infection. Sigmoidoscopy or colonoscopy can be helpful in diagnosing inflammatory bowel disease or ischemia. However, if the patient has abdominal tenderness, particularly with peritoneal signs, or any other evidence of perforation, endoscopy is contraindicated. For chronic diarrhea tests for malabsorption and metabolic investigations should be conducted along with colonoscopy. Biopsies should be taken even if the colonic mucosa appears grossly normal. (See Schwartz 10th ed., p. 1184.)

10. A 76-year-old man undergoes an emergent sigmoidectomy for a perforated colon mass. The surgeon performs a Hartmann procedure and brings up a colostomy. In an emergency setting, where is the most appropriate location to seat a colostomy?
    A. Above the beltline, within the rectus abdominus muscle, away from the costal margin
    B. Below the beltline, within the rectus abdominus muscle, near the iliac crest
    C. Above the beltline, within the rectus abdominus muscle, near the costal margin
    D. Below the beltline, within the rectus abdominus muscle, away from the iliac crest

Answer: A
In an emergency operation, like this one, where the stoma site has not been marked, an attempt should be made to place a stoma within the rectus muscle and away from both the costal margin and iliac crest. In emergencies, placement high on the abdominal wall is preferred to a low-lying site. (See Schwartz 10th ed., p. 1192.)

11. A previously healthy 46-year-old woman with a history of rectal adenocarcinoma, first discovered on colonoscopy 1 year ago who is status post low anterior resection with a diverting loop ileostomy returns to clinic 3 months after her low anterior resection for a preoperative appointment for her ileostomy reversal. Over the past 3 months she has had good ileostomy output as well as occasional loose stools per rectum. What workup does she need to have prior to ileostomy reversal?
    A. A digital rectal examination to palpate the anastomosis and check for patency.
    B. No examination is needed as this was a simple diversion and she has continued to pass stool per rectum.
    C. A flexible sigmoidoscopy or contrast enema to check for patency.
    D. A colonoscopy to evaluate for polyps not previously seen on previous colonoscopy.

Answer: C
A flexible endoscopic examination and a contrast enema (Gastrografin) are recommended prior to closure to ensure that the anastomosis has not leaked and is patent. (See Schwartz 10th ed., p. 1193.)

12. A 75-year-old woman undergoes a right hemicolectomy and end ileostomy for right-sided perforated diverticulitis. What is the most concerning adverse outcome in the short term of this procedure and will require revision?
    A. Skin breakdown caused by succus entericus.
    B. Stoma necrosis above the level of the fascia.
    C. Stoma necrosis below the level of the fascia.
    D. Stomal retraction below the level of the fascia.

Answer: C
Stoma necrosis may occur in the early postoperative period and is usually caused by skeletonizing the distal small bowel and/or creating an overly tight fascial defect. Limited mucosal necrosis above the fascia may be treated expectantly, but necrosis below the level of the fascia requires surgical revision. Stoma retraction may occur early or late and may be exacerbated by obesity. Local revision may be necessary. (See Schwartz 10th ed., p. 1193.)

13. A 19-year-old man with medically refractor ulcerative colitis undergoes a total colectomy with J-pouch creation. What are some of the late complications of ileal pouch-anal reconstruction?
    A. More than eight bowel movements per day
    B. Nocturnal incontinence
    C. Pouchitis
    D. Small bowel obstruction
    E. All of the above

Answer: E
The functional outcome of ileal pouch-anal reconstruction is not always perfect. Patients should be counseled to expect 8 to 10 bowel movements per day. Up to 50% have some degree of nocturnal incontinence. Pouchitis occurs in nearly 50% of patients who undergo the operation for chronic ulcerative colitis, and small bowel obstruction is common. Pouches fail in 5 to 10% of patients. (See Schwartz 10th ed., p. 1194.)

14. A 50-year-old woman who underwent a total colectomy with ileal pouch-anal reconstruction 5 years ago presents to the emergency room with diarrhea, fever, 2 weeks of malaise, and severe abdominal pain. What is the most appropriate differential diagnosis?
    A. Parasitic infection, ulcerative colitis of the remaining rectal cuff, undiagnosed Crohn disease.
    B. Bacterial or viral infection, undiagnosed Crohn disease, and pouchitis.
    C. Rectal cancer of remaining rectal cuff, bacterial or viral infection, and undiagnosed Crohn disease.
    D. Parasitic infection, bacterial or viral infection, and pouchitis.

Answer: B
This patient is likely presenting with pouchitis. Pouchitis is an inflammatory condition that affects both ileoanal pouches and continent ileostomy reservoirs. The incidence of pouchitis ranges from 30 to 55%. Symptoms include increased diarrhea, hematochezia, abdominal pain, fever, and malaise. Diagnosis is made endoscopically with biopsies. Differential diagnosis includes infection and undiagnosed Crohn disease. (See Schwartz 10th ed., p. 1194.)

15. A 68-year-old man is undergoing a right hemicolectomy for a cecal mass. He asks what the current research has shown about decreasing postoperative infection after this procedure. When should antibiotics always be used for this procedure?
    A. Oral antibiotics should be used in combination with bowel preparation.
    B. Parenteral antibiotic prophylaxis at the time of surgery after the skin incision is made and redosed as needed during the procedure.
    C. Parenteral antibiotic prophylaxis at the time of surgery before the skin incision is made.
    D. Oral antibiotics should be used postoperatively to decrease risk of anastomosis leak.

Answer: C
Prospective randomized trials are needed to better understand the role of oral antibiotic prophylaxis in colorectal surgery. In contrast, long-standing, convincing data support the efficacy of parenteral antibiotic prophylaxis at the time of surgery. Broad-spectrum parenteral antibiotic(s) with activity against aerobic and anaerobic enteric pathogens should be administered just prior to the skin incision and redosed as needed depending on the length of the operation. There is no proven benefit to using antibiotics postoperatively after an uncomplicated colectomy. (See Schwartz 10th ed., p. 1194.)

16. A 22-year-old woman presents to the clinic with a 3-year history of bloody diarrhea, abdominal pain, and anorectal fistulas. Her father had similar symptoms during his 20's and has had multiple abdominal surgeries. What is the percentage of patients with this disease who have family members with the same disease?
    A. 5–10%
    B. 10–20%
    C. 10–30%
    D. 20–40%

Answer: C
Family history may play a role in inflammatory bowel disease as 10 to 30% of patients with inflammatory bowel disease report a family member with the same disease. (See Schwartz 10th ed., p. 1195.)

17. A 25-year-old man is undergoing workup to determine if he has ulcerative colitis, Crohn disease, or indeterminate colitis. What diagnostic findings would indicate that he has Crohn disease?
    A. Atrophic mucosa, crypt abscesses, inflammatory pseudopolyps, scarred and shortened colon, continuous involvement of rectum and colon.
    B. Mucosal ulcerations, noncaseating granulomas, fibrosis, strictures, and fistulas in the colon with deep serpiginous ulcers.
    C. Atrophic mucosa, noncaseating granulomas, strictures, "cobblestone" appearance on endoscopy.
    D. Mucosal ulcerations, crypt abscesses, inflammatory pseudopolyps, continuous involvement of colon and rectum.

Answer: B
Ulcerative colitis is a mucosal process in which the colonic mucosa and submucosa are infiltrated with inflammatory cells. The mucosa may be atrophic, and crypt abscesses are common. Endoscopically, the mucosa is frequently friable and may possess multiple inflammatory pseudopolyps. In long-standing ulcerative colitis, the colon may be foreshortened and the mucosa replaced by scar. A key feature of ulcerative colitis is the continuous involvement of the rectum and colon; rectal sparing or skip lesions suggest a diagnosis of Crohn disease. Crohn disease is a transmural inflammatory process that can affect any part of the gastrointestinal tract from mouth to anus. Mucosal ulcerations, an inflammatory cell infiltrate, and noncaseating granulomas are characteristic pathologic findings. Chronic inflammation may ultimately result in fibrosis, strictures, and fistulas in either the colon or small intestine. The endoscopic appearance of Crohn colitis is characterized by deep serpiginous ulcers and a "cobblestone" appearance. (See Schwartz 10th ed., p. 1195.)

230

18. What structures are most likely to be site of extracolonic disease in inflammatory bowel disease?
    A. Liver, biliary tree, joints, skin, eyes
    B. Biliary tree, lungs, heart, spleen
    C. Joints, skin, biliary tree, bladder
    D. Skin, liver, pancreas, joints, eyes

Answer: A

The liver is a common site of extracolonic disease in inflammatory bowel disease. Fatty infiltration of the liver is present in 40 to 50% of patients, and cirrhosis is found in 2 to 5%. Primary sclerosing cholangitis is a progressive disease characterized by intra- and extrahepatic bile duct strictures. Forty to 60% of patients with primary sclerosing cholangitis have ulcerative colitis. Pericholangitis is also associated with inflammatory bowel disease and may be diagnosed with a liver biopsy. Bile duct carcinoma is a rare complication of long-standing inflammatory bowel disease. Arthritis also is a common extracolonic manifestation of inflammatory bowel disease, and the incidence is 20 times greater than in the general population. Erythema nodosum is seen in 5 to 15% of patients with inflammatory bowel disease and usually coincides with clinical disease activity. Pyoderma gangrenosum is an uncommon but serious condition that occurs almost exclusively in patients with inflammatory bowel disease. Up to 10% of patients with inflammatory bowel disease will develop ocular lesions. These include uveitis, iritis, episcleritis, and conjunctivitis. (See Schwartz 10th ed., p. 1196.)

19. An 18-year-old woman is undergoing workup to determine if she has ulcerative colitis, Crohn disease, or indeterminate colitis. What diagnostic findings would indicate that she has ulcerative colitis?
    A. Atrophic mucosa, crypt abscesses, inflammatory pseudopolyps, scarred and shortened colon, continuous involvement of rectum and colon.
    B. Mucosal ulcerations, noncaseating granulomas, fibrosis, strictures, and fistulas in the colon with deep serpiginous ulcers.
    C. Atrophic mucosa, noncaseating granulomas, strictures, "cobblestone" appearance on endoscopy.
    D. Mucosal ulcerations, crypt abscesses, inflammatory pseudopolyps, continuous involvement of colon and rectum.

Answer: A

Ulcerative colitis is a mucosal process in which the colonic mucosa and submucosa are infiltrated with inflammatory cells. The mucosa may be atrophic, and crypt abscesses are common. Endoscopically, the mucosa is frequently friable and may possess multiple inflammatory pseudopolyps. In long-standing ulcerative colitis, the colon may be foreshortened and the mucosa replaced by scar. A key feature of ulcerative colitis is the continuous involvement of the rectum and colon; rectal sparing or skip lesions suggest a diagnosis of Crohn disease. Crohn disease is a transmural inflammatory process that can affect any part of the gastrointestinal tract from mouth to anus. Mucosal ulcerations, an inflammatory cell infiltrate, and noncaseating granulomas are characteristic pathologic findings. Chronic inflammation may ultimately result in fibrosis, strictures, and fistulas in either the colon or small intestine. The endoscopic appearance of Crohn colitis is characterized by deep serpiginous ulcers and a "cobblestone" appearance. (See Schwartz 10th ed., p. 1195.)

20. The goals of medical therapy for inflammatory bowel disease are to decrease inflammation and alleviate symptoms. Mild to moderate flares are treated in the clinic and more severe symptoms may require hospitalization. What is the first-line therapy for inflammatory bowel disease in the outpatient setting?
    A. Salicylates, such as sulfasalazine and 5-acetyl salicylic acid
    B. Antibiotics, such as metronidazole and fluoroquinolones
    C. Corticosteroids
    D. Azathioprine and 6-mercaptopurine

Answer: A

Sulfasalazine (Azulfidine), 5-acetyl salicylic acid (5-ASA), and related compounds are first-line agents in the medical treatment of mild to moderate inflammatory bowel disease. These compounds decrease inflammation by inhibition of cyclooxygenase and 5-lipoxygenase in the gut mucosa. They require direct contact with affected mucosa for efficacy. Multiple preparations are available for administration to different sites in the small intestine and colon. Antibiotics are often used to decrease the intraluminal bacterial load in Crohn disease. Metronidazole has been reported to improve Crohn colitis and perianal disease, but the evidence is weak. Fluoroquinolones may also be effective in some cases. In the absence of fulminant colitis or toxic megacolon, antibiotics are not used to treat ulcerative colitis. Corticosteroids (either oral or parenteral) are a key component of treatment for an acute exacerbation of either ulcerative colitis or Crohn disease.

Corticosteroids are nonspecific inhibitors of the immune system, and 75 to 90% of patients will improve with the administration of these drugs. Azathioprine and 6-mercatopurine (6-MP) are antimetabolite drugs that interfere with nucleic acid synthesis and thus decrease proliferation of inflammatory cells. These agents are useful for treating ulcerative colitis and Crohn disease in patients who have failed salicylate therapy or who are dependent on, or refractory to, corticosteroids. (See Schwartz 10th ed., p. 1196.)

21. A thin and ill appearing 26-year-old man presents to the emergency department (ED) with fevers, chills, severe abdominal pain, and a rigid abdomen. While doing a history and physical, it is noted that he has a history of ulcerative colitis. What would be indications that stoma creation would be more appropriate than a primary anastomosis in this patient?
    A. Long-standing history of ulcerative colitis with multiple colon polyps.
    B. A prealbumin of 6.0 in a patient who has been on corticosteroids.
    C. A blood glucose level of 300 in a patient who finished a corticosteroid course 3 weeks ago.
    D. Diarrhea more than 10 times per day for months with albumin of 3.6.

Answer: B
Patients with inflammatory bowel disease are often malnourished. Abdominal pain and obstructive symptoms may decrease oral intake. Diarrhea can cause significant protein loss. Ongoing inflammation produces a catabolic physiologic state. Parenteral nutrition should be strongly considered early in the course of therapy for either Crohn disease or ulcerative colitis. The nutritional status of the patient also should be considered when planning operative intervention, and nutritional parameters such as serum albumin, prealbumin, and transferrin should be assessed. In extremely malnourished patients, especially those who are also being treated with corticosteroids, creation of a stoma is often safer than a primary anastomosis. (See Schwartz 10th ed., p. 1197.)

22. A 24-year-old woman presents to the ED with fever, severe abdominal pain with guarding on palpation, and a history of 5 days of bloody stools. She has a history of ulcerative colitis. What are the indications for emergency surgery for ulcerative colitis?
    A. Hemorrhage with continued decrease in hematocrit levels in spite of blood transfusion.
    B. Hemodynamic instability requiring transfer to the ICU with decline in status over a 48-hour period after admission.
    C. Severe abdominal pain and diarrhea that does not respond to bowel rest, hydration, and parenteral corticosteroids.
    D. Cecum measured at 9 cm in diameter on computed tomography (CT) scan.
    E. All of the above.

Answer: E
Emergency surgery is required for patients with massive life-threatening *hemorrhage, toxic megacolon,* or *fulminant colitis* who fail to respond rapidly to medical therapy. Patients with signs and symptoms of fulminant colitis should be treated aggressively with bowel rest, hydration, broad-spectrum antibiotics, and parenteral corticosteroids. Colonoscopy and barium enema are contraindicated, and antidiarrheal agents should be avoided. Deterioration in clinical condition or failure to improve within 24 to 48 hours mandates surgery. (See Schwartz 10th ed., p. 1197.)

23. A 55-year-old woman with a history of long-standing Crohn disease presents to the clinic with a 1-month history of abdominal pain and a new area of induration, fluctuance, and foul-smelling drainage from a former midline incision. What are the most common indications for surgery for Crohn disease?
    A. Internal fistula or abscess
    B. Obstruction
    C. Toxic megacolon
    D. Strictures

Answer: A
The most common indications for surgery are *internal fistula or abscess* (30–38% of patients) and *obstruction* (35–37% of patients). Crohn disease of the large intestine may present as *fulminant colitis* or *toxic megacolon*. In this setting, treatment is identical to treatment of fulminant colitis and toxic megacolon secondary to ulcerative colitis. Resuscitation and medical therapy with bowel rest, broad-spectrum antibiotics, and parenteral corticosteroids should be instituted. If the patient's condition worsens or fails to rapidly improve, total abdominal colectomy with end ileostomy is recommended. (See Schwartz 10th ed., p. 1199.)

24. A 23-year-old man presents to the clinic with severe pain on defecation that began 2 months ago. He has tried conservative management at home with sitz baths but his pain has become so severe that he has started to restrict how much he eats to prevent having bowel movements. On rectal examination, a fissure is found. What would indicate that this fissure from Crohn disease?
    A. Deep and broad ulcer located in the lateral position.
    B. Shallow and broad ulcer located in the anterior position.
    C. Deep and narrow ulcer located in the posterior midline position.
    D. Shallow and narrow ulcer located in the lateral position.

Answer: A

The most common perianal lesions in Crohn disease are *skin tags* that are minimally symptomatic. *Fissures* are also common. Typically, a fissure from Crohn disease is particularly deep or broad and perhaps better described as an anal ulcer. These fissures are often multiple and located in a lateral position rather than anterior or posterior midline as seen in an idiopathic fissure in ano. A classic-appearing fissure in ano located laterally should raise the suspicion of Crohn disease. (See Schwartz 10th ed., p. 1200.)

25. A 65-year-old man presents to the ED with fevers, abdominal pain, and bloody stools for the past 2 days. On CT scan he is found to have diverticulitis with scant free air and a small fluid collection associated with the sigmoid colon. What is the etiology of diverticulosis?
    A. Lack of dietary fiber causes smaller stools volume requiring higher intraluminal pressure.
    B. Chronic contraction causes muscular hypertrophy and causes colon to act as segments rather than a continuous tube.
    C. The mucosa and muscularis mucosa herniate through the colon wall.
    D. All of the above.

Answer: D

The majority of colonic diverticula are *false diverticula* in which the mucosa and muscularis mucosa have herniated through the colonic wall. These diverticula occur between the teniae coli, at points where the main blood vessels penetrate the colonic wall (presumably creating an area of relative weakness in the colonic muscle). They are thought to be *pulsion* diverticula resulting from high intraluminal pressure. The most accepted theory is that a lack of dietary fiber results in smaller stool volume, requiring high intraluminal pressure and high colonic wall tension for propulsion. Chronic contraction then results in muscular hypertrophy and development of the process of segmentation in which the colon acts like separate segments instead of functioning as a continuous tube. As segmentation progresses, the high pressures are directed radially toward the colon wall rather than to development of propulsive waves that move stool distally. The high radial pressures directed against the bowel wall create pulsion diverticula. (See Schwartz 10th ed., p. 1201.)

26. A 72-year-old woman presents to the clinic to discuss surgical management of her long-standing diverticulosis. What would be an indication for a colectomy in this patient?
    A. Three episodes of diverticulitis requiring hospitalization in an otherwise asymptomatic patient.
    B. A single episode of diverticulitis in an immunosuppressed patient.
    C. A current episode of complicated diverticulitis resulting in feculent peritonitis.
    D. Inability to exclude malignancy in a patient who was recently hospitalized for her first episode of complicated diverticulitis.

Answer: B

Many surgeons now will not advise colectomy even after two documented episodes of diverticulitis assuming the patient is completely asymptomatic and that carcinoma has been excluded by colonoscopy. Immunosuppressed patients are generally still advised to undergo colectomy after a single episode of documented diverticulitis. Medical comorbidities should be considered when evaluating a patient for elective resection, and the risks of recurrent disease should be weighed against the risks of the operation. Because colon carcinoma may present in an identical fashion to diverticulitis (either complicated or uncomplicated), all patients must be evaluated for malignancy after resolution of the acute episode. Colonoscopy is recommended 4 to 6 weeks after recovery. Inability to exclude malignancy is another indication for resection. (See Schwartz 10th ed., p. 1202.)

27. A 63-year-old woman presents to the ED with a 2-day history of left lower quadrant abdominal pain and is found to be febrile to 38.6°C. Her white blood cell (WBC) count is 15,000. On CT scan she is found to have colonic inflammation with an associated pericolic abscess. What is her Hinchey stage?
    A. Stage I
    B. Stage II
    C. Stage III
    D. Stage IV

Answer: A
The *Hinchey staging system* is often used to describe the severity of complicated diverticulitis: Stage I includes colonic inflammation with an associated pericolic abscess; stage II includes colonic inflammation with a retroperitoneal or pelvic abscess; stage III is associated with purulent peritonitis; and stage IV is associated with fecal peritonitis. (See Schwartz 10th ed., p. 1202.)

28. A 68-year-old woman presents to the ED with a 2-day history of left lower quadrant abdominal pain and is found to be febrile to 39°C. Her WBC count is 12,000. On CT scan she is found to have colonic inflammation with an associated retroperitoneal abscess. What is her Hinchey stage?
    A. Stage I
    B. Stage II
    C. Stage III
    D. Stage IV

Answer: B
The *Hinchey staging system* is often used to describe the severity of complicated diverticulitis: Stage I includes colonic inflammation with an associated pericolic abscess; stage II includes colonic inflammation with a retroperitoneal or pelvic abscess; stage III is associated with purulent peritonitis; and stage IV is associated with fecal peritonitis. (See Schwartz 10th ed., p. 1202.)

29. A 62-year-old woman presents to the ED with a 2-day history of severe left lower quadrant abdominal pain and is found to be febrile to 39°C. On physical examination her abdomen is rigid. Her WBC count is 21,000. On CT scan she is found to have diverticula and gross intra-abdominal free air and free fluid. She is taken to the operating room (OR) for an emergent exploratory laparotomy and she is found to have feculent material intra-abdominally. What is her Hinchey stage?
    A. Stage I
    B. Stage II
    C. Stage III
    D. Stage IV

Answer: D
The *Hinchey staging system* is often used to describe the severity of complicated diverticulitis: Stage I includes colonic inflammation with an associated pericolic abscess; stage II includes colonic inflammation with a retroperitoneal or pelvic abscess; stage III is associated with purulent peritonitis; and stage IV is associated with fecal peritonitis. (See Schwartz 10th ed., p. 1202.)

30. A 58-year-old man presents to the clinic with a 2-month history of the sensation of urinating air. He has a history of diverticulitis, with his last episode requiring hospitalization being 6 months ago. What are the most common fistulas that develop in complicated diverticulitis?
    A. Colovaginal fistulas
    B. Coloenteric fistulas
    C. Colocutaneous fistulas
    D. Colovesical fistulas

Answer: D
Approximately 5% of patients with complicated diverticulitis develop fistulas between the colon and an adjacent organ. *Colovesical* fistulas are most common, followed by *colovaginal* and *coloenteric* fistulas. *Colocutaneous* fistulas are a rare complication of diverticulitis. (See Schwartz 10th ed., p. 1203.)

31. A 32-year-old man presents to the ED with a 2-month history of alternating diarrhea and constipation, rectal bleeding, a 20-lb weight loss, and worsening fatigue. What are the most common genetic mutations that could have led to the development of this patient's colon cancer?
    A. *APC*, deleted in colorectal carcinoma (DCC), *p53*
    B. *APC*, *BRCA1*, *K-ras*
    C. *DCC*, *p53*, and *MYH* gene on chromosome 6p
    D. *MYH* gene on chromosome 1p, *APC*, *K-ras*

Answer: A
Mutations may cause *activation of oncogenes (K-ras)* and/or *inactivation of tumor suppressor genes (APC,* deleted in colorectal carcinoma [*DCC*], *p53*). Colorectal carcinoma is thought to develop from adenomatous polyps by accumulation of these mutations in what has come to be known as the *adenoma-carcinoma sequence*. The *APC* gene is a *tumor suppressor gene*. Mutations in both alleles are necessary to initiate polyp formation. Mutation of *K-ras* results in an inability to hydrolyze guanosine triphosphate (GTP), thus leaving the G-protein permanently in the active form. It is thought that this then leads to uncontrolled cell division. *MYH* is a base excision repair gene, and biallelic deletion results in changes in other downstream

molecules. Since its discovery, *MYH* mutations have been associated with an AFAP phenotype in addition to sporadic cancers. The tumor suppressor gene *p53* has been well characterized in a number of malignancies. The p53 protein appears to be crucial for initiating apoptosis in cells with irreparable genetic damage. Mutations in *p53* are present in 75% of colorectal cancers. (See Schwartz 10th ed., pp. 1204–1205.)

32. A 64-year-old man presents to the clinic with a 1-month history of 10-lb weight loss and rectal bleeding. His hematocrit is found to be 27. On colonoscopy he is found to have a large cecal mass. What risk factors should he have modified to prevent development of colon cancer?
    A. Eating a high-fat, high-protein, and low-carbohydrate diet and drinking a bottle of wine a day.
    B. Eating a high-fiber, low-fat, and low-protein diet, drinking a six packs of beer a day.
    C. Eating a high-fiber, low-fat, and high-protein diet and drinking only on holidays.
    D. Eating a high-fat, low-fiber diet and drinking only on holidays.

Answer: C

A diet high in saturated or polyunsaturated fats increases risk of colorectal cancer, while a diet high in oleic acid (olive oil, coconut oil, fish oil) does not increase risk. Animal studies suggest that fats may be directly toxic to the colonic mucosa and thus may induce early malignant changes. In contrast, a diet high in *vegetable fiber* appears to be protective. A correlation between alcohol intake and incidence of colorectal carcinoma has also been suggested. Ingestion of calcium, selenium, vitamins A, C, and E, carotenoids, and plant phenols may decrease the risk of developing colorectal cancer. Obesity and sedentary lifestyle dramatically increase cancer-related mortality in a number of malignancies, including colorectal carcinoma. This knowledge is the basis for primary prevention strategies to eliminate colorectal cancer by altering diet and lifestyle. (See Schwartz 10th ed., p. 1204.)

33. A 63-year-old man undergoes a screening colonoscopy and is found to have a polyp in his sigmoid colon. Which type of polyp is most associated with malignancy?
    A. Tubular adenoma
    B. Villous adenoma
    C. Tubulovillous adenoma
    D. 1 cm polyp

Answer: B

Adenomatous polyps are common, occurring in up to 25% of the population older than 50 years of age in the United States. By definition, these lesions are dysplastic. The risk of malignant degeneration is related to both the size and type of polyp. Tubular adenomas are associated with malignancy in only 5% of cases, whereas villous adenomas may harbor cancer in up to 40%. Tubulovillous adenomas are at intermediate risk (22%). Invasive carcinomas are rare in polyps smaller than 1 cm; the incidence increases with size. The risk of carcinoma in a polyp larger than 2 cm is 35 to 50%. Although most neoplastic polyps do not evolve to cancer, most colorectal cancers originate as a polyp. (See Schwartz 10th ed., p. 1205.)

34. A 50-year-old woman presents to the ED after having her first colonoscopy on her birthday. She endorses left lower quadrant abdominal pain and is febrile to 38.5°C. What complications after a colonoscopy require emergent laparotomy?
    A. Small perforation in a stable patient.
    B. Hypotension and temperature of 38°C in an otherwise stable patient.
    C. Rigid abdomen and severe abdominal pain in a patient with poor bowel preparation.
    D. Findings of a large, flat sessile polyp.

Answer: C

Complications of polypectomy include *perforation* and *bleeding*. A small perforation (*microperforation*) in a fully prepared, stable patient may be managed with bowel rest, broad-spectrum antibiotics, and close observation. Signs of sepsis, peritonitis, or deterioration in clinical condition are indications for laparotomy. Bleeding may occur immediately after polypectomy or may be delayed. The bleeding will usually stop spontaneously, but colonoscopy may be required to resnare a bleeding stalk or cauterize the lesion. Occasionally angiography and infusion of vasopressin may be necessary. Rarely, colectomy is required. (See Schwartz 10th ed., p. 1206.)

35. A 36-year-old woman with a complicated family history including her grandmother, mother, and sister who were diagnosed with colon cancer and a younger sister who was recently diagnosed with pancreatic cancer presents to the clinic for genetic counseling. What is a correct statement about this syndrome?
   A. It is the result of mismatch repair genes such as *FAP* and screening criteria look for three family members who have related cancers or two family members diagnosed before age 50.
   B. It is the result of an autosomal dominant condition and screening criteria look for three family members with the diagnosis of adenocarcinoma or two relatives diagnosed before age 50.
   C. It is the result of mismatch repair genes such as *PMS2* or *MSH6 and* three affected relatives with histologically verified adenocarcinoma of the large bowel in two successive generations of a family with one patient diagnosed before age 50.
   D. It is the result of an autosomal dominant condition *and* three affected relatives with histologically verified adenocarcinoma of the large bowel in two successive generations of a family with one patient diagnosed before age 50.

Answer: C

Hereditary nonpolyposis colorectal cancer (HNPCC; Lynch syndrome) is extremely rare (1–3% of all colon cancers). The genetic defects associated with HNPCC arise from errors in *mismatch repair*, the phenotypic result being MSI. HNPCC is inherited in an autosomal dominant pattern and is characterized by the development of colorectal carcinoma at an early age (average age, 40–45 years). Approximately 70% of affected individuals will develop colorectal cancer. Cancers appear in the proximal colon more often than in sporadic colorectal cancer and have a better prognosis regardless of stage. The risk of synchronous or metachronous colorectal carcinoma is 40%. HNPCC may also be associated with extracolonic malignancies, including endometrial carcinoma, which is most common, and ovarian, pancreas, stomach, small bowel, biliary, and urinary tract carcinomas. The diagnosis of HNPCC is made based on family history. The *Amsterdam criteria* for clinical diagnosis of HNPCC are three affected relatives with histologically verified adenocarcinoma of the large bowel (one must be a first-degree relative of one of the others) in two successive generations of a family with one patient diagnosed before age 50 years. HNPCC results from mutations in mismatch repair genes, and like *FAP*, specific mutations are associated with different phenotypes. For example, mutations in *PMS2* or *MSH6* result in a more attenuated form of HNPCC when compared to mutations in other genes. *MSH6* inactivation also appears to be associated with a higher risk for endometrial cancer. Further significance of these specific mutations remains to be determined. (See Schwartz 10th ed., p. 1207.)

36. A 67-year-old man presents to the ED with a 2-month history of nausea, emesis, 20-lb weight loss, and worsening diarrhea until 4 days ago, when he stopped passing flatus and having bowel movements. A CT scan shows a large obstructing right colon mass that may be involving the omentum with two liver lesions. What should be resected in this case?
   A. Right hemicolectomy, involved omentum, and as many of the peritoneal masses you can.
   B. Right hemicolectomy with arterial supply and as many nodes as you can.
   C. Right hemicolectomy with arterial supply, at least 12 nodes, the involved omentum, and resectable liver masses.
   D. Don't do a colon resection. This patient has distant metastases and should be diverted for palliation.

Answer: C

The objective in treatment of carcinoma of the colon is to remove the primary tumor along with its lymphovascular supply. Because the lymphatics of the colon accompany the main arterial supply, the length of bowel resected depends on which vessels are supplying the segment involved with the cancer. Any adjacent organ or tissue, such as the omentum, that has been invaded should be resected en bloc with the tumor. If all of the tumor cannot be removed, a palliative procedure should be considered, although it important to note that "debulking" is rarely effective in colorectal adenocarcinoma. If the metastatic disease is low volume (isolated or potentially resectable liver lesions) and the resection of the primary tumor is straightforward (segmental abdominal colectomy), it is probably reasonable to proceed with resection. On the other hand, if the metastatic disease is high volume (carcinomatosis), especially if the primary tumor is minimally symptomatic, the operation should be aborted in order to facilitate early systemic chemotherapy. (See Schwartz 10th ed., p. 1212.)

37. A 30-year-old man presents to the ED after a witnessed syncopal episode. He has been having bloody diarrhea and intermittent crampy abdominal pain for the past 3 months. A week later he has a colonoscopy and is found to have ulcerative colitis based on colonoscopy findings and mucosal biopsies. Which feature of listed below is NOT seen in ulcerative colitis?
   A. The terminal ileum shows inflammatory changes.
   B. The colon is shortened and mucosa is replaced by scars.
   C. Rectal sparing with inflammation seen in the transverse and descending colon.
   D. Atrophic mucosa with crypt abscesses.

Answer: C

Ulcerative colitis is a mucosal process in which the colonic mucosa and submucosa are infiltrated with inflammatory cells. The mucosa may be atrophic, and crypt abscesses are common. In long-standing ulcerative colitis, the colon may be foreshortened and the mucosa replaced by scar. Ulcerative colitis does not involve the small intestine, but the terminal ileum may demonstrate inflammatory changes ("backwash ileitis"). A key feature of ulcerative colitis is the continuous involvement of the rectum and colon; rectal sparing or skip lesions suggest a diagnosis of Crohn disease. (See Schwartz 10th ed., p. 1195.)

CHAPTER 30

The Appendix

1. The incidence of appendectomy for acute appendicitis was decreasing in the United Status until the 1990s, at which point the frequency of appendectomy for nonperforated appendicitis began to rise. What is one potential explanation for this observation?
   A. Increased use of diagnostic imaging and detection of appendicitis that otherwise would have resolved.
   B. Increased incidence of obesity and the impact of peri-appendicular fat on luminal obstruction.
   C. Increasing incidence of inflammatory bowel disease and the potential mitigation of ulcerative colitis symptoms seen with appendectomy.
   D. Reimbursement patterns have changed in the United States, favoring aggressive surgical decision making.

Answer: A
While the true reason is unknown, some have suggested that the quality and usage of diagnostic imaging in the past 20 to 30 years has resulted in the detection of acute appendicitis that would have otherwise spontaneously resolved. While appendectomy may mitigate the clinical symptoms of ulcerative colitis, this is likely not responsible for the broad reduction in observed appendectomy. Obesity is not known to impact appendicitis incidence. Reimbursement patterns should hopefully not impact surgical decision making so directly. (See Schwartz 10th ed., p. 1243.)

2. What imaging finding would exclude appendicitis?
   A. A computed tomographic (CT) scan with a nonvisualized appendix.
   B. A barium enema where a short (2 cm) appendix was clearly identified.
   C. An ultrasound study with a compressible appendix that is <5 mm in diameter.
   D. A CT scan showing an edematous but retrocecal appendix.

Answer: C
Graded compression ultrasonography is inexpensive and rapid. The appendix is identified as a nonperistaltic, blind ending loop of bowel. The compressibility and anteroposterior dimensions are measured. Thickening of the wall as well as peri-appendiceal fluid with a noncompressible appendix are suggestive of appendicitis while an easily compressible, narrow appendix excludes the diagnosis. Failure to identify the appendix on imaging does not definitely rule out appendicitis. A fecalith in the mid appendix may allow proximal filling of the appendix with barium in the presence of appendicitis. Sonographic sensitivity for appendicitis is 55 to 96% while specificity is 85 to 98%. (See Schwartz 10th ed., p. 1245.)

3. A 25-year-old man presents with migratory right lower quadrant (RLQ) pain, leukocytosis, and a CT scan consistent with acute, uncomplicated appendicitis. He is physiologically normal and it is 2 AM. You are planning an appendectomy, what difference might be expected in his outcome if his operation is delayed until the next morning?
   A. Increased risk of an intra-abdominal abscess.
   B. Increased risk of surgical-site infection.
   C. Decreased operative time.
   D. Increased risk of perforation.
   E. No difference in perforation rates, surgical-site infection, abscess, conversion rate or operative time.

Answer: E
There have been three retrospective studies comparing urgent versus emergent appendectomy. No difference was found in the incidence of complicated appendicitis, surgical-site infections, abscess formation, or conversion to an open procedure. While hospital length of stay was longer in the urgent group (as might be anticipated given the delay in definitive surgical care) this was not statistically or clinically different from the emergent group. It may be safe in physiologically normal patients with uncomplicated appendicitis to wait 12 to 24 hours and book them as an "urgent" case. (See Schwartz 10th ed., p. 1250.)

4. A 55-year-old man has CT evidence of complicated appendicitis with a contained abscess in the RLQ. He is mildly tachycardic, afebrile, and normotensive with focal RLQ tenderness but no peritonitis. What is the optimal approach to this patient?
   A. Immediate laparotomy.
   B. Laparoscopic exploration and abscess drainage.
   C. Percutaneous drainage, intravenous (IV) fluids, bowel rest, and broad spectrum antibiotics.
   D. IV fluids, bowel rest, and broad spectrum antibiotics.

Answer: C
Conservative management of the physiologically stable patient with complicated appendicitis has been shown to be associated with fewer overall complications, fewer bowel obstructions, fewer intra-abdominal abscesses, and fewer reoperations. While patients with peritonitis or hemodynamic instability should proceed to the operating room, conservative management of more stable patients with complicated appendicitis is favored. This may not necessarily be true in the pediatric population, however, as two prospective randomized trials in children demonstrate equivalent or superior outcomes with early operative intervention. (See Schwartz 10th ed., p. 1251.)

5. A 23-year-old woman who is 28 weeks pregnant presents with right-sided abdominal pain, leukocytosis, and an abdominal ultrasound that does not visualize the appendix. What intervention would you recommend?
   A. Exploratory laparoscopy.
   B. Abdominal CT scan.
   C. Abdominal magnetic resonance imaging (MRI) scan.
   D. Serial clinical observations.

Answer: C
Appendicitis complicates 1/766 births and is rare in the third trimester. The rate of negative appendectomy in the pregnant patient appears to be about 25% higher than in nonpregnant patients. This is not, however, a benign procedure as a negative appendectomy is associated with a 4% risk of fetal loss and a 10% risk of early delivery. The American College of Radiology recommends the use of nonionizing radiation techniques as front-line imaging in pregnant women. Serial examinations would be inappropriate as rates of fetal loss are considerably higher in patients with complicated appendicitis and the greatest opportunity to improve fetal outcomes is to improve diagnostic accuracy. (See Schwartz 10th ed., p. 1256.)

6. A 34-year-old man presents to your clinic asking about an elective appendectomy. He has no history of appendicitis. What are possible indications for appendectomy in this patient?
   A. Planned travel to a remote place with no surgical care.
   B. Patients with Crohn disease where the cecum is free of gross disease.
   C. As part of Ladd procedure.
   D. All of the above.

Answer: D
Incidental appendectomy is generally not indicted. A few select indications could be considered and they include children about to undergo chemotherapy, the disabled who cannot describe pain or react normally to pain, patients with Crohn disease when the cecum is free of macroscopic disease, and those patients planning to travel to remote areas with limited surgical care. While part of the traditional teaching, the ubiquity of antibiotics and the evolving understanding of our ability to treat at least some appendicitis nonoperatively may further limit the indications for elective, incidental appendectomy. (See Schwartz 10th ed., p. 1257.)

7. While reviewing pathology of a recent laparoscopic appendectomy, you note that in addition to acute appendicitis, the patient had a 1.5-cm carcinoid tumor located at the base of the appendix. The patient is otherwise healthy and recovering well from surgery. What would you recommend?
   A. No additional therapy necessary.
   B. Right hemicolectomy.
   C. Radical appendectomy.
   D. Adjuvant chemotherapy.

Answer: B
Appendiceal carcinoid is one of the most common neoplasms to identify in an appendectomy specimen. Lesions that are <1 cm generally do not require additional therapy. Lesions larger than 1 or 2 cm, involving the appendiceal base or with lymph node metastasis of mesenteric invasion warrant right hemicolectomy. A radical appendectomy is not a described operation and adjuvant chemotherapy could be considered but only after definitive surgical care. (See Schwartz 10th ed., p. 1258.)

8. An 8-year-old boy presents to the emergency department complaining of generalized abdominal pain for the past 24 hours. Laboratory tests reveal a leukocytosis of 13,000 and he is tender in the RLQ on physical examination. He is taken to the operating room for laparoscopic appendectomy. Removal of the appendix has been associated with a protective effect of which of the following?
   A. Crohn colitis
   B. Ulcerative colitis
   C. *Clostridium difficile*
   D. Carcinoid

Answer: B
The appendix is an immunologic organ involved in secretion of immunoglobulins. An inverse association between appendectomy and development of ulcerative colitis has been reported. Routine resection of the normal appendix to improve the clinical course of ulcerative colitis is not generally indicated. (See Schwartz 10th ed., p. 1243.)

9. Which of the following physical signs is associated with the correct definition suggestive of acute appendicitis?
   A. Rovsing sign: pain in the RLQ on palpation of the left lower quadrant
   B. Dunphy sign: pain in the RLQ with palpation on the left
   C. Obturator sign: pain with extension of the leg
   D. Iliopsoas sign: pain on internal rotation of the right hip

Answer: A
Appendicitis usually starts with periumbilical pain that migrates to the RLQ. Patients often have associated gastrointestinal symptoms such as anorexia, nausea, and vomiting. On physical examination, patients often prefer to remain lying supine and often guard due to peritoneal irritation. Rebound tenderness is when the examiner presses on the RLQ and the patient experiences a sudden pain upon removal of the hand. Rovsing sign is RLQ pain that is induced by palpation of the left lower quadrant and is highly suggestive of a RLQ inflammatory process. Dunphy sign elicits pain with coughing and is related to inflammation of the peritoneum. The obturator sign occurs with internal rotation of the right hip. Lastly, the iliopsoas sign is pain with extension of the right hip, attributed to a retrocecal appendix. (See Schwartz 10th ed., p. 1244.)

10. A 29-year-old woman presents with RLQ pain, fever, and leukocytosis. Prior to imaging studies the Alvarado score is used to determine the patient's likelihood of having appendicitis. All of the following variables make up the Alvarado score EXCEPT
   A. Anorexia
   B. Left shift of neutrophils
   C. Iliopsoas sign
   D. RLQ pain
   E. Fever

Answer: C
The Alvarado score is the most widespread scoring system useful for ruling out appendicitis and selecting patients for further imaging or intervention (Table 30-1). The Alvarado score is calculated using RLQ tenderness, elevated temperature, rebound tenderness, migration of pain, anorexia, nausea/vomiting, leukocytosis, and a left shift on leukocyte differential as predictive factors. Several online calculators are freely available. (See Schwartz 10th ed., Table 30-2, p. 1245.)

TABLE 30-1	Scoring systems			
Alvarado Score[37]			**Appendicitis Inflammatory Response Score**[38,39]	
Findings	**Points**	**Findings**		**Points**
Migratory right iliac fossa pain	1	Vomiting		1
Anorexia	1	Pain in the right inferior fossa		1
Nausea or vomiting	1	Rebound tenderness or muscular defense		
Tenderness: right iliac fossa	2		Light	1
Rebound tenderness right iliac fossa	1		Medium	2
Fever ≥36.3°C	1		Strong	3
Leukocytosis ≥10 × 10^9 cells/L	2	Body temperature ≥38.5°C		1
Shift to the left of neutrophils	1	Polymorphonuclear leukocytes		
			70%–84%	1
			≥85%	2
		White blood cell count		
			10.0–14.9 × 10^9 cells/L	1
			≥15.0 × 10^9 cells/L	2
		C-reactive protein concentration		
			10–49 g/L	1
			≥50 g/L	2

Score: <3: Low likelihood of appendicitis.
4–6: Consider further imaging.
≥7: High likelihood of appendicitis.

Score: 0–4: Low probability. Outpatient follow-up.
5–8: Indeterminate group. Active observation or diagnostic laparoscopy.
9–12: High probability. Surgical exploration.

11. A 34-year-old man undergoes an uneventful appendectomy for acute, nonperforated appendicitis. The pathology report notes reads: acute inflammation with a 1-cm adenocarcinoma of the mid appendix. This patient should have
    A. No further treatment
    B. Chemotherapy
    C. Regional radiation
    D. Right hemicolectomy
    E. Ileocecectomy

Answer: D
Primary adenocarcinoma of the appendix is rare. Three types of adenocarcinoma exist; mucinous, colonic, and adenocarcinoid. The most common presentation of adenocarcinoma is acute appendicitis. The recommended treatment for all patients diagnosed with adenocarcinoma is a formal right hemicolectomy. Patients are at risk for both synchronous and metachronous neoplasms—half of which will originate in the GI tract. (See Schwartz 10th ed., p. 1258.)

12. A 45-year-old woman presents with RLQ pain. A CT scan is performed. What finding on CT scan is most suggestive of appendiceal lymphoma?
    A. Appendiceal diameter >2.5 cm or surrounding soft tissue thickening
    B. Lack of contrast filling the appendix
    C. 1-cm mass at the base of the appendix
    D. Prominent aortic lymph nodes

Answer: A
Lymphoma of the appendix is uncommon. The most common types of appendiceal lymphoma in decreasing order are non-Hodgkin, Burkitt, and leukemia. Findings on CT scan include appendiceal diameter of >2.5 cm or surrounding soft tissue thickening. The management is confined to appendectomy. Right hemicolectomy is indicated if the tumor extends beyond the appendix onto the cecum or into the mesentery. If requiring a right hemicolectomy, postoperatively the patient will require a staging workup and possible adjuvant chemotherapy. (See Schwartz 10th ed., p. 1259.)

Liver

1. With regard to hepatic anatomy, the falciform ligament divides the _____ from the _____.
   A. Caudate lobe, quadrate lobe
   B. Right lobe, left lobe
   C. Left medial section, left lateral section
   D. Left medial section, right lobe

Answer: C
The falciform ligament divides the left lateral section from the left medial section. The plane between the gallbladder fossa and the inferior vena cava (IVC—referred to as *Cantlie's line*) divides the right and left lobes. The falciform ligament, along with the round, triangular, and coronary ligaments may be divided in a bloodless plane during liver resection (Figs. 31-1 to 31-3). (See Schwartz 10th ed., p. 1265.)

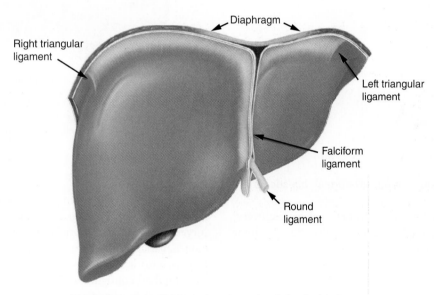

FIG. 31-1. Hepatic ligaments suspending the liver to the diaphragm and anterior abdominal wall.

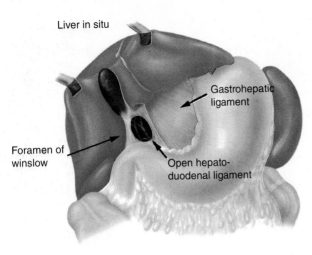

FIG. 31-2. In situ liver hilar anatomy with hepatoduodenal and gastrohepatic ligaments. Foramen of Winslow is depicted.

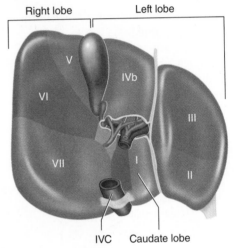

FIG. 31-3. Couinaud liver segments (I through VIII) numbered in a clockwise manner. The left lobe includes segments II to IV, the right lobe includes segments V to VIII, and the caudate lobe is segment I. IVC = inferior vena cava.

2. The most common variant of normal hepatic artery anatomy is
   A. Replaced left hepatic artery from the left gastric artery
   B. Completely replaced common hepatic artery from the superior mesenteric artery (SMA)
   C. Replaced right and left hepatic arteries
   D. Replaced right hepatic artery from the SMA

Answer: D

Understanding the anatomic variants of the hepatic arterial supply is important to avoid complications during liver surgery. The standard arterial anatomy is as follows: the common hepatic artery arises from the celiac trunk, and then divides into the gastroduodenal and proper hepatic artery. In a standard configuration, the proper hepatic artery gives rise to the right gastric artery, but this is variable. The proper hepatic artery then divides into the right and left hepatic artery (Fig. 31-4). However, this standard arterial configuration only occurs in 76% of patients. The most common variants include replaced right hepatic artery from the SMA (10–15%), replaced left hepatic artery from the left gastric artery (3–10%), replaced right and left hepatic arteries (1–2%), and the completely replaced common hepatic artery from the SMA (1–2%) (Fig. 31-5). (See Schwartz 10th ed., p. 1266.)

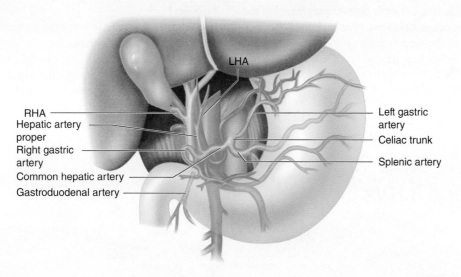

FIG. 31-4. Arterial anatomy of the upper abdomen and liver, including the celiac trunk and hepatic artery branches. a. = artery; LHA = left hepatic artery; RHA = right hepatic artery.

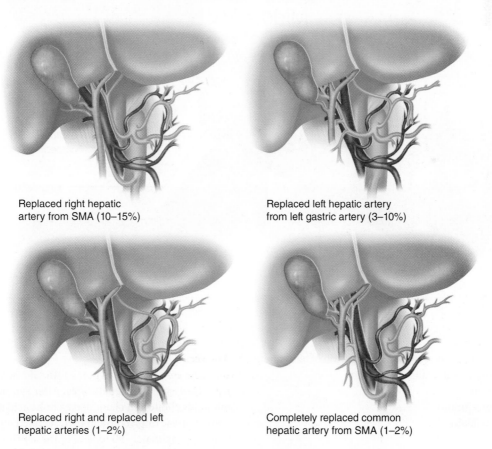

Replaced right hepatic
artery from SMA (10–15%)

Replaced left hepatic artery
from left gastric artery (3–10%)

Replaced right and replaced left
hepatic arteries (1–2%)

Completely replaced common
hepatic artery from SMA (1–2%)

FIG. 31-5. Common hepatic artery anatomic variants. SMA = superior mesenteric artery.

3. Which of the following correctly pairs the segments of the liver and their associated systemic venous drainage?
   A. Segments I, II, III: Right hepatic vein
   B. Segment IV: Right hepatic vein
   C. Segment I: IVC
   D. Segment V, VI, VII, VIII: Left hepatic vein

Answer: C

There are three hepatic veins (right, middle, and left) that serve as the outflow for the hepatic circulation and drain into the suprahepatic IVC. The right hepatic vein drains segments V to VIII; the middle hepatic vein drains segment IV, as well as segments V and VIII; and the left hepatic vein drains segments II and III (Fig. 31-6). The caudate lobe (segment I) drains directly in to the IVC. (See Schwartz 10th ed., Figure 31–8, p. 1267.)

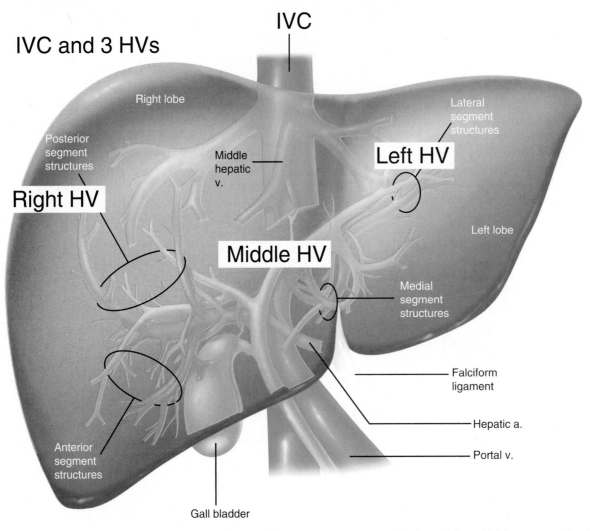

FIG. 31-6. Confluence of the three hepatic veins (HVs) and the inferior vena cava (IVC). Note that the middle and left hepatic veins (HVs) drain into a common trunk before entering the IVC. a. = artery; v. = vein. (Adapted with permission from Cameron JL, ed. *Atlas of Surgery. Vol. I, Gallbladder and Biliary Tract, the Liver, Portosystemic Shunts, the Pancreas.* Toronto: BC Decker; 1990, p. 153.)

4. With respect to the enterohepatic circulation of bile, where are the majority of bile salts reabsorbed?
   A. Duodenum
   B. Proximal jejunum
   C. Terminal ileum
   D. Colon

Answer: C

Bile salts are sodium and potassium salts of bile acids derived from cholesterol by hepatocytes. After synthesis, the primary bile acids cholic and chenodeoxycholic acid are conjugated to either taurine or glycine and then secreted into the biliary system. Approximately 90 to 95% of these primary bile salts and acids are absorbed by active transport at the terminal ileum, while the remainder enter the colon and are converted to secondary bile acids (deoxycholic and lithocholic acids) and their associated salts by resident bacteria. Bile acids and salts reabsorbed in the terminal ileum are reabsorbed through the portal circulation, while those lost in the stool are replaced by hepatic synthesis. (See Schwartz 10th ed., p. 1270.)

5. Which of the following compounds is not synthesized predominantly by the liver?
   A. Albumin
   B. Factor VIII
   C. Factor VII
   D. Factor II

Answer: B
The liver is the largest gland in the body, and responsible for synthesis of the majority of plasma proteins. The liver produces approximately 10 g of albumin per day, and albumin measurement can therefore be used as a surrogate for liver synthetic function. This must be interpreted with caution, as albumin levels can be influenced by a host of factors unrelated to hepatic function, and albumin's long half-life (15–20 days) makes it a poor marker for acute hepatic dysfunction. Most clotting factors are synthesized predominantly in the liver, except for factor VIII. Due to this fact the prothrombin time (PT) and international normalized ratio (INR) may also be used as markers of hepatic synthetic function. However, these too should be interpreted with caution as other conditions, including vitamin K deficiency and warfarin use, may prolong a patient's PT/INR. (See Schwartz 10th ed., p. 1271.)

6. The gold standard for identifying liver lesions by imaging is
   A. Intraoperative ultrasound
   B. Computed tomography (CT) with triple-phase contrast
   C. Magnetic resonance imaging (MRI) with gadoxetate-based contrast
   D. Positron emission tomography (PET) scan

Answer: A
The use of intraoperative ultrasound of the liver has rapidly expanded over the years with the increasing number and complexity of hepatic resections being performed. It has the ability to provide the surgeon with real-time accurate information useful for surgical planning. Intraoperative ultrasound is considered the gold standard for detecting liver lesions, and studies have shown that it can identify 20% to 30% more lesions than other preoperative imaging modalities. Importantly, it has been shown to influence surgical management in almost 50% of planned liver resections for malignancies. Applications for intraoperative ultrasound of the liver include tumor staging, visualization of intrahepatic vascular structures, and guidance of resections plane by assessment of the relationship of a mass to the vessels. In addition, biopsy of lesions and ablation of tumors can be guided by intraoperative ultrasound. (See Schwartz 10th ed., p. 1273.)

7. The most common cause of acute liver failure (ALF) in the United States is
   A. Acute viral hepatitis
   B. Cardiogenic shock
   C. Autoimmune hepatitis
   D. Drug/toxin-induced (including acetaminophen)

Answer: D
Acute liver failure (ALF) is defined as development of hepatic encephalopathy within 26 weeks of severe liver injury in a patient with no history of liver disease or portal hypertension. In developing countries, the most common etiology of ALF is viral infections, including hepatitis B, A, and E. In the West (including the United States, Australia, United Kingdom, and most of Europe), 65% of ALF cases are related to drugs and toxins, especially acetaminophen. (See Schwartz 10th ed., pp. 1275–1276.)

8. A patient presents with painless jaundice, and is found to have cirrhosis. They have no history of alcohol abuse, but do note a history of diabetes mellitus and pseudogout. They also mention that multiple members of their family have suffered from cirrhosis. What is the most likely etiology for their cirrhosis?
   A. Alcohol abuse
   B. Wilson disease
   C. α₁-antitrypsin deficiency
   D. Hemochromatosis

Answer: D
Chronic hepatitis C infection is the most common cause of chronic liver disease in the United States. Other etiologies include alcohol abuse, nonalcoholic steatohepatitis (NASH), and autoimmune diseases (primary biliary cirrhosis, primary sclerosing cholangitis, and autoimmune hepatitis). Hereditary hemochromatosis is the most common metabolic cause of cirrhosis, and should be suspected if a patient presents with skin hyperpigmentation, diabetes mellitus, pseudogout, cardiomyopathy, or a family history of cirrhosis. (See Schwartz 10th ed., p. 1278.)

9. Which of the following is not one of the physiologic changes noted in patients with cirrhosis?
   A. Reduced resting energy expenditure
   B. Reduced muscle and fat stores
   C. Increased cardiac output
   D. Decreased systemic vascular resistance

Answer: A

The clinical manifestations of cirrhosis are the result of numerous physiologic changes associated with a patient's progressive liver failure. Hypoalbuminemia results in finger clubbing, while spider angiomata and palmar erythema are thought to be caused by alterations in sex hormones. The physiologic basis for feminization of males (gynecomastia, loss of chest/axillary hair, testicular atrophy) with cirrhosis is less well understood. Portal hypertension manifests as caput medusa and varices. Cirrhotic patients suffer from chronic malnutrition, which may be associated with weakness, weight loss, and decreased fat and muscle stores. Despite this fact, patients with cirrhosis have elevated resting energy expenditure. Also noted are increased cardiac output and heart rate with decreased systemic vascular resistance and blood pressure. (See Schwartz 10th ed., p. 1279.)

10. Clinically significant portal hypertension is evident when the _____ exceeds _____ mm Hg.
    A. Wedged hepatic venous pressure, 10
    B. Free hepatic venous pressure, 20
    C. Hepatic venous pressure gradient, 10
    D. Hepatic venous pressure gradient, 20

Answer: C

Portal hypertension occurs when the pressure in the portal system is increased due to factors that may be divided into three categories. Presinusoidal causes of portal hypertension include sinistral/extrahepatic (splenic vein thrombosis, splenomegaly, splenic atrioventricular fistula) and intrahepatic (schistosomiasis, congenital hepatic fibrosis, idiopathic portal fibrosis, myeloproliferative disorder, sarcoid, graft-versus-host disease) etiologies. Sinusoidal portal hypertension is a consequence of cirrhosis of any etiology. Postsinusoidal hypertension can also be divided into intrahepatic (vascular occlusive disease) and posthepatic (Budd-Chiari, congestive heart failure [CHF], IVC webs) etiologies. In evaluating patients with suspected portal hypertension, an enlarged portal vein on routine abdominal ultrasonography may suggest portal hypertension but this is not diagnostic. Doppler ultrasound allows identification of vascular occlusion and the direction of portal venous flow. CT and MR angiography are useful for evaluating portal venous patency and anatomy. The most accurate method for measuring portal hypertension is hepatic venography. This procedure introduces a balloon catheter directly into the hepatic vein where free hepatic venous pressure (FHVP) is measured. The hepatic vein is then occluded by inflation of the balloon allowing measurement of the wedged hepatic venous pressure (WHVP). The hepatic venous pressure gradient (HVPG) may then be calculated by subtracting the FHVP from the WHVP (HVPG = WHVP–FHVP). Clinically significant portal hypertension is defined as HVPG greater than 10 mm Hg. (See Schwartz 10th ed., pp. 1280–1281.)

11. All of the following therapies are considered appropriate during the management of an acute variceal hemorrhage EXCEPT?
    A. Endoscopy with variceal band ligation
    B. Short-term antibiotic prophylaxis
    C. Somatostatin analogues
    D. Recombinant factor VIIa

Answer: D

Variceal bleeding is the leading cause of morbidity and mortality in those with portal venous hypertension. Approximately 30% of patients with compensated cirrhosis and 60% of those with decompensated cirrhosis will have varices, and one-third of these patients will experience a variceal bleed. These episodes carry a 20 to 30% risk of mortality. Prevention of variceal bleeding may be accomplished through administration of nonselective β-blockers (eg, propranolol) and routine endoscopic surveillance and variceal band ligation. In the case of acute variceal bleeding, patients should be admitted to an ICU for resuscitation and management. While prompt resuscitation is critical, administration of both blood products and crystalloid should be done with care. A target of hemoglobin of 8 g/dL is appropriate, and administration of platelets and fresh frozen plasma may be considered for patients with thrombocytopenia or severe coagulopathy. However, over-resuscitation with both blood products and crystalloid solution has been associated with increased risk of re-bleeding and morbidity. Use of recombinant factor VIIa has not been shown to be better than standard therapy, and is not recommended. Patients with cirrhosis who experience a variceal bleed are at high risk for developing bacterial infection, including spontaneous bacterial peritonitis (~50% of infectious complications), pneumonia, and urinary tract infection. These bacterial infections not only carry their own risk of morbidity and mortality, but also are associated with increased risk of re-bleeding. For this reason short-term antibiotic prophylaxis (eg, ceftriaxone) is recommended for patients with acute variceal bleeding. Management of the bleeding can be accomplished with vasoactive medications, including vasopressin and somatostatin analogues (eg, octreotide). These therapies cause splanchnic vasoconstriction and slow the flow of blood to the varices. Though vasopressin is the most potent vasoconstrictor, it is limited by its systemic effects. Thus, somatostatin analogues are the preferred agent. Further therapy for bleeding varices should include endoscopy with variceal band ligation. (See Schwartz 10th ed., pp. 1281–1282.)

12. A cirrhotic patient is admitted with variceal bleeding. The bleeding is controlled with pharmacologic therapy, and the patient recovers from the acute episode. Assuming they receive no other therapies to treat their varices or their underlying cause, what is the likelihood that they will experience a recurrent variceal bleed within 2 years
    A. 20%
    B. 40%
    C. 70%
    D. 100%

Answer: C
The risk of re-bleed for patients is 70% over 2 years if they receive no further treatment. Patients who recover from an episode of variceal bleeding should be treated with follow-up endoscopy and variceal band ligation. In appropriate patients, transjugular intrahepatic portosystemic shunt (TIPS) or orthotopic liver transplant should be considered. (See Schwartz 10th ed., p. 1282.)

13. Which of the following INCORRECTLY matches a grading scale for patients with liver disease and one of its components?
    A. Model for End-Stage Liver Disease (MELD): Serum creatinine
    B. Child-Turcotte-Pugh (CTP): Bilirubin
    C. CTP: INR
    D. MELD: Albumin

Answer: D
The Child-Turcotte-Pugh (CTP) was initially derived for use in predicting the risk of portocaval shunt procedures, and comprises five components: bilirubin, albumin, INR, presence of encephalopathy, presence of ascites. The Model for End-Stage Liver Disease (MELD) score was developed as a model to predict mortality after TIPS, but has been adapted and validated for use as the method of organ allocation for orthotopic liver transplantation (OLT) in the United States. It is a linear regression model based on the serum creatinine, total bilirubin, and INR. (See Schwartz 10th ed., p. 1280.)

14. Which of the following INCORRECTLY pairs the CTP class with overall risk of mortality following an intra-abdominal operation?
    A. Class A: 10%
    B. Class B: 30%
    C. Class C: 50%
    D. Class C: 75%

Answer: C
The overall mortality for patients with cirrhosis undergoing intra-abdominal surgery has consistently been shown to correlate with the CTP classification. The estimated mortality is 10%, 30% and 75 to 80% for those with CTP class A, B, and C cirrhosis, respectively. MELD score also predicts postoperative mortality in cirrhotic patients, and has been shown to

correlate well with estimates based on CTP classification. In general, those patients with a MELD below 10 should be considered appropriate for surgery, while those with scores above 15 should not be considered for elective procedures. (See Schwartz 10th ed., p. 1280.)

15. What is the most common complication following TIPS?
    A. Encephalopathy
    B. Hepatic ischemia
    C. Infection
    D. Life-threatening hemorrhage

Answer: A

TIPS is a percutaneous procedure used for treatment of patients who have gastroesophageal varices in the setting of portal hypertension. It has largely replaced surgical portosystemic shunts due to the fact that it is both safe and effective while also providing a minimally invasive alternative to major abdominal surgery. TIPS functions by creating an intrahepatic shunt between the portal and systemic circulation which causes a reduction in the portal pressure and ultimately in the blood flow through varices. It is accomplished by endovascular access through the jugular vein to a hepatic vein radical and subsequent creation of a needle tract that connects it to a branch of the portal vein. After dilation of the tract, a metallic stent is deployed to hold the new portosystemic connection open. Because this shunt reduces first pass metabolism of the liver, the most common complication of TIPS is encephalopathy which occurs in 25 to 30% of patients. Other complications such as hepatic ischemia, infection, renal failure, and hemorrhage may occur, but are rare. (See Schwartz 10th ed., p. 1282.)

16. Initial management of a pyogenic liver may include all of the following EXCEPT?
    A. Treatment of the underlying cause
    B. Broad-spectrum intravenous antibiotics
    C. Surgical drainage and/or resection
    D. Percutaneous fine-needle aspiration and culture

Answer: A

Pyogenic abscesses are the most common liver abscesses seen in the United States. Though traditionally a result of intra-abdominal infections such as appendicitis and diverticulitis, earlier diagnosis of these conditions in patients has reduced prevalence of these conditions as causes for pyogenic liver abscess. Other etiologies include impaired biliary drainage, subacute bacterial endocarditis, dental work, infected indwelling catheters, or direct extension from abscesses related to inflammatory bowel disease. Pyogenic liver abscesses are most commonly seen in the right lobe of the liver, and *Escherichia coli* is the most commonly isolated pathogen. Approximately 40% of abscesses are polymicrobial, while 20% of culture negative. Treatment of pyogenic liver abscesses include correction of the underlying cause and intravenous antibiotics for at least 8 weeks, which is effective in approximately 80 to 90% of patients. Empiric antibiotic coverage should include gram-negative and anaerobic organisms, with percutaneous aspiration and culture used to tailor long-term antibiotic therapy. Placement of a percutaneous drainage catheter may be considered, though it is often ineffective due to the viscous nature of the collection. Surgical drainage or resection is reserved for patients who fail nonoperative management. (See Schwartz 10th ed., p. 1284.)

17. The most common benign hepatic lesion is the
    A. Hemangioma
    B. Simple cyst
    C. Adenoma
    D. Bile duct hamartoma

Answer: B

While hemangiomas are the most common solid benign masses found in the liver, the simple hepatic cyst is still the most common overall. Simple cysts have a prevalence of approximately 2.8 to 3.6%, and are more common in women by a ratio of 4:1. Cysts are generally found incidentally during abdominal imaging, and small, asymptomatic cysts may be managed conservatively. Large cysts may begin to cause abdominal pain, epigastric fullness, and early satiety. These patients may be treated with percutaneous cyst aspiration and sclerotherapy which is effective in approximately 90% of patients. For those who fail percutaneous treatment, or where percutaneous treatment is not available, surgical cyst fenestration may be considered. If surgical fenestration is performed, the cyst wall should be sent for pathologic analysis to exclude carcinoma. (See Schwartz 10th ed., p. 1288.)

18. Which of the following liver lesions carry a significant risk of spontaneous rupture?
    A. Hemangioma
    B. Hepatic cyst
    C. Adenoma
    D. Bile duct hamartoma

Answer: C
Hemangiomas are congenital vascular lesions that may range in size from less than 1 to 25 cm or greater. They are predominantly found in women, and are generally asymptomatic. Large lesions may result in discomfort from compression of nearby organs. Though hemangiomas are at risk for bleeding if they are biopsied, spontaneous rupture is rare. Adenomas, on the other hand, carry a significant risk for spontaneous rupture with intraperitoneal bleeding. For this reason, along with their potential for malignant degeneration, it is generally recommended that hepatic adenomas be resected once discovered. (See Schwartz 10th ed., pp. 1290–1291.)

19. A patient presents with results from a contrast-enhanced CT scan that describe a well-circumscribed lesion that demonstrates homogenous enhancement during arterial phase, isodensity on the venous phase, and a central scar. In general, what would be the recommended treatment?
    A. Reassurance and observation
    B. Percutaneous radio frequency ablation
    C. Resection
    D. Transarterial chemoembolization

Answer: A
On contrast-enhanced imaging, a focal nodular hyperplasia (FNH) can be recognized as a well-circumscribed mass that demonstrates enhancement on the arterial phase and isodensity on the venous phase. FNH also demonstrates a characteristic central scar. FNH are solid benign lesions, are similar to adenomas, and are more common in women of childbearing age. Unlike adenomas, however, they are not prone to malignant degeneration or spontaneous rupture. For this reason, asymptomatic FNHs may be managed conservatively unless adenoma or HCC cannot be definitively excluded. Gadolinium-enhanced MRI may allow better visualization of the fibrous septa extending from the FNH's central scar. While FNH and adenomas may appear similar on CT or standard MRI, new MRI contrast agents, such as gadobenate dimeglumine (MultiHance), allow superior discrimination between these two lesions. (See Schwartz 10th ed., p. 1291.)

20. What is the annual conversion rate to HCC for patients with cirrhosis?
    A. Less than 1%
    B. 1–2%
    C. 2–6%
    D. 6–10%

Answer: C
HCC is the fifth most common malignancy worldwide, and its risk factors include viral hepatitis, alcoholic cirrhosis, hemochromatosis, and NASH. Cirrhosis is present in 70 to 90% of patients who develop HCC, and the annual conversion rate from cirrhosis is 2 to 6%. (See Schwartz 10th ed., p. 1291.)

21. Patient's eligible for the Mayo Clinical protocol to treat hilar cholangiocarcinoma do NOT include
    A. Patients with hilar cholangiocarcinoma and primary sclerosing cholangitis (PSC).
    B. Patients with unresectable cholangiocarcinoma.
    C. Patients with tumors less than 3 cm.
    D. Patients who have had prior radiotherapy.

Answer: D
Cholangiocarcinoma is an adenocarcinoma of the bile ducts, and represents the second most common primary liver malignancy. Cholangiocarcinoma may be intra- or extrahepatic, and the latter may be divided into proximal or distal. Proximal cholangiocarcinoma is also known as *hilar cholangiocarcinoma* or *Klatskin tumor*. The only curative treatment option for hilar cholangiocarcinoma is surgical resection, for which the reported 5-year survival rates range from 25 to 40%. However, in the presence of primary sclerosing cholangitis (PSC, ~10% of patients with cholangiocarcinoma), the

results of surgical resection are poor due to associated liver dysfunction and portal hypertension. For this reason, the Mayo Clinic protocol was developed to treat patients with hilar cholangiocarcinoma and PSC. This treatment comprises external beam radiation, 5-FU-based chemotherapy, and iridium-192 brachytherapy followed by operative staging and OLT in patients without metastatic disease. The 5-year survival rate for patients completing this protocol is 70%. Current eligibility criteria for this protocol include patients with hilar cholangiocarcinoma with PSC or patients with unresectable hilar cholangiocarcinoma who have not received prior radiotherapy. Furthermore, the patient must have a primary tumor less than 3 cm in radial dimension and no evidence of intrahepatic or extrahepatic metastases. (See Schwartz 10th ed., pp. 1291–1292.)

22. A patient undergoes routine cholecystectomy and is incidentally found to have gallbladder carcinoma that is staged as T1. Further treatment should include
    A. No further treatment.
    B. External beam radiation with systemic chemotherapy.
    C. Reoperation with central liver resection and hilar lymphadenectomy.
    D. Reoperation with formal lobectomy and bile duct resection.

Answer: D
Gallbladder cancer is a rare and aggressive form of biliary malignancy. In approximately one-third of cases it is diagnosed incidentally following routine cholecystectomy. Treatment for these patients is guided by T stage of the tumor. In those patients with T1 tumors, no further treatment is necessary. In patients with T2 or greater tumors, reoperation with central liver resection and hilar lymphadenectomy is recommended. The role for more radical resections is unclear. (See Schwartz 10th ed., p. 1293.)

23. Which of the following is considered a primary determinant of suitability for resection when evaluating a patient with hepatic colorectal metastases?
    A. Number of metastatic tumors
    B. Size of metastatic tumors
    C. Predicted volume of hepatic remnant
    D. Prior therapy

Answer: C
The liver is a common site for metastatic disease in patients with colorectal disease, and approximately 50 to 60% of patients diagnosed with colorectal cancer will develop liver metastases within their lifetime. With the advent of more aggressive strategies for the management of metastatic colorectal cancer, including improved chemotherapeutic regimens and expanded use of metastasectomy, the 5-year survival for patients with isolated metastases to the liver may exceed 30%. Given these encouraging results, the paradigm for surgical evaluation and treatment of these patients has shifted to primarily consider the health of the background liver and volume of the hepatic remnant, and not tumor characteristics such as size and number. (See Schwartz 10th ed., pp. 1293–1294.)

24. Based on the standard Milan criteria, which of the following patients with HCC would be eligible for transplantation?
    A. One 4.5-cm lesion in segment VI with invasion of the right portal vein.
    B. Three lesions confined to the right lobe, with the largest being 2.5 cm.
    C. A single, 5.5-cm lesion in segment II.
    D. Three lesions spread throughout the liver, with the largest being 3.5 cm.

Answer: B
OTL was first attempted in the 1980s and 1990s, with initial series reporting 5-year survival rates of 20 to 50%. This led to the introduction of the Milan criteria which limited eligibility to patients with one tumor less than 5 cm or up to three tumors less than 3 cm and no evidence of gross intravascular or extrahepatic spread. Adoption of these guidelines resulted in significant improvement in 5-year survival for patients with HCC treated with OTL. (See Schwartz 10th ed., p. 1295.)

25. The only FDA-approved systemic chemotherapeutic agent for HCC is
    A. Epirubicin
    B. Cisplatin
    C. 5-Fluorouracil
    D. Sorafenib

Answer: D

Though systemic chemotherapy has not proven very effective in the treatment of HCC, the multikinase inhibitor sorafenib has been approved for use specifically in these patients. Based on results of the SHARP trial, the sorafenib demonstrated a 3-month survival benefit versus placebo. Though these results are modest, it remains a treatment option for patients with advanced, unresectable HCC. (See Schwartz 10th ed., p. 1296.)

26. Which of the following correctly pairs the Brisbane 2000 hepatic resection terminology with appropriate liver segments?
    A. Right posterior sectionectomy: Segments IV and IV
    B. Left hepatectomy: Segments I, II, III, and IV
    C. Right Hepatectomy: Segments VI, VII, and VIII
    D. Left lateral sectionectomy: Segments II and III

Answer: D

See Table 31-1. (See Schwartz 10th ed., Table 31-8, p. 1297.)

TABLE 31-1	Brisbane 2000 liver terminology
Older Hepatic Resection Terminology	**Brisbane 2000 Hepatic Resection Terminology**
Right hepatic lobectomy	Right hepatectomy or right hemihepatectomy (V, VI, VII, VIII)
Left hepatic lobectomy	Left hepatectomy or left hemihepatectomy (II, III, IV)
Right hepatic trisegmentectomy	Right trisectionectomy or extended right hepatectomy (or hemihepatectomy, IV, V, VII, VIII)
Left hepatic trisegmentectomy	Left trisectionectomy or extended left hepatectomy (or hemihepatectomy, II, III, IV, V, VIII)
Left lateral segmentectomy	Left lateral sectionectomy or bisegmentectomy (II, III)
Right posterior lobectomy	Right posterior sectionectomy (VI, VII)
Caudate lobectomy	Caudate lobectomy or segmentectomy (I)
	Alternative "Sector" Terminology
	Right anterior sectorectomy
	Right posterior sectorectomy or right lateral sectorectomy
	Left medial sectorectomy or left paramedian sectorectomy (bisegmentectomy, III, IV)
	Left lateral sectorectomy (segmentectomy, II)

CHAPTER 32

The Gallbladder and Extrahepatic Biliary System

1. The arterial supply of the common bile duct is derived from
   A. The left hepatic artery
   B. The right hepatic artery
   C. The gastroduodenal artery
   D. The right hepatic and gastroduodenal arteries
   E. The left hepatic and gastroduodenal arteries

2. Anomalies of the hepatic artery and cystic artery are present in what percent of individuals
   A. 15%
   B. 25%
   C. 35%
   D. 50%
   E. 75%

3. The treatment of choice for a type I choledochal cyst is
   A. Observation.
   B. Cyst resection and primary re-anastomosis of the common bile duct.
   C. Resection of the common bile duct, cholecystectomy, and hepatico-jejunostomy.
   D. Resection of the cyst and choledocho-duodenostomy.

Answer: D
The majority of the blood flow to the human common bile duct originates from the right hepatic artery and gastroduodenal arteries, with major trunks running along the medial and lateral aspects of the common duct (often referred to as the *3 o'clock* and *9 o'clock* positions). (See Schwartz 10th ed., p. 1311.)

Answer: D
Variations in the anatomy of the cystic and hepatic arteries are exceedingly common, the "classical" anatomy only appearing in 50 to 60% of the population. The cystic artery is a branch of the right hepatic artery in 90% of individuals. The most common arterial anomaly of the portal arterial system is a replaced right hepatic artery originating from the superior mesenteric artery; this happens in 20% of persons. (See Schwartz 10th ed., p. 1312.)

Answer: C
Choledochal cysts are rare congenital cystic dilations of the extrahepatic and/or intrahepatic biliary tree. Females are affected three to eight times more commonly than men. Though they are commonly diagnosed in childhood, as many as one half of patients are not diagnosed until adulthood. The most common presentations in adulthood are jaundice and cholangitis, and less than one-half of patients present with the classic clinical triad of abdominal pain, jaundice, and a mass. Ultrasonography (US) or computed tomographic (CT) scanning will confirm the diagnosis, but a more definitive imaging technique such as endoscopic retrograde cholangiopancreatography (ERCP), percutaneous transhepatic cholangiography, or magnetic resonance cholangiopancreatography (MRCP) is required to assess the biliary anatomy and plan the appropriate surgical treatment. The risk of cancer development in these patients is up to 15%, and can largely be mitigated by excision of the biliary tree. Types I, II, and IV cysts are treated with excision of the extrahepatic biliary tree with a Roux-en-Y hepaticojejunostomy. Type IV may also require a segmental liver resection. Sphincterotomy is recommended for type III cysts. (See Schwartz 10th ed., p. 1330.)

4. Relaxation of the sphincter of Oddi in response to a meal is largely under the control of which hormone?
   A. Gastrin
   B. Cholecystokinin (CCK)
   C. Motilin
   D. Secretin
   E. Ghrelin

Answer: B

The sphincter of Oddi is a complex structure that is functionally independent from the duodenal musculature and creates a high-pressure zone between the bile duct and the duodenum. The sphincter of Oddi is about 4 to 6 mm in length and has a basal resting pressure of about 13 mm Hg above the duodenal pressure. On manometry, the sphincter shows phasic contractions with a frequency of about 4/min and an amplitude of 12 to 140 mm Hg. The spontaneous motility of the sphincter of Oddi is regulated by the interstitial cells of Cajal through intrinsic and extrinsic inputs from hormones and neurons acting on the smooth muscle cells. Relaxation occurs with a rise in cholecystokinin (CCK), leading to diminished amplitude of phasic contractions and reduced basal pressure, allowing increased flow of bile into the duodenum. During fasting, the sphincter of Oddi activity is coordinated with the periodic partial gallbladder emptying and an increase in bile flow that occurs during phase II of the migrating myoelectric motor complexes. (See Schwartz 10th ed., p. 1313.)

5. What percentage of the bile acid pool is reabsorbed in the ileum through the enterohepatic circulation?
   A. 25%
   B. 50%
   C. 75%
   D. 90%
   E. 95%

Answer: E

Bile is mainly composed of water, electrolytes, bile salts, proteins, lipids, and bile pigments. Sodium, potassium, calcium, and chlorine have the same concentration in bile as in plasma or extracellular fluid. The pH of hepatic bile is usually neutral or slightly alkaline, but varies with diet; an increase in protein shifts the bile to a more acidic pH. The primary bile salts, cholate and chenodeoxycholate, are synthesized in the liver from cholesterol. They are conjugated there with taurine and glycine and act within the bile as anions (bile acids) that are balanced by sodium. Bile salts are excreted into the bile by the hepatocyte and aid in the digestion and absorption of fats in the intestines. In the intestines, about 80% of the conjugated bile acids are absorbed in the terminal ileum. The remainder is de-hydroxylated (de-conjugated) by gut bacteria, forming secondary bile acids deoxycholate and lithocholate. These are absorbed in the colon, transported to the liver, conjugated, and secreted into the bile. Eventually, about 95% of the bile acid pool is reabsorbed and returned via the portal venous system to the liver, the so-called enterohepatic circulation. Five percent is excreted in the stool, leaving the relatively small amount of bile acids to have maximum effect. (See Schwartz 10th ed., p. 1312.)

6. The solubility of cholesterol in bile is determined by
   A. Cholesterol, calcium, bilirubin
   B. Cholesterol, bile salts, lecithin
   C. Bile salts, cholesterol, bilirubin
   D. Calcium, cholesterol, bile salts

Answer: B

Pure cholesterol stones are uncommon and account for <10% of all stones. They usually occur as single large stones with smooth surfaces. Most other cholesterol stones contain variable amounts of bile pigments and calcium, but are always >70% cholesterol by weight. These stones are usually multiple, of variable size, and may be hard and faceted or irregular, mulberry-shaped, and soft. Colors range from whitish yellow and green to black. Most cholesterol stones are radiolucent; <10% are radiopaque. Whether pure or of mixed nature, the common primary event in the formation of cholesterol stones is supersaturation of bile with cholesterol. Therefore, high bile cholesterol levels and cholesterol gallstones are considered one disease. Cholesterol is highly nonpolar and insoluble in water and bile. Cholesterol solubility depends on the relative concentration of cholesterol, bile salts, and lecithin (the main phospholipid in bile). Supersaturation almost always is caused by cholesterol hypersecretion rather than by a reduced secretion of phospholipid or bile salts. (See Schwartz 10th ed., p. 1318.)

7. Acute cholecystitis is considered
   A. A primary infectious process with secondary inflammation.
   B. A sterile primary inflammatory process.
   C. A primary inflammatory process with occasional bacterial contamination.
   D. A primary autoimmune process.

Answer: C
Obstruction of the cystic duct by a gallstone is the initiating event that leads to gallbladder distention, inflammation, and edema of the gallbladder wall. Why inflammation develops only occasionally with cystic duct obstruction is unknown. It is probably related to the duration of obstruction of the cystic duct. Initially, acute cholecystitis is an inflammatory process, probably mediated by the mucosal toxin lysolecithin, a product of lecithin, as well as bile salts and platelet-activating factor. Increase in prostaglandin synthesis amplifies the inflammatory response. Secondary bacterial contamination is documented in 15 to 30% of patients undergoing cholecystectomy for acute uncomplicated cholecystitis. In acute cholecystitis, the gallbladder wall becomes grossly thickened and reddish with subserosal hemorrhages. Pericholecystic fluid often is present. The mucosa may show hyperemia and patchy necrosis. In severe cases, about 5 to 10%, the inflammatory process progresses and leads to ischemia and necrosis of the gallbladder wall. More frequently, the gallstone is dislodged and the inflammation resolves. (See Schwartz 10th ed., p. 1320.)

8. A 54-year-old otherwise healthy woman presents to the emergency department with abdominal pain, fever, chills, and confusion. Blood pressure is 95/50, heart rate 110, and temperature 39°C. Laboratory tests demonstrate a white blood cell count of 15,000, normal hematocrit and platelets, as well as a direct bilirubin of 7.2. Initial management should be
   A. Emergency biliary decompression endoscopically or transhepatically.
   B. Emergent cholecystectomy.
   C. Intravenous (IV) fluid resuscitation and antibiotics.
   D. Observation and pain control.
   E. Discharge home with oral antibiotics with planned cholecystectomy in the coming weeks.

Answer: C
The initial treatment of patients with cholangitis includes intravenous (IV) antibiotics and fluid resuscitation. These patients may require intensive care unit monitoring and vasopressor support. Most patients will respond to these measures. However, the obstructed bile duct must be drained as soon as the patient has been stabilized. About 15% of patients will not respond to antibiotics and fluid resuscitation, and an emergency biliary decompression may be required. Biliary decompression may be accomplished endoscopically, via the percutaneous transhepatic route, or surgically. The selection of procedure should be based on the level and the nature of the biliary obstruction. Patients with choledocholithiasis or periampullary malignancies are best approached endoscopically, with sphincterotomy and stone removal, or by placement of an endoscopic biliary stent. In patients in whom the obstruction is more proximal or perihilar, or when a stricture in a biliary-enteric anastomosis is the cause or the endoscopic route has failed, percutaneous transhepatic drainage is used. When neither ERCP nor percutaneous transhepatic cholangiography (PTC) is available, an emergent operation for decompression of the common bile duct with a T tube may be necessary and lifesaving. Definitive operative therapy should be deferred until the cholangitis has been treated and the proper diagnosis established. Patients with indwelling stents and cholangitis usually require repeated imaging and exchange of the stent over a guidewire. (See Schwartz 10th ed., p. 1323.)

9. Risk factors for acalculous cholecystitis include
   A. Sepsis
   B. Severe burns
   C. Prolonged parenteral nutrition
   D. Multiple trauma
   E. All of the above

Answer: E

Acute inflammation of the gallbladder can occur without gallstones. Acalculous cholecystitis typically develops in critically ill patients in the intensive care unit. Patients on parenteral nutrition with extensive burns, sepsis, major operations, multiple trauma, or prolonged illness with multiple organ system failure are at risk for developing acalculous cholecystitis. The cause is unknown, but gallbladder distention with bile stasis and ischemia has been implicated as causative factors. Pathologic examination of the gallbladder wall reveals edema of the serosa and muscular layers, with patchy thrombosis of arterioles and venules. US is the diagnostic test of choice. Percutaneous US or CT-guided cholecystostomy is typically the intervention of choice, as they are often unfit for surgery. After recovery from the systemic disease, cholecystectomy may be indicated. (See Schwartz 10th ed., pp. 1327–1330.)

10. Appropriate management of a patient with cirrhosis secondary to sclerosing cholangitis includes
    A. Systemic immunosuppression with corticosteroids and calcineurin inhibitors
    B. Anti-tumor necrosis factor (TNF) monoclonal antibodies (infliximab)
    C. Consideration for transplantation
    D. Ursodeoxycholic acid
    E. Excision of the extrahepatic biliary tree (Kasai procedure)

Answer: C

Sclerosing cholangitis (primary or secondary) is an uncommon disease characterized by inflammatory strictures involving the intrahepatic and extrahepatic biliary tree. It is a progressive disease which can lead to biliary cirrhosis. Medical therapy has long been attempted with immunosuppressants, antibiotics, steroids, and ursodeoxycholic acid, and has been disappointing. Surgical management with resection of the extrahepatic biliary tree and hepaticojejunostomy has produced reasonable results in patients with extrahepatic and bifurcation strictures, but without cirrhosis or significant hepatic fibrosis. In patients with sclerosing cholangitis and advanced liver disease, liver transplantation is the only option. It offers excellent results, with overall 5-year survival as high as 85%. Primary sclerosing cholangitis recurs in 10 to 20% of patients and may require retransplantation. (See Schwartz 10th ed., p. 1331.)

11. All of the following patients should be referred to for cholecystectomy EXCEPT
    A. A 45-year-old woman with recurrent bouts of biliary colic and documented gallstones.
    B. A 60-year-old man with biliary pancreatitis.
    C. A 78-year-old man with choledocholithiasis and cholelithiasis.
    D. A 30-year-old woman with acute cholecystitis in her second trimester of pregnancy.

Answer: C

Patients older than 70 years presenting with bile duct stones should have their ductal stones cleared endoscopically. Studies comparing surgery to endoscopic treatment have documented less morbidity and mortality for endoscopic treatment in this group of patients. They do not need to be submitted for a cholecystectomy, as only about 15% will become symptomatic from their gallbladder stones, and such patients can be treated as the need arises by a cholecystectomy. (See Schwartz 10th ed., p. 1322.)

12. Over a 10-year period, what percentage of patients with asymptomatic gallstones will remain symptom-free?
    A. 10%
    B. 25%
    C. 50%
    D. 66%
    E. 90%

Answer: D

Gallstones in patients without biliary symptoms are commonly diagnosed incidentally on US, CT scans, or abdominal radiography or at laparotomy. Several studies have examined the likelihood of developing biliary colic or developing significant complications of gallstone disease. Approximately 3% of asymptomatic individuals become symptomatic per year (ie, develop biliary colic). Once symptomatic, patients tend to have recurring bouts of biliary colic. Complicated gallstone disease develops in 3 to 5% of symptomatic patients per year. Over a 20-year period, about two-thirds of asymptomatic patients with gallstones remain symptom-free. (See Schwartz 10th ed., p. 1317.)

13. All of the following increase risk for the development of gallbladder cancer EXCEPT
    A. Female gender
    B. History of cholelithiasis
    C. History of choledochal cysts
    D. Smoking
    E. Gallbladder polyps

Answer: D

Cholelithiasis is the most important risk factor for gallbladder carcinoma, and up to 95% of patients with carcinoma of the gallbladder have gallstones. However, the 20-year risk of developing cancer for patients with gallstones is <0.5% for the overall population and 1.5% for high-risk groups. The pathogenesis has not been defined but is probably related to chronic inflammation. Larger stones (>3 cm) are associated with a 10-fold increased risk of cancer. The risk of developing cancer of the gallbladder is higher in patients with symptomatic than asymptomatic gallstones.

Polypoid lesions of the gallbladder are associated with increased risk of cancer, particularly in polyps >10 mm. The calcified "porcelain" gallbladder is associated with >20% incidence of gallbladder carcinoma. These gallbladders should be removed, even if the patients are asymptomatic. Patients with choledochal cysts have an increased risk of developing cancer anywhere in the biliary tree, but the incidence is highest in the gallbladder. (See Schwartz 10th ed., p. 1334.)

14. The most common type of gallbladder cancer is
    A. Oat cell
    B. Adenocarcinoma
    C. Adenosquamous
    D. Anaplastic
    E. Squamous cell

Answer: B

Between 80 and 90% of the gallbladder tumors are adenocarcinomas. Squamous cell, adenosquamous, oat cell, and other anaplastic lesions occur rarely. The histologic subtypes of gallbladder adenocarcinomas include papillary, nodular, and tubular. Less than 10% are of the papillary type, but these are associated with an overall better outcome, as they are most commonly diagnosed while localized to the gallbladder. (See Swartz 10th ed., p. 1334.)

15. The gallbladder lymphatics drain into which of the following liver segments?
    A. III and IV
    B. V and VI
    C. IV and V
    D. III and V
    E. I and IV

Answer: C

Lymphatic flow from the gallbladder drains first to the cystic duct node (Calot), then the pericholedochal and hilar nodes, and finally the peripancreatic, duodenal, periportal, celiac, and superior mesenteric artery nodes. The gallbladder veins drain directly into the adjacent liver, usually segments IV and V, where tumor invasion is common. (See Schwartz 10th ed., p. 1334.)

16. Adequate treatment for a gallbladder lesion involving the lamina propria of the gallbladder includes
    A. Cholecystectomy followed by adjuvant chemotherapy.
    B. Neoadjuvant chemoradiotherapy followed by surgical resection.
    C. Segmental liver resection and lymphadenectomy alone.
    D. Cholecystectomy alone.
    E. Extended right hepatectomy.

Answer: D

Tumors limited to the muscular layer of the gallbladder (T1) are usually identified incidentally, after cholecystectomy for gallstone disease. There is near universal agreement that simple cholecystectomy is an adequate treatment for T1 lesions and results in a near 100% overall 5-year survival rate. (See Schwartz 10th ed., p. 1335.)

17. All of the following are different morphological classifications of bile duct adenocarcinomas EXCEPT
    A. Nodular
    B. Scirrhous
    C. Diffusely infiltrating
    D. Serous
    E. Papillary

Answer: D

Over 95% of bile duct cancers are adenocarcinomas. Morphologically, they are divided into nodular (the most common type), scirrhous, diffusely infiltrating, or papillary. (See Schwartz 10th ed., p. 1335.)

18. According to the Bismuth-Corlette classification system, perihilar cholangiocarcinomas extending into the right secondary intrahepatic ducts are classified as
    A. Type II
    B. Type IIIb
    C. Type IIIa
    D. Type IV
    E. Type I

Answer: C
Perihilar cholangiocarcinomas, also referred to as *Klatskin tumors,* are further classified based on anatomic location by the Bismuth-Corlette classification. Type I tumors are confined to the common hepatic duct, but type II tumors involve the bifurcation without involvement of the secondary intrahepatic ducts. Type IIIa and IIIb tumors extend into the right and left secondary intrahepatic ducts, respectively. Type IV tumors involve both the right and left secondary intrahepatic ducts. (See Schwartz 10th ed., pp. 1335–1336.)

19. The best initial imaging test for evaluating for suspected cholangiocarcinoma includes
    A. Percutaneous cholangiography
    B. Endoscopic retrograde cholangiopancreatography
    C. Ultrasound
    D. MRCP
    E. Hepatobiliary iminodiacetic acid (HIDA) scan

Answer: C
The initial tests are usually ultrasound or CT scan. A perihilar tumor causes dilatation of the intrahepatic biliary tree, but normal or collapsed gallbladder and extrahepatic bile ducts distal to the tumor. Distal bile duct cancer leads to dilatation of the extra- and intrahepatic bile ducts as well as the gallbladder. Ultrasound can establish the level of obstruction and rule out the presence of bile duct stones as the cause of the obstructive jaundice. It is usually difficult to visualize the tumor itself on ultrasound or on a standard CT scan. Either ultrasound or spiral CT can be used to determine portal vein patency. The biliary anatomy is defined by cholangiography. PTC defines the proximal extent of the tumor, which is the most important factor in determining resectability. ERCP is used, particularly in the evaluation of distal bile duct tumors. For the evaluation of vascular involvement, celiac angiography may be necessary. With the newer types of MRI, a single noninvasive test has the potential of evaluating the biliary anatomy, lymph nodes, and vascular involvement, as well as the tumor growth itself. (See Schwartz 10th ed., p. 1336.)

20. All of the following examples are considered resectable lesions EXCEPT
    A. Nodular type cholangiocarcinoma limited to the distal common bile duct.
    B. Lesions requiring resection of the portal vein as part of the dissection.
    C. Lesions involving the caudate lobe and positive portahepatis nodes.
    D. Klatskin tumors requiring resection of segments IV and V.
    E. Mid common bile duct lesion with positive celiac lymph nodes.

Answer: E
Patients should undergo surgical exploration if they have no signs of metastasis or locally unresectable disease. However, despite improvements in US, CT scanning, and MRI, more than one-half of patients who are explored are found to have peritoneal implants, nodal or hepatic metastasis, or locally advanced disease that precludes resection. For these patients, surgical bypass for biliary decompression and cholecystectomy to prevent the occurrence of acute cholecystitis should be performed. (See Schwartz 10th ed., p. 1336.)

21. Patients with a history of choledochal cysts are at increased risk of developing biliary cancer
    A. In the gallbladder alone.
    B. Predominantly intrahepatic portions of the biliary tree.
    C. In the distal common bile duct.
    D. At the site of the previous cyst.
    E. Throughout the biliary tree.

Answer: E
Patients with choledochal cysts have an increased risk of developing cancer anywhere in the biliary tree, but the incidence is highest in the gallbladder. Sclerosing cholangitis, anomalous pancreaticobiliary duct junction, and exposure to carcinogens (azotoluene, nitrosamines) also are associated with cancer of the gallbladder. (See Schwartz 10th ed., p. 1334.)

22. What percentage of bile duct injuries are identified intraoperatively?
    A. 85%
    B. 5%
    C. 25%
    D. 50%
    E. 10%

Answer: C

Only about 25% of major bile duct injuries (common bile duct or hepatic duct) are recognized at the time of operation. Most commonly, intraoperative bile leakage, recognition of the correct anatomy, and an abnormal cholangiogram lead to the diagnosis of a bile duct injury. (See Schwartz 10th ed., p. 1332.)

23. The best initial test for a suspected postoperative bile leak includes
    A. PTC
    B. ERCP
    C. MRI
    D. US
    E. Plain film X-ray

Answer: D

Bile leak, most commonly from the cystic duct stump, a transected aberrant right hepatic duct, or a lateral injury to the main bile duct, usually presents with pain, fever, and a mild elevation of liver function tests. A CT scan or an ultrasound will show either a collection (biloma) in the gallbladder area or free fluid (bile) in the peritoneum. (See Schwartz 10th ed., p. 1332.)

24. What is the best initial management for an intraoperatively identified minor lateral injury to the common bile duct?
    A. Placement of a T-tube through the site of injury in the duct.
    B. Primary oversew of the injury intraoperatively.
    C. Resection of the injured portion of the duct with end-to-end anastomosis.
    D. Intraoperative placement of endoscopic biliary stent.
    E. Resection of the bile duct and a Roux-en-Y hepatico-jejunostomy reconstruction.

Answer: A

Lateral injury to the common bile duct or the common hepatic duct, recognized at the time of surgery, is best managed with a T-tube placement. If the injury is a small incision in the duct, the T tube may be placed through it as if it were a formal choledochotomy. In more extensive lateral injuries, the T tube should be placed through a separate choledochotomy and the injury closed over the T-tube end to minimize the risk of subsequent stricture formation. (See Schwartz 10th ed., p. 1333.)

25. After identification of a postoperative biliary stricture, what is the best initial management?
    A. Operative resection of the involved biliary segment and reconstruction with an end-to-end Roux-en-Y hepaticojejunostomy.
    B. ERCP with sphincterotomy and stenting of the pancreatic duct.
    C. Transhepatic catheter placement for biliary decompression.
    D. HIDA scan.
    E. Operative placement of a T tube at site of biliary stricture.

Answer: C

Patients with bile duct stricture from an injury or as a sequela of previous repair usually present with either progressive elevation of liver function tests or cholangitis. The initial management usually includes transhepatic biliary drainage catheter placement for decompression as well as for defining the anatomy and the location and the extent of the damage. These catheters will also serve as useful technical aids during subsequent biliary enteric anastomosis. An anastomosis is performed between the duct proximal to the injury and a Roux loop of jejunum. Balloon dilatation of a stricture usually requires multiple attempts and rarely provides adequate long-term relief. Self-expanding metal or plastic stents, placed either percutaneously or endoscopically across the stricture, can provide temporary drainage and, in the high-risk patient, permanent drainage of the biliary tree. (See Schwartz 10th ed., p. 1333.)

26. In the early postoperative period, what is the most common presentation of a patient with a biliary injury?
    A. Fever
    B. Abdominal pain
    C. Steatorrhea
    D. Elevated transaminases
    E. Nausea

Answer: D

In the early postoperative period, patients present either with progressive elevation of liver function tests due to an occluded or a stenosed bile duct, or with a bile leak from an injured duct. (See Schwartz 10th ed., p. 1333.)

Pancreas

1. The percentage of patients who will have an occurrence of a replaced right hepatic artery is
   A. 1–2%
   B. 5–10%
   C. 15–20%
   D. 20–25%

Answer: C

In 15 to 20% of patients, the right hepatic artery will arise from the superior mesenteric artery and travel upward toward the liver along the posterior aspect of the head of the pancreas (referred to as a *replaced right hepatic artery*). It is important to look for this variation on preoperative computed tomographic (CT) scans and in the operating room (OR) so the replaced hepatic artery is recognized and injury is avoided. (See Schwartz 10th ed., p. 1345.)

2. The most common complication of chronic pancreatitis is
   A. Pseudocysts
   B. Duct strictures and/or stones
   C. Pancreatic necrosis
   D. Duodenal obstruction

Answer: A

A chronic collection of pancreatic fluid surrounded by a non-epithelialized wall of granulation tissue and fibrosis is referred to as a *pseudocyst*. Pseudocysts occur in up to 10% of patients with acute pancreatitis, and in 20 to 38% of patients with chronic pancreatitis, and thus, they comprise the most common complication of chronic pancreatitis. (See Schwartz 10th ed., pp. 1375–1376.)

3. Insulinomas associated with the multiple endocrine neoplasia (MEN)1 syndrome
   A. Do not usually require resection
   B. Are sporadic in nature
   C. Have a lower rate of recurrence
   D. Are more likely to be malignant

Answer: B

Approximately 90% of insulinomas are sporadic, and 10% are associated with the multiple endocrine neoplasia (MEN)1 syndrome. Insulinomas associated with the MEN1 syndrome are more likely to be multifocal and have a higher rate of recurrence. (See Schwartz 10th ed., p. 1391.)

4. A pancreatic cystic neoplasms that is <3 cm, has atypical cells present, and has a solid component
   A. Requires a repeat CT scan in 3 to 6 months
   B. Requires a repeat CT scan in 1 year
   C. Requires continued observation
   D. Requires resection

Answer: D

See Figure 33-1. (See Schwartz 10th ed., Figure 33-75, p. 1409.)

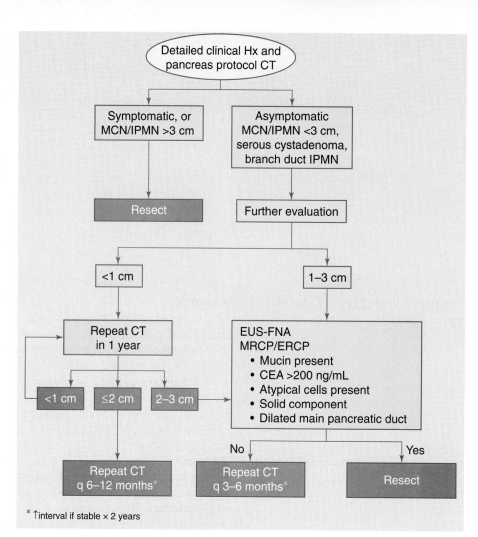

FIG. 33-1. Algorithm for management of pancreatic cystic neoplasms. CEA = carcinoembryonic antigen; CT = computed tomography; ERCP = endoscopic retrograde cholangiopancreatography; EUS = endoscopic ultrasound; FNA = fine-needle aspiration; Hx = history; IPMN = intraductal papillary mucinous neoplasm of the pancreas; MCN = mucinous cystic neoplasm; mo = month(s); MRCP = magnetic resonance cholangiopancreatography; y = year(s).

5. According to Ranson criteria a 67-year-old female patient suspected of acute pancreatitis presenting to the OR with sudden onset of severe abdominal pain, a serum aspartate transaminase (AST) >250 U/dL, a white blood cell (WBC) >16,000/mm³, and a blood glucose >200 mg/dL would receive a disease classification of
    A. Predicted severe
    B. Predicted mild, uncomplicated
    C. Predicted moderate
    D. A mortality of 10%

Answer: A
See Table 33-1. (See Schwartz 10th ed, Table 33-7, p. 1356.)

TABLE 33-1	Ranson's prognostic signs of pancreatitis

Criteria for Acute Pancreatitis Not due to Gallstones

At admission	During the initial 48 h
Age >55 y	Hematocrit fall >10 points
WBC >16,000/mm³	BUN elevation >5 mg/dL
Blood glucose >200 mg/dL	Serum calcium <8 mg/dL
Serum LDH >350 IU/L	Arterial PO_2 <60 mm Hg
Serum AST >250 U/dL	Base deficit >4 mEq/L
	Estimated fluid sequestration >6 L

Criteria for Acute Gallstone Pancreatitis

At admission	During the initial 48 h
Age >70 y	Hematocrit fall >10 points
WBC >18,000/mm³	BUN elevation >2 mg/dL
Blood glucose >220 mg/dL	Serum calcium <8 mg/dL
Serum LDH >400 IU/L	Base deficit >5 mEq/L
Serum AST >250 U/dL	Estimated fluid sequestration >4 L

AST = aspartate transaminase; BUN = blood urea nitrogen; LDH = lactate dehydrogenase; PO_2 = partial pressure of oxygen; WBC = white blood cell count.
Note: Fewer than 3 positive criteria predict mild, uncomplicated disease whereas more than 6 positive criteria predict severe disease with a mortality risk of 50%.
Sources: Data from Ranson JHC. Etiological and prognostic factors in human acute pancreatitis: A review. *Am J Gastroenterol* 77:633, 1982, and From Ranson JH, Rifkind KM, Roses DF, et al. Prognostic signs and the role of operative management in acute pancreatitis. *Surg Gynecol Obstet* 139:69, 1974.

6. Which of the following is the most common presenting symptom in patients with a somatostatinoma?
   A. Cholelithiasis
   B. Constipation
   C. Hypoglycemia
   D. Hypocalcemia

Answer: A

Because somatostatin inhibits pancreatic and biliary secretions, patients with a somatostatinoma present with gallstones due to bile stasis, diabetes due to inhibition of insulin secretion, and steatorrhea due to inhibition of pancreatic exocrine secretion and bile secretion. Most somatostatinomas originate in the proximal pancreas or the pancreatoduodenal groove, with the ampulla and periampullary area as the most common site (60%). The most common presentations are abdominal pain (25%), jaundice (25%), and cholelithiasis (19%). This rare type of pancreatic endocrine tumor is diagnosed by confirming elevated serum somatostatin levels, which are usually above 10 ng/mL. Although most reported cases of somatostatinoma involve metastatic disease, an attempt at complete excision of the tumor and cholecystectomy is warranted in fit patients. (See Schwartz 10th ed., p. 1393.)

7. The etiology associated with chronic calcific pancreatitis is
   A. Hyperparathyroidism
   B. Hyperlipidemia
   C. Alcohol abuse
   D. All of the above

Answer: D

This type is the largest subgroup in the classification scheme proposed by Singer and Chari, and includes patients with calcific pancreatitis of most etiologies (Table 33-2). Although the majority of patients with calcific pancreatitis have a history of alcohol abuse, stone formation and parenchymal calcification can develop in a variety of etiologic subgroups; hereditary pancreatitis and tropical pancreatitis are particularly noteworthy for the formation of stone disease. The clinician should therefore avoid the assumption that calcific pancreatitis confirms the diagnosis of alcohol abuse. (See Schwartz 10th ed., Table 33-11, p. 1365.)

TABLE 33-2	Classification of chronic pancreatitis based on etiologic causes			
Chronic Calcific Pancreatitis	**Chronic Obstructive Pancreatitis**	**Chronic Inflammatory Pancreatitis**	**Chronic Autoimmune Pancreatitis**	**Asymptomatic Pancreatic Fibrosis**
Alcohol	Pancreatic tumors	Unknown	Associated with autoimmune disorders (e.g., primary sclerosing cholangitis)	Chronic alcoholic
Hereditary	Ductal stricture			Endemic in asymptomatic residents in tropical climates
Tropical	Gallstone- or trauma-induced or pancreas divisum			
Hyperlipidemia			Sjögren syndrome	
Hypercalcemia			Primary biliary cirrhosis	
Drug-induced				
Idiopathic				

Source: Reproduced with permission from Singer MV, Chari ST. Classification of chronic pancreatitis, in Beger HG et al, eds. *The Pancreas.* London: Blackwell-Science, 1998, p. 665. Copyright Wiley Blackwell.

8. In patients undergoing endoscopic retrograde cholangio-pancreatography (ERCP) for diagnosis and staging of chronic pancreatitis, the population most at risk of developing procedure-induced pancreatitis is
   A. One with calculus disease
   B. One with intraductal lesions
   C. One with sphincter of Oddi dysfunction
   D. One with a high percentage of parenchymal calcification

Answer: C

Endoscopic retrograde cholangiopancreatography (ERCP) is considered to be the gold standard for the diagnosis and staging of chronic pancreatitis. It also serves as a vehicle that enables other diagnostic and therapeutic maneuvers, such as biopsy or brushing for cytology, or the use of stents to relieve obstruction or drain a pseudocyst (Fig. 33-2). Unfortunately, ERCP also carries a risk of procedure-induced pancreatitis that occurs in approximately 5% of patients. Patients at increased risk include those with sphincter of Oddi dysfunction and those with a previous history of post-ERCP pancreatitis. Post-ERCP pancreatitis occurs after uncomplicated procedures, as well as after those that require prolonged manipulation. Severe pancreatitis and deaths have occurred after ERCP, it should be reserved for patients in whom the diagnosis is unclear despite the use of other imaging methods, or in whom a diagnostic or therapeutic maneuver is specifically indicated. (See Schwartz 10th ed., Figure 33-29, pp. 1370–1371.)

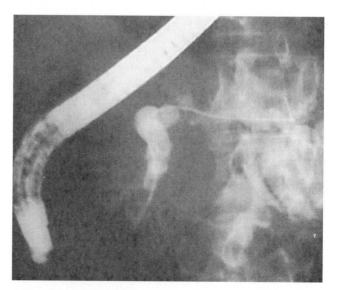

FIG. 33-2. Pancreatic duct stenting. At endoscopic retrograde cholangiopancreatography, a stent is placed in the proximal pancreatic duct to relieve obstruction and reduce symptoms of pain. Pancreatic duct stents are left in place for only a limited time to avoid further inflammation.

9. Treatment of a 1-cm gastrinoma in the wall of the duodenum is best accomplished by
   A. Enucleation
   B. Full-thickness resection
   C. Duodenectomy
   D. Whipple procedure

Answer: B

Fifty percent of gastrinomas metastasize to lymph nodes or the liver, and are therefore considered malignant. Patients who meet criteria for operability should undergo exploration for possible removal of the tumor. Although the tumors are submucosal, a full-thickness excision of the duodenal wall is performed if a duodenal gastrinoma is found. All lymph nodes in Passaro triangle are excised for pathologic analysis. If the gastrinoma is found in the pancreas and does not involve the main pancreatic duct, it is enucleated. Pancreatic resection is justified for solitary gastrinomas with no metastases. A highly selective vagotomy can be performed if unresectable disease is identified or if the gastrinoma cannot be localized. This may reduce the amount of expensive proton pump inhibitors required. In cases in which hepatic metastases are identified, resection is justified if the primary gastrinoma is controlled and the metastases can be safely and completely removed. Debulking or incomplete removal of multiple hepatic metastases is probably not helpful, especially in the setting of MEN1. The application of new modalities such as radiofrequency ablation seems reasonable, but data to support this approach are limited. Postoperatively, patients are followed with fasting serum gastrin levels, secretin stimulation tests, octreotide scans, and CT scans. In patients found to have inoperable disease, chemotherapy with streptozocin, doxorubicin, and 5-fluorouracil (5-FU) is used. Other approaches such as somatostatin analogues, interferon, and chemoembolization also have been used in gastrinoma with some success. (See Schwartz 10th ed., p. 1392.)

10. The ERCP finding that is virtually diagnostic of intraductal papillary mucinous neoplasms (IPMNs) is
    A. A fish-eye lesion
    B. Calcification
    C. Beaded or chain-of-lakes appearance of the duct
    D. Cysts that resemble serous cystadenomas

Answer: A

Intraductal papillary mucinous neoplasms (IPMNs) usually occur within the head of the pancreas and arise within the pancreatic ducts. The ductal epithelium forms a papillary projection into the duct, and mucin production causes intraluminal cystic dilation of the pancreatic ducts (Fig. 33-3). Imaging studies demonstrate diffuse dilation of the pancreatic duct, and the pancreatic parenchyma is often atrophic due to chronic duct obstruction. However, classic features of chronic pancreatitis, such as calcification and a beaded appearance of the duct, are not present. At ERCP, mucin can be seen extruding from the ampulla of Vater, a so-called *fish-eye lesion*, that is virtually diagnostic of IPMN (Fig. 33-4). (See Schwartz 10th ed., Figures 33-77 and 33-8, pp. 1411–1412.)

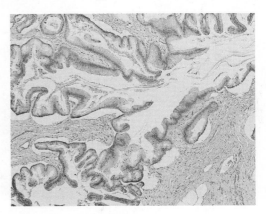

FIG. 33-3. Intraductal papillary mucinous neoplasm histology. Papillary projections of ductal epithelium resemble villous morphology and contain mucin-filled vesicles. (From Asiyanbola B, Andersen DK. *IPMN*. Editorial Update. AccessSurgery, McGraw-Hill, 2008, with permission. Copyright The McGraw-Hill Companies, Inc.)

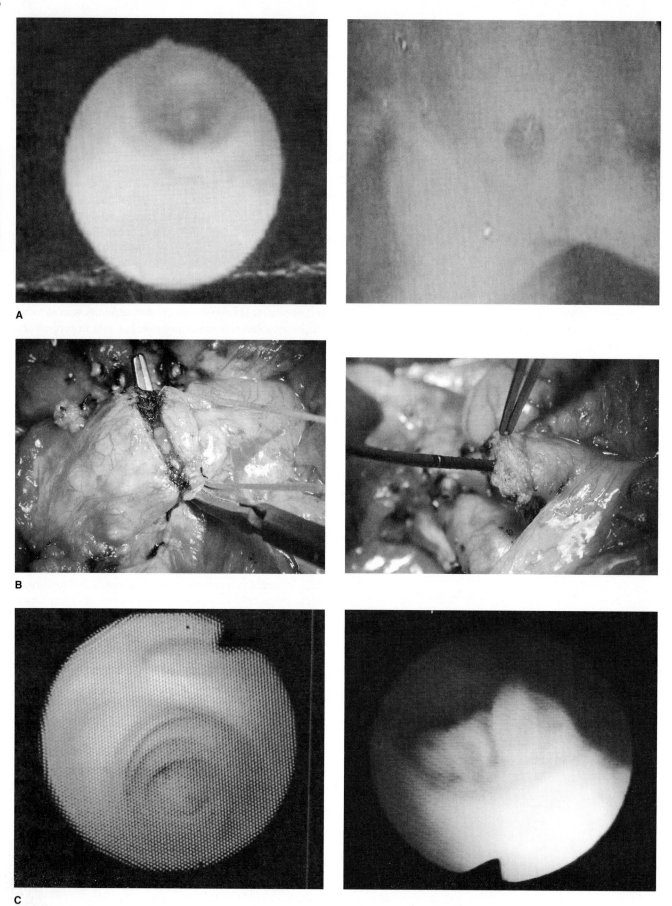

FIG. 33-4. Intraductal papillary mucinous neoplasm (IPMN). **A.** Examples of "fish-eye deformity" of IPMN. Mucin is seen extruding from the ampulla. **B.** Mucin coming from pancreatic duct when neck of pancreas is transected during Whipple procedure (left). Intraoperative pancreatic ductoscopy to assess the pancreatic tail (right). **C.** Views of pancreatic duct during ductoscopy; normal (left) and IPMN (right).

11. Pain from chronic pancreatitis can be caused by
    A. Ductal hypertension
    B. Parenchymal disease
    C. Obstructive pancreatopathy
    D. All of the above

12. A patient undergoing the Frey procedure to relieve pain from obstructive pancreatopathy is found to have 85% parenchymal fibrosis. The percentage of pain relief the patient is likely to experience is
    A. 50%
    B. 10%
    C. 100%
    D. 60%

Answer: D

Pain from chronic pancreatitis has been ascribed to three possible etiologies. Ductal hypertension, due to strictures or stones, may predispose to pain that is initiated or exacerbated by eating. Chronic pain without exacerbation may be related to parenchymal disease or retroperitoneal inflammation with persistent neural involvement. Acute exacerbations of pain in the setting of chronic pain may be due to acute increases in duct pressure or recurrent episodes of acute inflammation in the setting of chronic parenchymal disease. Nealon and Matin have described these various pain syndromes as being predictive of the response to various surgical procedures. Pain that is found in association with ductal hypertension is most readily relieved by pancreatic duct decompression, through endoscopic stenting or surgical decompression. (See Schwartz 10th ed., p. 1371.)

Answer: C

The surgical relief of pain due to obstructive pancreatopathy may be dependent on the degree of underlying fibrosis rather than the presence of ductal obstruction, per se, according to a recent study from Johns Hopkins by Cooper et al. Thirty-five patients with chronic pain associated with evidence of duct obstruction were treated with local resection of the pancreatic head and longitudinal pancreatico-jejunostomy (LR-LPJ), or Frey procedure, and the degree of pain resolution after surgery was compared to the degree of underlying parenchymal fibrosis. After a follow-up that averaged 22 months, patients with more than 80% fibrosis had 100% pain relief, whereas only 60% patients with less than 10% fibrosis experienced substantial or complete pain relief (Fig. 33-5). These findings suggest that minimal fibrosis, or "minimal change chronic pancreatitis," may produce chronic pain due to extra-pancreatic or "peri-pancreatic" inflammatory events which are not ameliorated by decompression. (See Schwartz 10th ed., Figure 33-31, pp. 1371–1372.)

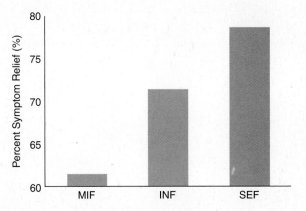

FIG. 33-5. Pain relief from chronic pancreatitis treated with the Frey procedure correlates with the degree of underlying fibrosis. Percent of patients with pain relief for those with mild or minimal fibrosis (MIF, n=13), intermediate fibrosis (INF, n=7), and severe or extensive fibrosis (SEF, n=14). P<0.05 for MIF versus SEF by chi-square analysis. (Reproduced with permission from Cooper M, Makary MA, Ng Y, et al. Extent of pancreatic fibrosis as a determinant of symptom resolution after the Frey procedure: A clinicopathologic analysis. *J Gastrointest Surg* 17:682-687;2013.)

13. The only therapy shown to prevent the progression of chronic pancreatitis is
    A. Pancreatic duct decompression
    B. Major resection
    C. Transduodenal sphincteroplasty
    D. Roux-en-Y pancreaticojejunostomy

Answer: A

The traditional approach to surgical treatment of chronic pancreatitis and its complications has maintained that surgery should be considered only when the medical therapy of symptoms has failed. Nealon and Thompson published a landmark study in 1993, however, that showed that the progression of chronic obstructive pancreatitis could be delayed or prevented by pancreatic duct decompression. No other therapy has been shown to prevent the progression of chronic pancreatitis, and this study demonstrated the role of surgery in the early management of the disease (Table 33-3). Small-duct disease or "minimal change chronic pancreatitis" are causes for uncertainty over the choice of operation, however. Major resections have a high complication rate, both early and late, in chronic alcoholic pancreatitis, and lesser procedures often result in symptomatic recurrence. So the choice of operation and the timing of surgery are based on each patient's pancreatic anatomy, the likelihood (or lack thereof) that further medical and endoscopic therapy will halt the symptoms of the disease, and the chance that a good result will be obtained with the lowest risk of morbidity and mortality. Finally, preparation for surgery should include restoration of protein-caloric homeostasis, abstinence from alcohol and tobacco, and a detailed review of the risks and likely outcomes to establish a bond of trust and commitment between the patient and the surgeon. (See Schwartz 10th ed., Table 33-20, p. 1382.)

TABLE 33-3	Effect of surgical drainage on progression of chronic pancreatitis
Treatment Group	**24-Month Evaluation**
Operated ($n = 47$)	Mild to moderate 48 (87%); severe 6 (13%)
Nonoperated ($n = 36$)	Mild to moderate 8 (22%); severe 28 (78%)

Eighty-three patients with chronic pancreatitis were evaluated by exocrine, endocrine, nutritional, and endoscopic retrograde cholangiopancreatography studies, and all had mild to moderate disease and dilated pancreatic ducts. A Puestow-type duct decompression procedure was performed in 47 patients, and all subjects were restaged by the same methods 24 months later.

Source: Reproduced with permission from Nealon WH, Thompson JC. Progressive loss of pancreatic function in chronic pancreatitis is delayed by main pancreatic duct decompression. A longitudinal prospective analysis of the modified puestow procedure. *Ann Surg* 217:458, discussion 466, 1993.

14. The part of the pancreas resected in order to ensure successful resolution of pain long-term for patients with chronic pancreatitis is
    A. The head
    B. The body
    C. The neck
    D. The tail

Answer: A
The common element of these variations on the theme of LR-LPJ remains the excavation or "coring out" of the central portion of the pancreatic head. It remains uncertain, however, whether and to what degree the dichotomy needs to be extended into the body and tail. The logical conclusion of all of these efforts is that the head of the pancreas is the nidus of the chronic inflammatory process in chronic pancreatitis, and that removal of the central portion of the head of the gland is the key to the successful resolution of pain long-term. (See Schwartz 10th ed., pp. 1342 and 1387.)

15. In pylorus-preserving resections of the pancreas, the technique with the lowest rate of pancreatic leakage is
    A. Stent
    B. Glue
    C. Octreotide
    D. All of the above

Answer: D
The preservation of the pylorus has several theoretical advantages, including prevention of reflux of pancreaticobiliary secretions into the stomach, decreased incidence of marginal ulceration, normal gastric acid secretion and hormone release, and improved gastric function. Patients with pylorus-preserving resections have appeared to regain weight better than historic controls in some studies. Return of gastric emptying in the immediate postoperative period may take longer after the pylorus-preserving operation, and it is controversial whether there is any significant improvement in long-term quality of life with pyloric preservation.

Techniques for the pancreaticojejunostomy include end-to-side or end-to-end and duct-to-mucosa sutures or invagination (Fig. 33-6). Pancreaticogastrostomy has also been investigated.

Some surgeons use stents, glue to seal the anastomosis, or octreotide to decrease pancreatic secretions. No matter what combination of these techniques is used, the pancreatic leakage rate is always about 10%. Therefore, the choice of techniques depends more on the surgeon's personal experience. (See Schwartz 10th ed., Figure 33-73, p. 1403.)

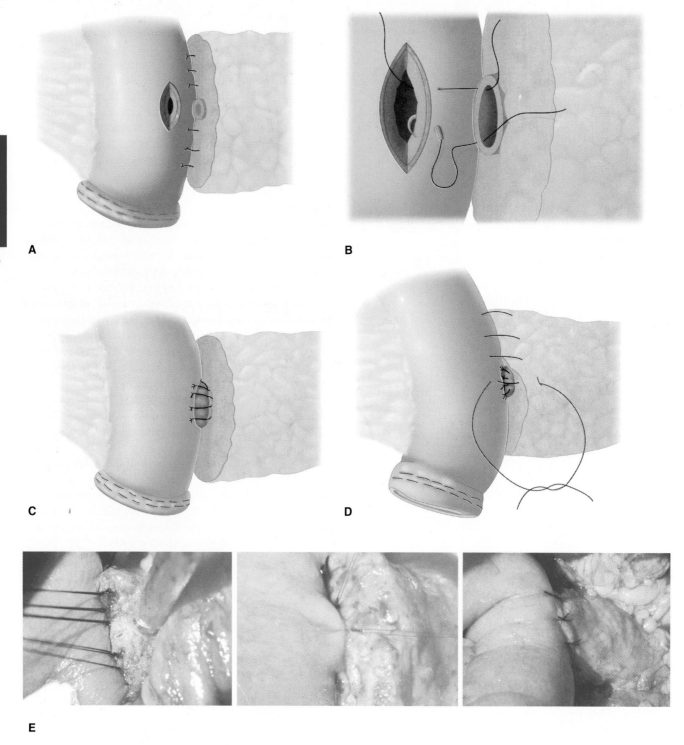

A

B

C

D

E

FIG. 33-6. Techniques for pancreaticojejunostomy. **A** to **D.** Duct-to-mucosa, end-to-side. **E.** Intraoperative photographs of end-to-side pancreaticojejunostomy. **F** to **J.** End-to-end invagination. **K** to **O.** End-to-side invagination.

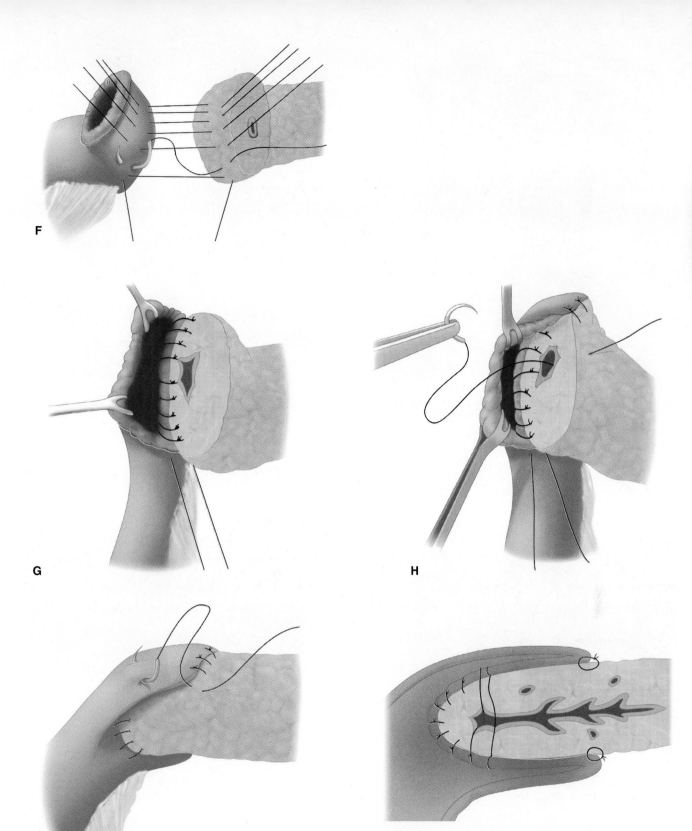

FIG. 33-6. (*Continued*)

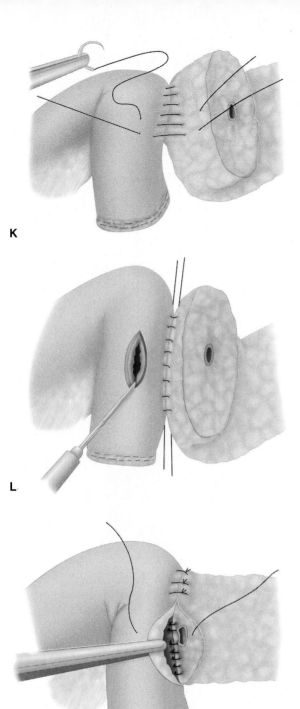

K

L

M

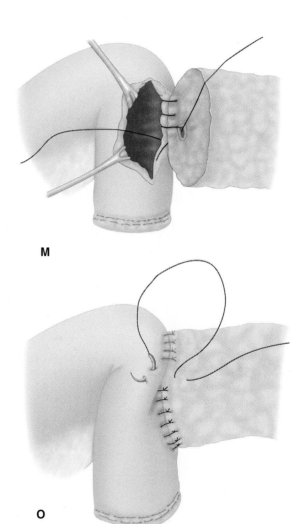

N

O

FIG. 33-6. *(Continued)*

16. The prognosis factor that does NOT decrease survival rates in patients with gastrinomas is
    A. Liver metastases
    B. Absence of MEN1
    C. Lymph node metastases
    D. Primary tumor located outside of Passaro triangle

Answer: C

Fifty percent of gastrinomas metastasize to lymph nodes or the liver, and are therefore considered malignant. Patients who meet criteria for operability should undergo exploration for possible removal of the tumor. Although the tumors are submucosal, a full-thickness excision of the duodenal wall is performed if a duodenal gastrinoma is found. All lymph nodes in Passaro triangle are excised for pathologic analysis. If the gastrinoma is found in the pancreas and does not involve the main pancreatic duct, it is enucleated. Pancreatic resection is justified for solitary gastrinomas with no metastases. A highly selective vagotomy can be performed if unresectable disease is identified or if the gastrinoma cannot be localized. This may reduce the amount of expensive proton pump inhibitors required. In cases in which hepatic metastases are identified, resection is justified if the primary gastrinoma is controlled and the metastases can be safely and completely removed. Debulking or incomplete removal of multiple hepatic metastases is probably not helpful, especially in the setting of MEN1. The application of new modalities such as radiofrequency ablation seems reasonable, but data to support this approach are limited. Postoperatively, patients are followed with fasting serum gastrin levels, secretin stimulation tests, octreotide scans, and CT scans. In patients found to have inoperable disease, chemotherapy with streptozocin, doxorubicin, and 5-fluorouracil (5-FU) is used. Other approaches such as somatostatin analogues, interferon, and chemoembolization also have been used in gastrinoma with some success.

Unfortunately, a biochemical cure is achieved in only about one-third of the patients operated on for Zollinger-Ellison syndrome (ZES). Despite the lack of success, long-term survival rates are good, even in patients with liver metastases. The 15-year survival rate for patients without liver metastases is about 80%, while the 5-year survival rate for patients with liver metastases is 20 to 50%. Pancreatic tumors are usually larger than tumors arising in the duodenum, and more often have lymph node metastases. In gastrinomas, liver metastases decrease survival rates, but lymph node metastases do not. The best results are seen after complete excision of small sporadic tumors originating in the duodenum. Large tumors associated with liver metastases, located outside of Passaro triangle, have the worst prognosis. (See Schwartz 10th ed., p. 1392.)

CHAPTER 34

Spleen

1. Which of the following is NOT a location where accessory spleens can be found?
   A. Gastrocolic ligament
   B. Gerota's fascia
   C. Large bowel mesentery
   D. Broad ligament

Answer: B

The most common anomaly of splenic embryology is the accessory spleen. Present in up to 20% of the population, one or more accessory spleen(s) may occur in up to 30% of patients with hematologic disease. Over 80% of accessory spleens are found in the region of the splenic hilum and vascular pedicle. Other locations for accessory spleens in descending order of frequency are: the gastrocolic ligament, the tail of the pancreas, the greater omentum, the greater curve of the stomach, the splenocolic ligament, the small and large bowel mesentery, the left broad ligament in women, and the left spermatic cord in men. (See Schwartz 10th ed., p. 1424.)

2. Which of the following splenic ligaments is NOT an avascular plane?
   A. Gastrosplenic
   B. Splenocolic
   C. Phrenosplenic
   D. Splenorenal

Answer: A

Of particular clinical relevance, the spleen is suspended in position by several ligaments and peritoneal folds to the colon (splenocolic ligament); the stomach (gastrosplenic ligament); the diaphragm (phrenosplenic ligament); the kidney, the adrenal gland, and the tail of the pancreas (splenorenal ligament) (Fig. 34-1). Whereas the gastrosplenic ligament contains the short gastric vessels, the remaining ligaments are usually avascular, with rare exceptions, such as in a patient with portal hypertension. The relationship of the pancreas to the spleen also has important clinical implications. In cadaveric anatomic series, the tail of the pancreas has been demonstrated to lie within 1 cm of the splenic hilum 75% of the time and to actually abut the spleen in 30% of patients. (See Schwartz 10th ed., Figure 34-2, p. 1425.)

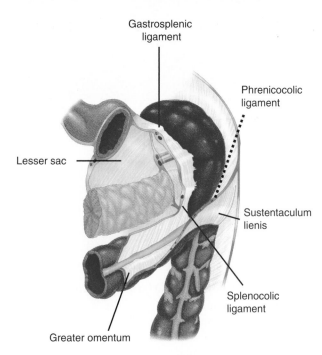

FIG. 34-1. Suspensory ligaments of the spleen. (Data from Poulin EC, Thibault C. The anatomical basis for laparoscopic splenectomy. *Can J Surg* 36:484;1993.)

3. All of the following are functions of the spleen EXCEPT
   A. Clearance of damaged or aged red blood cells (RBCs) from the blood.
   B. Extramedullary site for hematopoiesis and recycling iron.
   C. Initiation of adaptive immune response from filtration of lymph.
   D. Clearance of encapsulated bacteria from the bloodstream.

Answer: C

The spleen has both fast and slow circulation of blood. It is during slow circulation that blood travels through the reticular spaces and splenic cords where it is exposed to contact with splenic macrophages which remove senescent blood cells. Through this process the spleen is also able to remove erythrocyte inclusions such as Heinz bodies without lysing the cells. Through the reticuloendothelial system the spleen clears encapsulated bacteria such as pneumococcus and *Haemophilus influenzae* which are poorly opsonized from the hepatic reticuloendothelial system. In addition to these functions the spleen serves as an extramedullary site for hematopoiesis and plays a functional role in the recycling of iron. While the white pulp of the spleen is important in the initiation of the adaptive immune response, material is delivered to the spleen through the blood and not the lymph. (See Schwartz 10th ed., p. 1427.)

4. Which of the following proteins is not altered in hereditary spherocytosis (HS)?
   A. Pyruvate kinase
   B. Spectrin
   C. Ankyrin
   D. Band 3 protein

Answer: A

The underlying abnormality in hereditary spherocytosis (HS) is an inherited dysfunction or deficiency in one of the erythrocyte membrane proteins (spectrin, ankyrin, band 3 protein, or protein 4.2), which results in destabilization of the membrane lipid bilayer. This destabilization allows a release of lipids from the membrane, causing a reduction in membrane surface area and a lack of deformability, leading to sequestration and destruction of the spherocytic erythrocytes in the spleen.

Although less common than glucose-6-phosphate dehydrogenase (G6PD) deficiency overall, pyruvate kinase deficiency is the most common RBC enzyme deficiency to cause congenital chronic hemolytic anemia. (See Schwartz 10th ed., p. 1429.)

5. Splenectomy is indicated as a treatment in which of the following conditions?
   A. Cold-antibody autoimmune hemolytic anemia (AIHA)
   B. Hodgkin's disease
   C. G6PD deficiency
   D. Abscesses of the spleen

Answer: D

Autoimmune hemolytic anemias (AIHA) are characterized by destruction of RBCs due to autoantibodies against RBC antigens. AIHA is divided into warm and cold categories based on the temperature at which the autoantibodies exert their effect. In cold-agglutinin disease severe symptoms are uncommon and splenectomy is almost never indicated. Warm-agglutinin disease presents with mild jaundice as well as symptoms and signs of anemia with one-third to one-half of patients presenting with splenomegaly. Initial treatment is with corticosteroids with splenectomy being second-line therapy with failure of steroids. Although splenectomy has a 60 to 80% response rate recurrence is common. Hodgkin's disease is a disorder of the lymphoid system characterized by the presence of Reed-Sternberg cells. Most patients present with lympadenopathy above the diaphragm with adenopathy below the diaphragm rare on presentation. Adenopathy below the diaphragm can arise with disease progression and the spleen is often an occult site of spread although splenomegaly is uncommon. While splenectomy is performed for surgical staging in certain cases including clinical suspicion of lymphoma without evidence of peripheral disease or restaging for suspicion of failure after chemotherapy, staging laparotomy is less commonly performed in the current era of minimally invasive surgery and advanced imaging techniques. G6PD deficiency is the most common RBC enzyme deficiency and can be characterized by chronic hemolytic anemia, acute intermittent hemolytic episodes, or no hemolysis depending on the variant. Treatment for G6PD deficiency involves avoidance of drugs known to precipitate hemolysis. Treatment for splenic abscess involves initiation of broad-spectrum antibiotics with tailoring of antibiotic therapy once culture results become available as well as splenectomy. While splenectomy is the procedure of choice percutaneous or open drainage are options for patients unable to tolerate splenectomy. (See Schwartz 10th ed., p. 1431.)

6. The disproportionately high rate of overwhelming postsplenectomy infection (OPSI) in thalassemia patients is thought to be due to an immune deficiency. Which of the following strategies has been shown to reduce mortality?
   A. Partial splenectomy.
   B. Prophylactic antibiotic therapy.
   C. Delaying splenectomy until after 2 years of age.
   D. Transfusion to maintain a hemoglobin (HGB) of >9 mg/dL.

Answer: A

The increase in infectious complications associated with splenectomy in thalassemia patients is thought to be due to a coexisting immune deficiency that is caused by iron overload. Iron overload is associated with both thalassemia as well as the transfusions that accompany treatment for thalassemia. Some investigators have tried partial splenectomy with some success in reducing mortality associated with splenectomy in these patients. In addition, splenectomy should be delayed until the patient is older than 4 years unless absolutely necessary. While transfusion to maintain a hemoglobin (HGB) of >9 mg/dL is part of the treatment for thalassemia it does not reduce infectious complications associated with splenectomy in these patients. There is little evidence supporting efficacy of prophylactic antibiotics in asplenic patients in preventing infectious complications associated with splenectomy. (See Schwartz 10th ed., p. 1432.)

7. A 30-year-old woman presents to her primary care provider with complaints of bleeding gums while brushing her teeth as well as menorrhagia and several episodes of epistaxis within the past month. She has been previously healthy with no prior medical problems or surgeries. Examination reveals petechiae and ecchymosis over the lower extremities. Laboratory results show white blood cell (WBC) count 7000/mm³, HGB 14 g/dL, hematocrit (HCT) 42%, and platelet count 28,000/mm³ with numerous megakaryocytes on peripheral smear. First-line therapy for this condition would be
   A. Oral prednisone
   B. Intravenous (IV) immunoglobulin
   C. Rituximab
   D. Splenectomy

Answer: A
Idiopathic thrombocytopenic purpura (ITP) is an autoimmune disorder characterized by a low platelet count and mucocutaneous and petechial bleeding. The usual first line of therapy for ITP is oral prednisone with most responses occurring within the first 3 weeks after initiating therapy. Intravenous (IV) immunoglobulin is given for internal bleeding with platelet counts <5000/mm³, when extensive purpura exists, or to increase platelets preoperatively and is thought to work by impairing clearance of immunoglobulin G-coated platelets by competing for binding to tissue macrophage receptors. Both rituximab and thrombopoietin-receptor antagonists are second-line treatment options. Splenectomy is an option for refractory ITP and can provide a permanent response in about 75 to 85% of patients. (See Schwartz 10th ed., pp. 1432–1433.)

8. The most common physical finding in a patient with hairy cell leukemia (HCL) is
   A. Massive splenomegaly
   B. Shortness of breath
   C. Abdominal pain
   D. Joint pain

Answer: A
Hairy cell leukemia (HCL) is an uncommon blood disorder, representing only 2% of all adult leukemias. HCL is characterized by splenomegaly, pancytopenia, and large numbers of abnormal lymphocytes in the bone marrow. These lymphocytes contain irregular hair-like cytoplasmic projections identifiable on the peripheral smear. Most patients seek medical attention because of symptoms related to anemia, neutropenia, thrombocytopenia, or splenomegaly. The most common physical finding is splenomegaly, which occurs in 80% of patients with HCL and the spleen is often palpable 5 cm below the costal margin. Many patients with HCL have few symptoms and require no specific therapy. Treatment is indicated for those with moderate to severe symptoms related to cytopenias, such as repeated infections or bleeding episodes, or to splenomegaly, such as pain or early satiety. Splenectomy does not correct the underlying disorder, but does return cell counts to normal in 40 to 70% of patients and alleviates pain and early satiety. Newer chemotherapeutic agents (the purine analogues 2′-deoxycoformycin [2′-DCF] and 2-chlorodeoxyadenosine [2-CdA]) are able to induce durable complete remission in most patients. (See Schwartz 10th ed., p. 1434.)

9. Which of the following is an indication for splenectomy in a patient with chronic myelogenous leukemia (CML)?
   A. Failure of chemotherapy to decrease splenomegaly
   B. Sequestration requiring transfusion
   C. Symptomatic relief of early satiety
   D. Presence of *bcr* gene mutation

Answer: C
Chronic myelogenous leukemia (CML) is a disorder of the primitive pluripotent stem cells in the bone marrow, resulting in a significant increase in erythroid, megakaryotic, and pluripotent progenitors in the peripheral blood smear. The genetic hallmark is a transposition between the *bcr* gene on chromosome 9 and the *abl* gene on chromosome 22. CML accounts for 7 to 15% of all leukemias, with an incidence of 1.5 in 100,000 in the United States. CML is frequently asymptomatic in the chronic phase, but symptomatic patients often present with the gradual onset of fatigue, anorexia, sweating, and left upper quadrant pain and early satiety secondary to splenomegaly. Enlargement of the spleen is found in roughly one-half of patients with CML. Splenectomy is indicated to ease pain and early satiety. (See Schwartz 10th ed., p. 1435.)

10. Which of the following is an indication for splenectomy in polycythemia vera (PV)?
    A. Failure of aspirin to prevent thrombotic complications
    B. Frequent need for phlebotomy
    C. Symptoms related to splenomegaly
    D. Prevention of progression to myeloid metaplasia

Answer: C
Polycythemia vera (PV) is a clonal, chronic, progressive myeloproliferative disorder characterized by an increase in RBC mass, frequently accompanied by leukocytosis, thrombocytosis, and splenomegaly. Patients affected by PV typically enjoy prolonged survival compared to others affected by hematologic malignancies, but remain at risk for transformation to myelofibrosis or acute myeloid leukemia (AML). The disease is rare, with an annual incidence of 5 to 17 cases per million population. Although the diagnosis may be discovered by routine screening laboratory tests in asymptomatic individuals, affected patients may present with any number of nonspecific complaints, including headache, dizziness, weakness, pruritus, visual disturbances, excessive sweating, joint symptoms, and weight loss. Physical findings include ruddy cyanosis, conjunctival plethora, hepatomegaly, splenomegaly, and hypertension. The diagnosis is established by an elevated RBC mass (>25% of mean predicted value), thrombocytosis, leukocytosis, normal arterial oxygen saturation in the presence of increased RBC mass, splenomegaly, low serum erythropoietin (EPO) stores, and bone marrow hypercellularity. Treatment should be tailored to the risk status of the patient and ranges from phlebotomy and aspirin to chemotherapeutic agents. As in essential thrombocythemia (ET) splenectomy is not helpful in the early stages of disease and is best reserved for late-stage patients in whom myeloid metaplasia has developed and splenomegaly-related symptoms are severe. (See Schwartz 10th ed., pp. 1435–1436.)

11. Which of the following is the most common etiology of splenic cysts worldwide?
    A. Bacterial infection
    B. Trauma
    C. Parasitic infection
    D. Congenital anomaly

Answer: C
Splenic cysts are rare lesions. The most common etiology for splenic cysts worldwide is parasitic infestation, particularly echinococcal. Symptomatic parasitic cysts are best treated with splenectomy, though selected cases may be amenable to percutaneous aspiration, instillation of protoscolicidal agent, and reaspiration. Nonparasitic cysts most commonly result from trauma and are called *pseudocysts*; however, dermoid, epidermoid, and epithelial cysts have been reported as well. The treatment of nonparasitic cysts depends on whether or not they produce symptoms. Asymptomatic nonparasitic cysts may be observed with close ultrasound follow-up to exclude significant expansion. Patients should be advised of the risk of cyst rupture with even minor abdominal trauma if they elect nonoperative management for large cysts. Small symptomatic nonparasitic cysts may be excised with splenic preservation, and large symptomatic nonparasitic cysts may be unroofed. Both of these operations may be performed laparoscopically. (See Schwartz 10th ed., pp. 1436–1437.)

12. Which of the following is an indication for surgical treatment of a splenic aneurysm?
    A. Pregnancy
    B. Size >1.5 cm
    C. History of thrombocytopenia
    D. History of neutropenia

Answer: A
Although rare, splenic artery aneurysm (SAA) is the most common visceral artery aneurysm. Women are four times more likely to be affected than men. The aneurysm usually arises in the middle to distal portion of the splenic artery. The risk of rupture is between 3% and 9%; however, once rupture occurs, mortality is substantial (35–50%). According to a recent series, mortality is significantly higher in patients with underlying portal hypertension (>50%) than in those without it (17%). SAA is particularly worrisome when discovered

during pregnancy, as rupture imparts a high risk of mortality to both mother (70%) and fetus (95%). Most patients are asymptomatic and seek medical attention based on an incidental radiographic finding. About 20% of patients with SAA have symptoms of left upper quadrant pain. Indications for treatment include presence of symptoms, pregnancy, intention to become pregnant, and pseudoaneurysms associated with inflammatory processes. For asymptomatic patients, size greater than 2 cm constitutes an indication for surgery. Aneurysm resection or ligation alone is acceptable for amenable lesions in the mid-splenic artery, but distal lesions in close proximity to the splenic hilum should be treated with concomitant splenectomy. An excellent prognosis follows elective treatment. Splenic artery embolization has been used to treat SAA, but painful splenic infarction and abscess may follow. (See Schwartz 10th ed., p. 1438.)

13. A 45-year-old man presents to the emergency department with emesis of bright red blood. Laboratory results include HGB 10 g/dL, HCT 30%, platelets 300,000/mm³, international normalized ratio (INR) 1.0, aspartate transaminase (AST) 30 U/L, alanine transaminase (ALT) 45 U/L, and albumin 4.0 g/dL. After appropriate resuscitation he undergoes esophagogastroduodenoscopy (EGD) which is notable for gastric varices. What is the appropriate treatment for his condition?
    A. Transjugular intrahepatic portosystemic shunt
    B. Variceal band ligation
    C. Splenorenal shunt
    D. Splenectomy

Answer: D

While portal hypertension is most commonly a result of cirrhosis it can result from other causes such as splenic vein thrombosis. Patients with splenic vein thrombosis can present with bleeding from gastric varices in the setting of normal liver function test results. These patients also often have a history of pancreatic disease. Portal hypertension secondary to splenic vein thrombosis is potentially curable with splenectomy. (See Schwartz 10th ed., p. 1438.)

14. Which of the following is NOT part of the triad seen with Felty syndrome?
    A. Rheumatoid arthritis (RA)
    B. Splenomegaly
    C. Neutropenia
    D. Thrombocytopenia

Answer: D

The triad of rheumatoid arthritis (RA), splenomegaly, and neutropenia is called Felty syndrome. It exists in approximately 3% of all patients with RA, two-thirds of which are women. Immune complexes coat the surface of WBCs, leading to their sequestration and clearance in the spleen with subsequent neutropenia. This neutropenia (<2000/mm³) increases the risk for recurrent infections and often drives the decision for splenectomy. The size of the spleen is variable, from nonpalpable in 5 to 10% of patients, to massive enlargement in others. The spleen in Felty syndrome is four times heavier than normal. Corticosteroids, hematopoietic growth factors, methotrexate, and splenectomy have all been used to treat the neutropenia of Felty syndrome. Responses to splenectomy have been excellent, with over 80% of patients showing a durable increase in WBC count. More than one-half of patients who had infections prior to surgery did not have any infections after splenectomy. Besides symptomatic neutropenia, other indications for splenectomy include transfusion-dependent anemia and profound thrombocytopenia. (See Schwartz 10th ed., p. 1438.)

15. Which of the following is the most effective prevention strategy against OPSI?
    A. Vaccination 2 weeks after splenectomy
    B. Vaccination 2 weeks before splenectomy
    C. Daily antibiotic prophylaxis
    D. Carrying a reserve supply of antibiotics for self-administration

Answer: B

Asplenic patients have an increased susceptibility to infection for the remainder of their lives and although the overall lifetime risk of OPSI is low the consequences can be devastating. Patients undergoing splenectomy for hematologic or malignant indications have a greater risk of OPSI than patients undergoing splenectomy for trauma or iatrogenic injury, and OPSI is more common in children than adults. Providers need to have a high index of suspicion when evaluating asplenic patients for possible infection. Patient education and vaccinations against encapsulated pathogens is the mainstay of preventive therapy. Patients should be vaccinated 2 weeks prior to elective splenectomy in order to optimize antigen recognition and processing. If splenectomy is performed emergently vaccinations are given postoperatively with an attempt to delay administration for 2 weeks to avoid the transient immunosuppression associated with surgery. There is little evidence supporting efficacy of prophylactic antibiotics in asplenic patients and vaccination remains the most effective prevention strategy. (See Schwartz 10th ed., p. 1439.)

16. All of the following are true regarding laparoscopic splenectomy EXCEPT
    A. It is associated with shorter hospital stays.
    B. It is associated with increased intraoperative blood loss.
    C. It is associated with decreased morbidity.
    D. Patients are positioned in the right lateral decubitus position or the 45° right lateral decubitus position.

Answer: B

Laparoscopic splenectomy has become the favored procedure versus open splenectomy for elective splenectomy over the past two decades and is now considered the gold standard for elective splenectomy in patients with normal-sized spleens. With experienced surgeons laparoscopic splenectomy is associated with decreased intraoperative blood loss, shorter hospital length of stay, and lower morbidity rates as compared to open splenectomy. Laparoscopic splenectomy is often performed with the patient in the right lateral decubitus position, patients are sometimes placed in a 45° right lateral decubitus position to facilitate easier access for concomitant procedures such as laparoscopic cholecystectomy. (See Schwartz 10th ed., p. 1440.)

17. What is the most common complication following open splenectomy?
    A. Pancreatitis
    B. Left lower lobe atelectasis
    C. Pleural effusion
    D. Wound infection

Answer: B

Complications following splenectomy can be divided into pulmonary, hemorrhagic, infectious, pancreatic, and thromboembolic. Pulmonary complications include left lower lobe atelectasis, pleural effusion, and pneumonia with left lower lobe atelectasis being the most common complication overall. Hemorrhagic complications include intraoperative hemorrhage, postoperative hemorrhage, and subphrenic hematoma. Infectious complications include subphrenic abscess and wound infection. Placement of a drain in the left upper quadrant can be associated with postoperative subphrenic abscess and is therefore not routinely recommended. Pancreatic complications include pancreatitis, pseudocyst formation, and pancreatic fistula and often result from intraoperative trauma to the pancreas during dissection of the splenic hilum. Thromboembolic complications include deep vein thrombosis and portal vein thrombosis. (See Schwartz 10th ed., p. 1444.)

18. Which of the following patients is at highest risk for OPSI?
    A. A 30-year old who underwent splenectomy for ITP.
    B. A 25-year old who underwent splenectomy for iatrogenic bleeding after a total colectomy.
    C. A 3-year old who underwent splenectomy for hereditary spherocytosis.
    D. A 4-year old who underwent splenectomy due to bleeding after a motor vehicle crash.

Answer: C
While the all lifetime risk of OPSI is low (ranging from <1–5%) the consequences are serious. The reason for splenectomy is the single most influential determinant of OPSI risk. There is evidence that those who undergo splenectomy for hematologic disease are far more susceptible to OPSI than patients who undergo splenectomy for trauma or iatrogenic reasons. When taking age into consideration children who are 5 years of age or younger and adults who are 50 years of age or older seem to be at an elevated risk. The interval since splenectomy also seems to be a factor with the greatest risk occurring in the first 2 years after splenectomy, however, it is important to remember that cases of OPSI can occur decades later and asplenic patients remain at lifelong risk. (See Schwartz 10th ed., p. 1445.)

19. Which of the following asplenic patients should receive prophylactic antibiotic therapy to protect against OPSI?
    A. A 35-year-old man undergoing a tooth extraction.
    B. A 4-year-old child who recently underwent splenectomy.
    C. A 15-year-old boy who underwent splenectomy at age 13.
    D. There is little evidence supporting efficacy of prophylactic antibiotics.

Answer: D
Antibiotic therapy in asplenic patients falls into three categories: deliberate therapy for established or presumed infections, prophylaxis in anticipation of invasive procedures, and general prophylaxis. There is little evidence supporting efficacy of prophylactic antibiotics in anticipation of invasive procedures or efficacy of general prophylaxis and guidelines are not uniform. Common recommendations include daily antibiotics until 5 years of age or at least 5 years after splenectomy with some advocating continuing antibiotics until young adulthood, however, there is little evidence supporting efficacy. It is unlikely that randomized controlled trials on this issue will be performed due to the low incidence of overwhelming postsplenectomy infection as well as its serious consequences. (See Schwartz 10th ed., p. 1445.)

CHAPTER 35

Abdominal Wall, Omentum, Mesentery, and Retroperitoneum

1. A cutaneous malignancy of the anterior abdominal wall 2 inches above the umbilicus will drain to which lymphatic basin?
   A. Umbilical
   B. Axillary
   C. Retroperitoneal
   D. Inguinal

   Answer: B
   The lymphatic drainage of the anterior abdominal wall is principally to the axillary nodal basin and the inguinal nodal basin. The area of demarcation is roughly the arcuate line (semilunar line of Douglas) at the level of the anterior iliac spine. (See Schwartz 10th ed., p. 1450.)

2. The appropriate treatment of rectus abdominis diastasis is
   A. Observation
   B. Resection and primary repair
   C. Mesh overlay
   D. Lateral component separation

   Answer: A
   Rectus abdominis diastasis (or diastasis recti) is a separation of the two rectus abdominis muscular pillars. This results in a bulge of the abdominal wall that is sometimes mistaken for a ventral hernia despite the fact that the midline aponeurosis is intact and no hernia defect is present. Computed tomography (CT) scanning can provide an accurate measure of the distance between the rectus pillars and will differentiate rectus diastasis from a true ventral hernia. Surgical correction has been described for cosmetic reasons but is unnecessary and risks the formation of a true postoperative hernia. (See Schwartz 10th ed., p. 1453.)

3. Persistence of the vitelline duct can lead to which of the following?
   A. Colonic diverticulum
   B. Urachal cyst
   C. Umbilical cord hernia
   D. Omphalomesenteric duct cyst

   Answer: D
   During the third trimester of pregnancy, the vitelline duct regresses. Persistence of the vitelline duct remnant on the ileal border results in a Meckel diverticulum. Complete failure of the vitelline duct to regress results in a vitelline duct fistula which is associated with drainage of small intestinal contents from the umbilicus. If both the intestinal and umbilical ends of the vitelline duct regress into fibrous cords, a central vitelline duct (omphalomesenteric duct) cyst may occur. (See Schwartz 10th ed., p. 1453.)

4. The usual presentation of a rectus sheath hematoma is
   A. Unexplained anemia
   B. Abdominal wall bulge
   C. Sudden abdominal pain
   D. Inability to stand erect

   Answer: C
   Hemorrhage from the network of collateralizing vessels within the rectus sheath and muscles can result in a rectus sheath hematoma. Although a history of trauma may be present, a rectus sheath hematoma can follow vigorous coughing, sneezing, or extreme exertion. It typically occurs in elderly patients or those on anticoagulant therapy. Patients usually report the sudden onset of unilateral abdominal pain and have localized tenderness which is not accompanied by peritoneal signs. (See Schwartz 10th ed., p. 1453.)

5. A 40-year-old woman who underwent total abdominal colectomy for familial adenomatous polyposis (FAP) 5 years ago presents with a gradually expanding painless 4 cm mass of the anterior abdominal wall. A biopsy is returned as "desmoid tumor with no sign of malignancy." The correct management is
   A. Observation
   B. A course of doxorubicin, dacarbazine, or carboplatin
   C. Enucleation
   D. Wide local excision

Answer: D

Desmoid tumors of the abdominal wall are fibrous neoplasms that occur sporadically or in the setting of familial adenomatous polyposis (FAP). The condition can result in mortality due to aggressive local growth, so radical excision with confirmation of tumor-free margins of resection is required. Medical treatment with an antineoplastic agent such as doxorubicin, dacarbazine, or carboplatin can produce remission but the prognosis of advanced desmoids is poor. (See Schwartz 10th ed., p. 1454.)

6. Repair of a new 5-cm midline postoperative ventral hernia in an otherwise healthy patient is best accomplished with
   A. Primary suture repair
   B. Repair with synthetic mesh
   C. Repair with transposition of rectus muscle
   D. Lateral component separation with mesh overlay

Answer: B

Postincisional hernias have an unacceptably high incidence of recurrence after primary suture repair. Therefore, a mesh repair, performed either with an open surgical approach or laparoscopic approach, is preferred. Muscle transposition procedures are usually unnecessary in relatively small defects that are not recurrent or related to another abdominal wall defect. (See Schwartz 10th ed., p. 1455.)

7. Which of the following statements regarding umbilical hernias is true?
   A. Umbilical hernias are present in 10% of all newborns.
   B. Umbilical hernias should be repaired as soon as they are diagnosed.
   C. Adults with small, nonincarcerated umbilical hernias should undergo repair.
   D. Umbilical hernias are associated with disseminated carcinomatosis.

Answer: A

Umbilical hernias are present in 10% of all newborns, and are more common in premature infants. Most congenital umbilical hernias close spontaneously by 5 years of age, so repair should be delayed until examination shows persistence of the hernia before the child enters school. Adults with small, uncomplicated, unincarcerated umbilical hernias can be followed until symptoms occur. (See Schwartz 10th ed., p. 1455.)

8. Spigelian hernias usually occur
   A. On the lateral border of the rectus abdominis muscle
   B. In the linea alba
   C. In the medial wall of the inguinal canal
   D. In the posterior costovertebral angle

Answer: A

Spigelian hernias can occur anywhere along the length of the Spigelian line or zone—an aponeurotic band of variable width at the lateral border of the rectus abdominis. The most common location of these rare hernias is at the level of the arcuate line. These hernias are not always apparent on physical examination, and may cause local pain or incarceration. (See Schwartz 10th ed., p. 1455.)

9. Laparoscopic repair of incisional hernias is associated with which of the following?
   A. Reduced hospital cost
   B. Reduced recurrence rate
   C. Reduced wound infection rate
   D. Reduced seroma formation

Answer: C

A recent Cochrane database review concluded that short-term recurrence rates did not differ significantly and laparoscopic repairs were associated with higher in-hospital costs despite generally shorter lengths of stay. The major benefit for laparoscopic repairs compared with open repairs was a consistently lower risk of wound infections. (See Schwartz 10th ed., p. 1456.)

10. Which of the following statements about omental infarction are true?
    A. Patients usually present with fever and lassitude.
    B. Most cases are diagnosed on imaging studies.
    C. Most cases do not require surgery.
    D. Surgical resection is indicated in all cases.

Answer: C

Interruption of the blood supply to the omentum is a rare cause of symptoms of an acute abdomen. Depending on the location of the infarcted tissue, symptoms may mimic acute appendicitis, acute cholecystitis, acute diverticulitis, or perforated ulcer. The diagnosis is usually inferred from abdominal CT scan which shows a localized inflammatory-appearing mass of the omentum. Surgical resection can hasten recovery, but clinically stable patients can be managed conservatively. (See Schwartz 10th ed., p. 1457.)

11. A 60-year-old woman presents with abdominal pain, and a CT scan reveals an omental mass. The most likely diagnosis is
    A. Desmoid tumor
    B. Liposarcoma of the omentum
    C. Omental infarction
    D. Metastatic carcinoma

Answer: D
Primary tumors of the omentum are rare, as is omental infarction. Metastatic tumors of the omentum are common, with metastatic ovarian carcinoma having the highest preponderance of omental involvement. Cancers of any portion of the gastrointestinal tract, as well as melanoma, uterine, and renal cancer, can metastasize to the omentum. (See Schwartz 10th ed., p. 1457.)

12. Failure of fixation of the small intestinal and right colonic mesentery during gestation can result in
    A. Chronic constipation
    B. Intestinal malrotation
    C. Umbilical hernia
    D. Intussusception

Answer: B
During fetal development, after the midgut rotates and returns to the abdominal cavity, the mesentery of the duodenum, small intestine, and proximal colon become fixed to the retroperitoneum. Failure of fixation results in a spectrum of disorders associated with intestinal malrotation. (See Schwartz 10th ed., p. 1458.)

13. Which of the following statements about sclerosing mesenteritis is FALSE?
    A. It is always associated with diffuse abdominal pain.
    B. It can appear as a mass on CT scan.
    C. It can improve or resolve without surgical therapy.
    D. It can be mistaken for primary or metastatic tumor.

Answer: A
The etiology of sclerosing mesenteritis is unknown but its cardinal feature is increased tissue density within the mesentery. This can be associated with a discreet non-neoplastic mass or it can be more diffuse involving large swaths of thickened mesentery without well-defined borders. Many cases are discovered incidentally on CT scans performed for unrelated reasons. The process is self-limited and may demonstrate regression on follow-up imaging studies. (See Schwartz 10th ed., p. 1458.)

14. The primary treatment of retroperitoneal fibrosis is
    A. Corticosteroids
    B. Cyclosporine
    C. Radiation therapy
    D. Surgical resection

Answer: A
Once malignancy, drug-induced disease, and infectious etiologies are ruled out, corticosteroids are the mainstay of medical therapy. Surgical intervention is reserved for ureterolysis or ureteral stenting, or endovascular interventions for ileocaval obstruction. (See Schwartz 10th ed., p. 1462.)

CHAPTER 36

Soft Tissue Sarcomas

1. All of the following are true about soft tissue sarcoma EXCEPT
   A. Most common site is trunk and retroperitoneum.
   B. There are more than 11,000 new diagnoses of soft tissue sarcoma annually in the United States.
   C. Most soft tissue sarcoma-specific deaths are due to uncontrolled pulmonary metastases.
   D. The overall 5-year survival rate for all stages of soft tissue sarcoma approximates 50 to 60%.

Answer: A
Incidence rates are declining for most cancer sites, but they are increasing among both men and women for melanoma of the skin, cancers of the liver and thyroid. Incidence rates are decreasing for all four major cancer sites except for breast cancer in women. (See Schwartz 10th ed., p. 1465.)

2. Which of the following is NOT associated with the development of sarcoma?
   A. Radiation exposure
   B. Herbicide exposure
   C. Chronic lymphedema
   D. History of trauma

Answer: D
External radiation therapy is a rare but well-established risk factor for soft tissue sarcoma that may be associated with radiation-induced mutations of the *p53* gene. Exposure to herbicides, such as phenoxyacetic acids and to wood preservatives containing chlorophenols, has been linked to an increased risk of soft tissue sarcoma. In 1948, Stewart and Treves first described the association between chronic lymphedema after axillary dissection and subsequent lymphangiosarcoma. Although patients with sarcoma often report a history of trauma, no causal relationship has been established. More often, a minor injury calls attention to a pre-existing tumor. (See Schwartz 10th ed., p. 1466.)

3. Internationale Contre le Cancer (AJCC/UICC) sarcoma staging system?
   A. Tumor size
   B. Number of mitoses per high-powered microscopic field
   C. Lymph node metastatic status
   D. Retroperitoneal sarcoma nomograms

Answer: D
The seventh edition of the American Joint Committee on Cancer (AJCC) staging system for soft tissue sarcomas is based on histologic grade of aggressiveness, tumor size and depth, and the presence of nodal or distant metastases. Histologic grade is the most important prognostic factor for patients with soft tissue sarcoma. The features that define grade are cellularity, differentiation (good, moderate, or poor/anaplastic), pleomorphism, necrosis (absent, <50%, or ≥50%), and number of mitoses per high-power field (<10, 10–19, or ≥20). (See Schwartz 10th ed., p. 1470.)

4. All of the following are known molecular pathogenic events in sarcoma EXCEPT
   A. Chromosomal translocations
   B. Oncogene amplification
   C. Complex genomic rearrangements
   D. Epigenetic suppression

Answer: D

In general, sarcomas resulting from identifiable molecular events tend to occur in younger patients with histology suggesting a clear line of differentiation. The identifiable molecular events include point mutations, translocations causing overexpression of an autocrine grow factor, and oncogenic fusion transcription factor producing a cellular environment prone to malignant transformation. In contrast, sarcomas without identifiable genetic changes or expression profile signatures tend to occur in older patients and exhibit pleomorphic cytology and *p53* dysfunction. (See Schwartz 10th ed., pp. 1466–1467.)

5. For a T2G3NOMO sarcoma (stage II), treatment typically consists of
   A. Surgery alone
   B. Surgery and radiotherapy
   C. Surgery, radiotherapy, pre-surgical chemotherapy
   D. Surgery, radiotherapy, pre- and postsurgical chemotherapy

Answer: B

Recommendations for the management of soft tissue masses

1. Soft tissue tumors that are enlarging or greater than 3 cm should be evaluated with radiologic imaging (ultrasonography or computed tomography [CT]), and a tissue diagnosis should be made using core needle biopsy.
2. Once a sarcoma diagnosis is established, obtain imaging (magnetic resonance imaging for extremity lesions and CT for other anatomic locations) and evaluate for metastatic disease with chest CT for intermediate- or high-grade (grade 2 or 3) or large (T2) tumors.
3. A wide local excision with 1- to 2-cm margins is adequate therapy for low-grade lesions and T1 tumors.
4. Radiation therapy plays a critical role in the management of large (T2), intermediate- or high-grade tumors.
5. Patients with locally advanced high-grade sarcomas or distant metastases should be evaluated for chemotherapy.
6. An aggressive surgical approach should be taken in the treatment of patients with an isolated local recurrence or resectable distant metastases. (See Schwartz 10th ed., p. 1472.)

6. Which of the following is true about desmoid tumors?
   A. Local recurrence is observed in up to one-third of patients regardless of microscopic margin of resection status.
   B. A policy of watchful waiting for desmoids has been validated in prospective clinical trials.
   C. Analogous to other nonmetastasizing tumors, chemotherapy has no role in the treatment of desmoid tumors.
   D. Due to their propensity for local invasion, radiotherapy, when used, must be given at a dose of 75 Gy.

Answer: A

The primary therapy for desmoid tumors has long been considered surgical resection with wide local excision to achieve negative margins. However, local recurrence occurs in up to one-third of patients independently of the quality of surgical margins. Moreover, some authors advocate the possibility to observe patients at presentation, limiting surgery to those who progress or fail medical therapies. Radiation therapy may be effective in patients with unresectable tumors or as adjuvant therapy following surgery for recurrent disease although long-term side effects and the risk of radiation-induced sarcoma should always be considered. When used, a dose of 50 to 54 Gy is usually recommended. Systemic treatment is another option, when surgery is not indicated, although usually reserved for patients with tumor-associated symptoms who have not responded to other interventions. Combinations of methotrexate and vinblastine have been shown to have activity, as have single-agent pegylated liposomal doxorubicin and sorafenib. (See Schwartz 10th ed., p. 1485.)

CHAPTER 37

Inguinal Hernias

1. The incidence of inguinal hernias in men has a bimodal distribution, which peaks
   A. Before the second year of life and after age 50.
   B. Before the first year of life and after age 40.
   C. Before the eighth year of life and after age 40.
   D. Before the fifth year of life and after age 50.

Answer: B
Approximately 75% of abdominal wall hernias occur in the groin. The lifetime risk of inguinal hernia is 27% in men and 3% in women. Of inguinal hernia repairs, 90% are performed in men and 10% in women. The incidence of inguinal hernias in men has a bimodal distribution, with peaks before the first year of life and after age 40. Abramson demonstrated the age dependence of inguinal hernias in 1978. Those between ages 25 and 34 years had a lifetime prevalence rate of 15%, whereas those aged 75 years and over had a rate of 47% (Table 37-1). Approximately 70% of femoral hernia repairs are performed in women; however, inguinal hernias are five times more common than femoral hernias. The most common subtype of groin hernia in men and women is the indirect inguinal hernia. (See Schwartz 10th ed., p. 1495.)

TABLE 37-1	Inguinal hernia prevalence by age					
Age (y)	25–34	35–44	45–54	55–64	65–74	75+
Current prevalence (%)	12	15	20	26	29	34
Lifetime prevalence (%)	15	19	28	34	40	47

Current = repaired hernias excluded; lifetime = repaired hernias included.

2. The two types of collagen found to exist in a decreased ratio of the skin of inguinal hernia patients are
   A. Types I and II
   B. Types II and III
   C. Types I and III
   D. Types III and VI

Answer: C
Epidemiologic studies have identified risk factors that may predispose to a hernia. Microscopic examination of skin of inguinal hernia patients demonstrated significantly decreased ratios of type I to type III collagen. Type III collagen does not contribute to wound tensile strength as significantly as type I collagen. Additional analyses revealed disaggregated collagen tracts with decreased collagen fiber density in hernia patients' skin. Collagen disorders, such as Ehlers-Danlos syndrome, are also associated with an increased incidence of hernia formation (Table 37-2). Recent studies have found an association between concentrations of extracellular matrix elements and hernia formation. Although a significant amount of work remains to elucidate the biologic nature of hernias, current evidence suggests they have a multifactorial etiology with both environmental and hereditary influences. (See Schwartz 10th ed., Table 37-4, p. 1502.)

TABLE 37-2	Connective tissue disorders associated with groin herniation
Osteogenesis imperfecta	
Cutis laxa (congenital elastolysis)	
Ehlers-Danlos syndrome	
Hurler-Hunter syndrome	
Marfan syndrome	
Congenital hip dislocation in children	
Polycystic kidney disease	
α_1-Antitrypsin deficiency	
Williams syndrome	
Androgen insensitivity syndrome	
Robinow syndrome	
Serpentine fibula syndrome	
Alport syndrome	
Tel Hashomer camptodactyly syndrome	
Leriche syndrome	
Testicular feminization syndrome	
Rokitansky-Mayer-Kuster syndrome	
Goldenhar syndrome	
Morris syndrome	
Gerhardt syndrome	
Menkes syndrome	
Kawasaki disease	
Pfannenstiel syndrome	
Beckwith-Wiedemann syndrome	
Rubinstein-Taybi syndrome	
Alopecia-photophobia syndrome	

3. According to the Nyhus classification system that categorizes hernia defects by location, size, and type, type IIIC represents
   A. Indirect hernia; internal abdominal ring normal; typically in infants, children, small adults
   B. Direct hernia; size is not taken into account
   C. Recurrent hernia; modifiers A-D are sometimes added, which correspond to indirect, direct, femoral, and mixed.
   D. Femoral hernia

Answer: D
See Table 37-3. (See Schwartz 10th ed., Table 37-2, p. 1498.)

TABLE 37-3	Nyhus classification system
Type I	Indirect hernia; internal abdominal ring normal; typically in infants, children, small adults
Type II	Indirect hernia; internal ring enlarged without impingement on the floor of the inguinal canal; does not extend to the scrotum
Type IIIA	Direct hernia; size is not taken into account
Type IIIB	Indirect hernia that has enlarged enough to encroach upon the posterior inguinal wall; indirect sliding or scrotal hernias are usually placed in this category because they are commonly associated with extension to the direct space; also includes pantaloon hernias
Type IIIC	Femoral hernia
Type IV	Recurrent hernia; modifiers A–D are sometimes added, which correspond to indirect, direct, femoral, and mixed, respectively

4. Taxis
   A. Should be performed when strangulation is suspected.
   B. Refers to the method of securing mesh to the inguinal ligament.
   C. Should not be repeated more than five times.
   D. Should be used for incarcerated hernias without sequelae or strangulation.

Answer: D
Incarceration occurs when hernia contents fail to reduce; however, a minimally symptomatic, chronically incarcerated hernia may also be treated nonoperatively. Taxis should be attempted for incarcerated hernias without sequelae of strangulation, and the option of surgical repair should be discussed prior to the maneuver. To perform taxis, analgesics and light sedatives are administered, and the patient is placed in the Trendelenburg position. The hernia sac is elongated with both hands, and the contents are compressed in a milking fashion to ease their reduction into the abdomen.

The indication for emergent inguinal hernia repair is impending compromise of intestinal contents. As such, strangulation of hernia contents is a surgical emergency. Clinical signs that indicate strangulation include fever, leukocytosis, and hemodynamic instability. The hernia bulge is usually warm and tender, and the overlying skin may be erythematous or discolored. Symptoms of bowel obstruction in patients with sliding or incarcerated inguinal hernias may also indicate strangulation. Taxis should not be performed when strangulation is suspected, as reduction of potentially gangrenous tissue into the abdomen may result in an intra-abdominal catastrophe. Preoperatively, the patient should receive fluid resuscitation, nasogastric decompression, and prophylactic intravenous antibiotics. (See Schwartz 10th ed., p. 1505.)

5. A hernia sac that extends into the scrotum may
   A. Require extensive dissection and reduction
   B. Require division within the inguinal canal
   C. Require amputation of the sac
   D. Require the sac to be inverted into the preperitoneum

Answer: B
In cases where the viability of sac contents is in question, the sac should be incised, and hernia contents should be evaluated for signs of ischemia. The defect should be enlarged to augment blood flow to the sac contents. Viable contents may be reduced into the peritoneal cavity, while nonviable contents should be resected, and synthetic prostheses should be avoided in the repair. In elective cases, the sac may be amputated at the internal inguinal ring or inverted into the preperitoneum. Both methods are effective; however, patients undergoing sac excision had significantly increased postoperative pain in a prospective trial. Dissection of a densely adherent sac may result in injury to cord structures and should be avoided; however, sac ligation at the internal inguinal ring is necessary in these cases. A hernia sac that extends into the scrotum may require division within the inguinal canal, as extensive dissection and reduction risks injury to the pampiniform plexus, resulting in testicular atrophy and orchitis.

At this point, the inguinal canal is reconstructed, either with native tissue or with prostheses. The following sections describe the most commonly performed types of tissue-based and prosthetic-based reconstructions. (See Schwartz 10th ed., p. 1505.)

6. The technique indicated for femoral hernias in cases where prosthetic material is contraindicated is
   A. The Bassini repair
   B. The Shouldice repair
   C. The McVay repair
   D. Lichtenstein tension-free repair

Answer: C
The McVay repair addresses both inguinal and femoral ring defects. This technique is indicated for femoral hernias and in cases where the use of prosthetic material is contraindicated (Fig. 37-1). Once the spermatic cord has been isolated, an incision in the transversalis fascia permits entry into the preperitoneal space. The upper flap is mobilized by gentle blunt dissection of underlying tissue. Cooper ligament is bluntly dissected to expose its surface. A 2- to 4-cm relaxing incision

is made in the anterior rectus sheath vertically from the pubic tubercle. This incision is essential to reduce tension on the repair; however, it may result in increased postoperative pain and higher risk of ventral abdominal herniation. Using either interrupted or continuous suture, the superior transversalis flap is then fastened to Cooper ligament, and the repair is continued laterally along Cooper ligament to occlude the femoral ring. Lateral to the femoral ring, a transition stitch is placed, affixing the transversalis fascia to the inguinal ligament. The transversalis is then sutured to the inguinal ligament laterally to the internal ring. (See Schwartz 10th ed., Figure 37-17, pp. 1507–1508.)

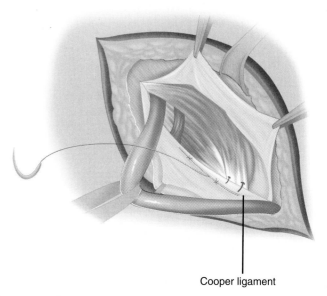

Cooper ligament

FIG. 37-1. McVay Cooper ligament repair.

7. General anesthesia induction resulting in reduction of an incarcerated or strangulated inguinal hernia during laparoscopic repair
   A. Requires no action
   B. Requires abdominal exploration for nonviable tissue
   C. Requires immediate conversion to an open repair
   D. Requires proceeding with a totally extraperitoneal (TEP) repair

Answer: B
Laparoscopic inguinal hernia repairs reinforce the abdominal wall via a posterior approach. Principal laparoscopic methods include the transabdominal preperitoneal (TAPP) repair, the totally extraperitoneal (TEP) repair, and the less commonly performed intraperitoneal onlay mesh (IPOM) repair. Although laparoscopic repairs in experienced hands are relatively expedient, they necessitate the administration of general anesthesia and its inherent risks. Any patient with a contraindication to the use of general anesthesia should not undergo laparoscopic hernia repair. Occasionally, general anesthesia induction may result in reduction of an incarcerated or strangulated inguinal hernia. If the surgeon suspects this might have occurred, the abdomen should be explored for nonviable tissue either via laparoscopy or upon conversion to an open laparotomy. (See Schwartz 10th ed., p. 1509.)

8. The medical issue NOT associated with hernia recurrence is
   A. Malnutrition
   B. Steroid use
   C. Smoking
   D. Alcohol use

Answer: D
When a patient develops pain, bulging, or a mass at the site of an inguinal hernia repair, clinical entities such as seroma, persistent cord lipoma, and hernia recurrence should be considered. Common medical issues associated with recurrence include malnutrition, immunosuppression, diabetes, steroid use, and smoking. Technical causes of recurrence include improper mesh size, tissue ischemia, infection, and tension in the reconstruction. A focused physical examination should be performed. As with primary hernias, ultrasound, (CT), or

magnetic resonance imaging (MRI) can elucidate ambiguous physical findings. When a recurrent hernia is discovered and warrants reoperation, an approach through a virgin plane facilitates its dissection and exposure. Extensive dissection of the scarred field and mesh may result in injury to cord structures, viscera, large blood vessels, and nerves. After an initial anterior approach, the posterior laparoscopic approach will usually be easier and more effective than another anterior dissection. Conversely, failed preperitoneal repairs should be approached using an open anterior repair. (See Schwartz 10th ed., p. 1514.)

9. Nociceptive pain is
   A. The result of ligamentous or muscular trauma and inflammation.
   B. The result of direct nerve damage or entrapment.
   C. The result of pain conveyed through afferent autonomic pain fibers.
   D. Characterized as acute.

Answer: A
Pain after inguinal hernia repair is classified into acute or chronic manifestations of three mechanisms: nociceptive (somatic), neuropathic, and visceral pain. Nociceptive pain is the most common of the three. Because it is usually a result of ligamentous or muscular trauma and inflammation, nociceptive pain is reproduced with abdominal muscle contraction. Treatment consists of rest, nonsteroidal anti-inflammatory drugs (NSAIDs), and reassurance, as it resolves spontaneously in most cases. Neuropathic pain occurs as a result of direct nerve damage or entrapment. It may present early or late, and it manifests as a localized, sharp, burning, or tearing sensation. It may respond to pharmacologic therapy and to local steroid or anesthetic injections when indicated. Visceral pain refers to pain conveyed through afferent autonomic pain fibers. It is usually poorly localized and may occur during ejaculation as a result of sympathetic plexus injury. (See Schwartz 10th ed., p. 1514.)

10. The triangle of pain is bordered by all of the following EXCEPT
    A. Iliopubic tract
    B. Ductus deferens
    C. Gonadal vessels
    D. Reflected peritoneum

Answer: B
The preperitoneal anatomy seen in laparoscopic hernia repair led to characterization of important anatomic areas of interest, known as the *triangle of doom*, the *triangle of pain*, and the *circle of death* (Fig. 37-2). The triangle of doom is bordered medially by the vas deferens and laterally by the vessels of the spermatic cord. The contents of the space include the external iliac vessels, deep circumflex iliac vein, femoral nerve, and genital branch of the genitofemoral nerve. The triangle of pain is a region bordered by the iliopubic tract and gonadal vessels, and it encompasses the lateral femoral cutaneous, femoral branch of the genitofemoral, and femoral nerves. The circle of death is a vascular continuation formed by the common iliac, internal iliac, obturator, inferior epigastric, and external iliac vessels. (See Schwartz 10th ed., Table 37-9, pp. 1499 and 1501.)

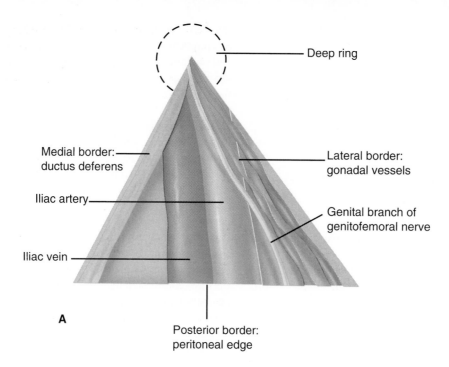

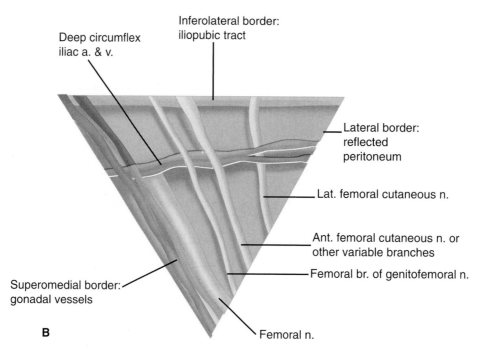

FIG. 37-2. Borders and contents of the **A.** triangle of doom and **B.** triangle of pain. a. = artery; Ant. = anterior; br. = branch; Lat. = lateral; n. = nerve; v. = vein. (Modified with permission from Colborn GL, Skandalakis JE. Laparoscopic cadaveric anatomy of the inguinal area. *Probl Gen Surg* 12:13;1995.)

11. The most common cause of urinary retention after hernia repair is
    A. General anesthesia
    B. Narcotic analgesia
    C. Pain
    D. Perioperative bladder distention

Answer: A

The most common cause of urinary retention after hernia repair is general anesthesia, which is routine in laparoscopic hernia repairs. Among 880 patients undergoing inguinal hernia repair with local anesthesia only 0.2% developed urinary retention, whereas the rate of urinary retention was 13% among 200 patients undergoing repair with general or spinal anesthesia. Other risk factors for postoperative urinary retention include pain, narcotic analgesia, and perioperative bladder distention. Initial treatment of urinary retention requires decompression of the bladder with short-term catheterization. Patients will generally require an overnight admission and trial of normal voiding before discharge. Failure to void normally requires reinsertion of the catheter for up to a week. Chronic requirement of a urinary catheter is rare, although older patients may require prolonged catheterization. (See Schwartz 10th ed., p. 1515.)

12. The outcome found more commonly with TAPP repair compared with TEP repair is
A. Length of stay
B. Time to recovery
C. Risk of intra-abdominal injuries
D. Higher short-term recurrence rates

Answer: C

Although controversy persists regarding the utility of TEP versus TAPP, reviews to date find no significant differences in operative duration, length of stay, time to recovery, or short-term recurrence rate between the two approaches. In TAPP repair, the risk of intra-abdominal injury is higher than in TEP repair. This finding prompted the International Endohernia Society (IEHS) to recommend that TAPP should only be attempted by surgeons with sufficient experience. A Cochrane systematic review found that rates of port-site hernias and visceral injuries were higher for the TAPP technique, whereas TEP may be associated with a higher rate of conversion to an alternative approach; however, neither finding was sufficiently compelling to recommend one technique over the other. (See Schwartz 10th ed., p. 1517.)

13. The ratio of inguinal hernias to femoral hernias is
A. 7:3
B. 5:1
C. 8:2
D. 10:1

Answer: B

Approximately 75% of abdominal wall hernias occur in the groin. The lifetime risk of inguinal hernia is 27% in men and 3% in women. Of inguinal hernia repairs, 90% are performed in men and 10% in women. The incidence of inguinal hernias in men has a bimodal distribution, with peaks before the first year of age and after age 40. Abramson demonstrated the age dependence of inguinal hernias in 1978. Those between 25 and 34 years had a lifetime prevalence rate of 15%, whereas those aged 75 years and over had a rate of 47% (Table 37-1). Approximately 70% of femoral hernia repairs are performed in women; however, inguinal hernias are five times more common than femoral hernias. The most common subtype of groin hernia in men and women is the indirect inguinal hernia. (See Schwartz 10th ed., p. 1495.)

14. The high incidence of inguinal hernias in preterm babies is most often due to
A. Failure of the peritoneum to close
B. Familial history
C. Female gender
D. Developmental dysplasia of the hip

Answer: A

Inguinal hernias may be congenital or acquired. Most adult inguinal hernias are considered acquired defects in the abdominal wall although collagen studies have demonstrated a heritable predisposition. A number of studies have attempted to delineate the precise causes of inguinal hernia formation; however, the best-characterized risk factor is weakness in the abdominal wall musculature (Table 37-4). Congenital hernias, which make up the majority of pediatric hernias, can be considered an impedance of normal development, rather than an acquired weakness. During the normal course of development, the testes descend from the intra-abdominal space into the scrotum in the third trimester. Their descent is preceded by the gubernaculum and a diverticulum of peritoneum, which protrudes through the inguinal canal and becomes the processus vaginalis. Between 36 and 40 weeks of gestation, the processus vaginalis closes and eliminates the peritoneal opening at the internal inguinal ring. Failure of the peritoneum to close results in a patent processus vaginalis (PPV), hence the high incidence of indirect inguinal hernias in preterm babies. Children with congenital indirect inguinal hernias will present with a PPV; however, a patent processus does not necessarily indicate an inguinal hernia (Fig. 37-3). In a study of nearly

600 adults undergoing general laparoscopy, bilateral inspection revealed that 12% had PPV. None of these patients had clinically significant symptoms of a groin hernia. In a group of 300 patients undergoing unilateral laparoscopic inguinal hernia repair, 12% were found to have a contralateral PPV, which was associated with a fourfold 5-year incidence of inguinal hernia. (See Schwartz 10th ed., Table 37-3 and Figure 37-10, pp. 1500 and 1502.)

TABLE 37-4	Presumed causes of groin herniation
Coughing	
Chronic obstructive pulmonary disease	
Obesity	
Straining	
Constipation	
Prostatism	
Pregnancy	
Birthweight <1500 g	
Family history of a hernia	
Valsalva's maneuver	
Ascites	
Upright position	
Congenital connective tissue disorders	
Defective collagen synthesis	
Previous right lower quadrant incision	
Arterial aneurysms	
Cigarette smoking	
Heavy lifting	
Physical exertion	

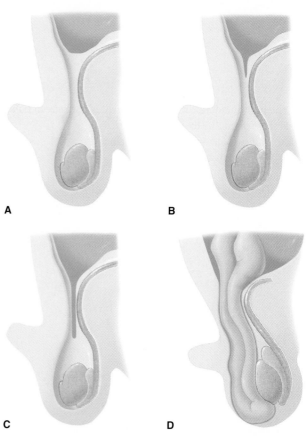

A

B

C

D

FIG. 37-3. Varying degrees of closure of the processus vaginalis (PV). **A.** Closed PV. **B.** Minimally patent PV. **C.** Moderately patent PV. **D.** Scrotal hernia.

15. Injury to the lateral femoral cutaneous nerve results in
    A. Inguinodynia
    B. Osteitis pubis
    C. Meralgia paresthetica
    D. Nerve entrapment

Answer: C

Other chronic pain syndromes include local nerve entrapment, meralgia paresthetica, and osteitis pubis. At greatest risk of entrapment are the ilioinguinal and iliohypogastric nerves in anterior repairs and the genitofemoral and lateral femoral cutaneous nerves in laparoscopic repairs. Clinical manifestations of nerve entrapment mimic acute neuropathic pain, and they occur with a dermatomal distribution. Injury to the lateral femoral cutaneous nerve results in meralgia paresthetica, a condition characterized by persistent paresthesias of the lateral thigh. Initial treatment of nerve entrapment consists of rest, ice, NSAIDs, physical therapy, and possible local corticosteroid and anesthetic injection. Osteitis pubis is characterized by inflammation of the pubic symphysis and usually presents as medial groin or symphyseal pain that is reproduced by thigh adduction. Avoiding the pubic periosteum when placing sutures and tacks reduces the risk of developing osteitis pubis. CT scan or MRI excludes hernia recurrence, and bone scan is confirmatory for the diagnosis. Initial treatment is identical to that of nerve entrapment; however, if pain remains intractable, orthopedic surgery consultation should be sought for possible bone resection and curettage. Irrespective of treatment, the condition often takes 6 months to resolve. (See Schwartz 10th ed., p. 1515.)

16. The hernia repair method associated with the lowest recurrence rate is the
    A. Lichtenstein tension-free repair
    B. Open elective tissue-based repair
    C. Bassini technique
    D. Shouldice repair

Answer: A

The incidence of recurrence is the most-cited measure of postoperative outcome following inguinal hernia repair. In evaluating the various available techniques, other salient signifiers of outcome include complication rates, operative duration, hospital stay, and quality of life. The following section summarizes the evidence-based outcomes of the various approaches to inguinal hernia repair.

Among tissue repairs, the Shouldice operation is the most commonly performed technique, and it is most frequently executed at specialized centers. A 2012 meta-analysis from the Cochrane Database demonstrated significantly lower rates of hernia recurrence (odds ratio [OR] 0.62, confidence interval [CI] 0.45–0.85) in patients undergoing Shouldice operations when compared with other open tissue-based methods. In experienced hands, the overall recurrence rate for the Shouldice repair is about 1%. Although it is an elegant procedure, its meticulous nature requires significant technical expertise to achieve favorable outcomes, and it is associated with longer operative duration and longer hospital stay. One study found the recurrence rate for Shouldice repairs decreased from 9.4 to 2.5% after surgeons performed the repair six times. Compared with mesh repairs, the Shouldice technique resulted in significantly higher rates of recurrence (OR 3.65, CI 1.79–7.47); however, it is the most effective tissue-based repair when mesh is unavailable or contraindicated.

Hernia recurrence is drastically reduced as a result of the Lichtenstein tension-free repair. Compared with open elective tissue-based repairs, mesh repair is associated with fewer recurrences (OR 0.37, CI 0.26–0.51) and with shorter hospital stay and faster return to usual activities. In a multi-institutional series, 3019 inguinal hernias were repaired using the Lichtenstein technique, with an overall recurrence rate of 0.2%. Among other tension-free repairs, the Lichtenstein technique remains the most commonly performed procedure worldwide. Meta-analysis demonstrates no significant differences in outcomes between the Lichtenstein and the plug and patch techniques; however, intra-abdominal plug migration and erosion into contiguous structures occurs in approximately 6% of cases. The Stoppa technique results in longer operative duration than the Lichtenstein technique. Nevertheless, postoperative acute pain, chronic pain, and recurrence rates are similar between the two methods. Perhaps the most compelling advantage of the Lichtenstein technique is that nonexpert surgeons rapidly achieve similar outcomes to their expert counterparts. Guidelines issued by the European Hernia Society recommend the Lichtenstein repair for adults with either unilateral or bilateral inguinal hernias as the preferred open technique. (See Schwartz 10th ed., p. 1516.)

17. A sliding hernia
    A. Has an abnormally high recurrence rate after repair
    B. Can involve the bladder
    C. Is more common in the right groin
    D. Occurs almost exclusively in women

Answer: B

Inguinal hernias may compress adjacent nerves, leading to generalized pressure, localized sharp pain, and referred pain. Pressure or heaviness in the groin is a common complaint, especially at the conclusion of the day or following prolonged activity. Sharp pain tends to indicate an impinged nerve and may not be related to the extent of physical activity performed by the patient. Neurogenic pain may be referred to the scrotum, testicle, or inner thigh. Questions should be directed to elicit and characterize extrainguinal symptoms. A change in bowel habits or urinary symptoms may indicate a sliding hernia consisting of intestinal contents or involvement of the bladder within the hernia sac. (See Schwartz 10th ed., p. 1503.)

CHAPTER 38

Thyroid, Parathyroid, and Adrenal

1. Which surgeon was awarded the Nobel Prize in Physiology or Medicine for his work on the "physiology, pathology, and surgery of the thyroid gland?"
   A. Theodore Billroth
   B. Emil Kocher
   C. John Hunter
   D. Harvey Cushing

Answer: B
The Nobel Prize in Physiology or Medicine was awarded to Emil Kocher in 1909. In addition to his research on the physiology of the thyroid, Kocher's operative methods greatly reduced the mortality risk of thyroidectomy. The Kocher clamp was designed to prevent hemorrhage from the hypervascular gland during thyroidectomy. (See Schwartz 10th ed., p. 1521.)

2. What congenital anomaly arises from the formation of the thyroid gland?
   A. The thyroid isthmus
   B. The cricothyroid arch
   C. A thyroglossal duct cyst
   D. An endobronchial cyst

Answer: C
The medial thyroid anlage descends from the base of the tongue through a channel called the *thyroglossal duct* at week 3 to 4 of gestation. The duct normally closes after its descent, but may remain patent and is susceptible to secondary infection and dilatation, referred to as a *thyroglossal duct cyst*. Removal is accomplished with the Sistrunk operation which also removes the central portion of the hyoid bone. (See Schwartz 10th ed., p. 1521.)

3. The arterial supply of the thyroid arises from which of the following vessels?
   A. The aorta
   B. The external carotid arteries
   C. The thyrocervical trunk
   D. All of the above

Answer: D
The superior thyroid arteries arise from the external carotid arteries, and the inferior thyroid arteries arise from the thyrocervical trunk shortly after their origin from the subclavian arteries. A thyroid ima artery arises directly from the aorta or innominate artery in 1 to 4% of cases. (See Schwartz 10th ed., p. 1523.)

4. In what location, relative to the inferior thyroid artery (ITA), is the recurrent laryngeal nerve (RLN) found?
   A. Medial or posterior to the ITA
   B. Lateral or anterior to the ITA
   C. Passing between the branches of the ITA
   D. All of the above

Answer: D
The RLN courses within the tracheoesophageal groove after emerging from the vagus nerve at the level of the aortic arch. As it ascends in the neck, the recurrent laryngeal nerve (RNL) may branch, and may pass anterior, posterior, or interdigitate with branches of the ITA. The location of the RLN must be confirmed before the ITA is divided. (See Schwartz 10th ed., p. 1524.)

5. Although injury to the RLN results in hoarseness (unilateral injury) or airway obstruction (bilateral injury), injury to the superior laryngeal nerve (SLN) results in a more subtle injury, affecting the ability to
   A. Speak loudly or sing high notes.
   B. Cough.
   C. Feel sensation in the anterior neck.
   D. Grimace.

Answer: A

The external branch of the superior laryngeal nerve (SLN) lies on the inferior pharyngeal constrictor muscle and descends alongside the superior thyroid vessels before innervating the cricothyroid muscle. Therefore the superior pole vessels should not be ligated en masse, but should be individually divided low on the thyroid gland. Injury to the SLN leads to inability to tense the ipsilateral vocal cord, and impairs the ability to "hit high notes" while singing, or projecting the voice loudly. (See Schwartz 10th ed., p. 1524.)

6. Thyroid hormones (T3 and T4) have regulatory roles in all of the following EXCEPT
   A. The hypoxia and hypercapnia drives of the respiratory center in the brain.
   B. Gastrointestinal motility.
   C. The speed of muscle contraction and relaxation.
   D. Visual acuity in low-light conditions ("night vision").

Answer: D

Thyroid hormones are responsible for maintaining the normal hypoxic and hypercapnic drive in the respiratory center of the brain, and regulate gastrointestinal motility which leads to diarrhea in hyperthyroidism and constipation in hypothyroidism. They also regulate bone and protein turnover and the speed of muscle contraction and regulation, hepatic gluconeogenesis, cholesterol synthesis, and intestinal glucose absorption. (See Schwartz 10th ed., p. 1528.)

7. In North America, hyperthyroidism is most often caused by
   A. Toxic multinodular goiter
   B. Diffuse toxic goiter (Graves disease)
   C. Thyroid cancer
   D. Thyroid stimulating hormone-secreting pituitary adenoma

Answer: B

Graves disease, named after Robert Graves, the Irish physician who described the disorder in three patients in 1835, is the most common cause of hyperthyroidism in North America, and accounts for 60 to 80% of cases. (See Schwartz 10th ed., p. 1531.)

8. Subtotal or total thyroidectomy is preferred for the treatment of Graves disease
   A. When radioactive iodine therapy is contraindicated.
   B. When the goiter is large or airway obstruction appears imminent.
   C. In patients with demonstrated poor compliance with anti-thyroid medications.
   D. All of the above.

Answer: D

Subtotal or total thyroidectomy is now preferred over subtotal thyroidectomy due to a lower recurrence rate. Surgery is preferred over medical therapy (radioactive iodine) in childbearing women who desire to have children in the near future, in noncompliant patients, or when airway obstruction appears likely. (See Schwartz 10th ed., p. 1533.)

9. What is the recommended course of action when fine needle aspiration biopsy (FNAB) of a thyroid nodule is "follicular neoplasm?"
   A. Repeat FNAB
   B. Lobectomy
   C. Lobectomy and isthmusectomy
   D. Total thyroidectomy

Answer: B

Follicular neoplasms of the thyroid are less aggressive than papillary neoplasms, and a fine needle aspiration biopsy (FNAB) may be unable to differentiate between a follicular adenoma and a follicular carcinoma. For this reason unilateral lobectomy is recommended for this FNAB diagnosis. (See Schwartz 10th ed., p. 1539.)

10. Which diseases are associated with germline mutations in the *RET* tyrosine kinase receptor gene?
    A. Multiple endocrine neoplasia type 2A (MEN2A)
    B. Multiple endocrine neoplasia type 2B (MEN2B)
    C. Hirschsprung disease
    D. All of the above

Answer: D

Mutations in the extracellular domain of the *RET* tyrosine kinase receptor are associated with multiple endocrine neoplasia type 2A (MEN2A), familial medullary thyroid cancer (FMTC), and Hirschsprung disease. Mutations in the intracellular domain are associated with MEN2B, FMTC, and Hirschsprung disease. (See Schwartz 10th ed., p. 1540.)

11. Children exposed to the Chernobyl disaster in 1986 subsequently demonstrated an increased incidence of which thyroid cancer?
    A. Papillary thyroid cancer (PTC)
    B. Follicular thyroid cancer (FTC)
    C. Medullary thyroid cancer (MTC)
    D. Anaplastic thyroid cancer (ATC)

Answer: A
Papillary thyroid cancer accounts for 80% of all thyroid malignancies and is the predominant thyroid cancer in children and individuals exposed to external radiation. (See Schwartz 10th ed., p. 1542.)

12. The recommended treatment for an otherwise healthy 50-year-old man with a 2-cm PTC in the left lobe diagnosed by FNAB is
    A. Left lobectomy
    B. Left lobectomy and isthmusectomy
    C. Total left lobectomy and subtotal right lobectomy
    D. Excisional biopsy with frozen section analysis

Answer: C
Total thyroidectomy or total lobectomy on the affected side with subtotal lobectomy on the nonaffected side is the recommended treatment of choice for unifocal PTC greater than 1 cm in diameter. Definitive operation can be performed without frozen section when the diagnosis is unequivocal on FNAB. (See Schwartz 10th ed., p. 1543.)

13. An adolescent patient with a thyroid mass undergoes FNAB which returns as MCT. What other diseases should be screened for before treatment is undertaken?
    A. Hyperparathyroidism
    B. Pheochromocytoma
    C. Mucocutaneous ganglioneuromas
    D. All of the above

Answer: D
MCT can be spontaneous (in 75%) or familial (in 25%) in MEN2. MEN2A is associated with pheochromocytoma and hyperparathyroidism, whereas MEN2B is associated with pheochromocytoma, Marfanoid habitus, and mucocutaneous ganglioneuromas. (See Schwartz 10th ed., p. 1550.)

14. An asymptomatic child with a normal physical examination is found to harbor a mutation in codon 918 of the *RET* tyrosine kinase receptor, compatible with MEN2B. Ultrasound of the neck is unremarkable and serum calcitonin levels are normal. What course is indicated?
    A. Repeat examination and ultrasound yearly
    B. Planned thyroidectomy in 3 to 5 years
    C. Total thyroidectomy
    D. Total thyroidectomy with bilateral neck dissection

Answer: C
Children with mutations at codon 634 of the *RET* tyrosine kinase receptor gene (MEN2A) are advised to undergo thyroidectomy before age 5, whereas children with mutations at codon 918 (MEN2B) should undergo thyroidectomy before age 1. If ultrasound of the neck is normal and calcitonin levels are normal, a formal neck dissection can be avoided. (See Schwartz 10th ed., p. 1550.)

15. Postoperative complications within 24 hours of thyroid surgery include
    A. Hypocalcemia
    B. Dyspnea
    C. Dystonia
    D. All of the above

Answer: D
Inadvertent injury (ischemia) or removal of the parathyroid glands can cause acute neuromuscular excitability due to hypocalcemia. An expanding hematoma in the neck may not cause bleeding from the wound, but can compress the membranous portion of the trachea and cause dyspnea. Nerve injuries can cause vocal cord paralysis or impaired speech. (See Schwartz 10th ed., p. 1556.)

16. A patient with primary hyperparathyroidism undergoes neck exploration where four small, normal appearing glands are found. What are the possible locations of an additional, supernumerary gland?
    A. In the thyroid gland
    B. In the thymus
    C. In the tracheoesophageal groove
    D. All of the above

Answer: D
Supernumerary parathyroid glands occur in 7 to 13% of people, and may be located in the thymus (most commonly), within the parenchyma of the thyroid gland, or in the tracheoesophageal groove, the mediastinum, or elsewhere in the neck. (See Schwartz 10th ed., p. 1557.)

17. A 70-year-old woman with early dementia but otherwise good physical health has an elevated parathyroid hormone (PTH) level and a sestamibi scan which localizes a single focus of increased activity to the left lower neck. An ultrasound confirms an enlarged gland in the same area. What treatment is likely to provide the best outcome?
    A. Bilateral neck exploration under general anesthesia.
    B. Unilateral, "mini-incision" parathyroidectomy under local anesthesia.
    C. Minimally invasive videoscopic parathyroidectomy from a left axillary approach under general anesthesia.
    D. Percutaneous alcohol ablation with ultrasound guidance under local anesthesia.

Answer: B

Localization studies such as sestamibi scans have been shown to allow more limited operations, including those utilizing "mini-incisions" under local anesthesia, for patients who are not good risks for general anesthesia. Improved cosmesis, shorter lengths of stay, and reduced complications are benefits from this approach. (See Schwartz 10th ed., p. 1564.)

18. Intraoperative, rapid PTH assays provide guidance that all hyperfunctioning glands have been removed during parathyroidectomy. What criterion is used to indicate satisfactory resolution of the hyperparathyroidism during the procedure?
    A. Greater than 50% fall in PTH level within 10 minutes of removal of parathyroid tissue.
    B. Greater than 25% fall in PTH level within 30 minutes of removal of parathyroid tissue.
    C. Greater than 75% fall in PTH level within 10 minutes of removal of parathyroid tissue.
    D. Greater than 90% fall in PTH level within 30 minutes of removal of parathyroid tissue.

Answer: A

When the PTH level falls by greater than 50% within 10 minutes after removal of parathyroid tissue, the cause of the hyperparathyroidism is likely to have been removed, and the operation can be stopped. (See Schwartz 10th ed., p. 1566.)

19. A patient with persistent ulcer disease is diagnosed with a gastrinoma. Serum chemistry studies indicate hypercalcemia, and an elevated PTH level is documented. What is the indicated course of treatment?
    A. Administration of mithramycin 25 mg/kg/day for 4 to 5 days to lower calcium levels.
    B. Administration of octreotide 100 mg TID to suppress gastrin secretion.
    C. Abdominal exploration for removal of the gastrinoma.
    D. Neck exploration for removal of the parathyroid adenoma.

Answer: D

In patients with MEN1, hyperparathyroidism should be corrected before treatment of the gastrinoma because resolution of hypercalcemia may allow gastrin levels to fall to normal. (See Schwartz 10th ed., p. 1567.)

20. Which of the following findings is suggestive of a parathyroid carcinoma?
    A. An elevated serum calcium level greater than 14 mg/dL.
    B. An elevated PTH level greater than five times normal.
    C. A palpable mass in the neck.
    D. All of the above.

Answer: A

Parathyroid carcinoma occurs in about 1% of patients with primary hyperparathyroidism, or in about 1000 patients per year in the United States. Findings include an elevated serum calcium level greater than 14 mg/dL, and elevated PTH level greater than five times normal, and a palpable mass in the neck, but none of these may be present. Complete surgical removal is the most effective therapy with radical neck dissection if lymphadenopathy is present; however, one-third of patients have metastatic disease when first diagnosed. (See Schwartz 10th ed., p. 1570.)

21. A 50-year-old, healthy-appearing man undergoes evaluation of persistent hypertension. Serum chemistries reveal hypokalemia (less than 3.2 mmol/L) and imaging studies reveal a unilateral adrenal mass. What is the likely diagnosis?
    A. Secondary hypercortisolism (Cushing disease)
    B. Primary hypercortisolism (Cushing syndrome)
    C. Hyperaldosteronism (Conn syndrome)
    D. Pheochromocytoma

Answer: C
Primary aldosteronism, or Conn syndrome, is seen in about 1% of hypertensive patients. It is more common in middle-aged individual and is usually associated with a single adenoma of the adrenal cortex. The hypertension is usually refractory to medical treatment, and is classically associated with hypokalemia, but may be seen in normokalemic individuals. (See Schwartz 10th ed., p. 1578.)

22. A 35-year-old woman undergoes an evaluation for infertility. She has gained almost 100 lb in the past year, is hypertensive, and is borderline diabetic. She also complains of easy bruising. Her serum chemistries are normal with the exception of an elevated glucose. Imaging studies reveal a unilateral adrenal mass. What is the likely diagnosis?
    A. Secondary hypercortisolism (Cushing disease)
    B. Primary hypercortisolism (Cushing syndrome)
    C. Hyperaldosteronism (Conn syndrome)
    D. Pheochromocytoma

Answer: B
Cushing syndrome refers to any cause of hypercortisolism caused by either an adrenal source or exogenous administration of steroids. Cushing disease refers only to an adrenocorticotropic hormone (ACTH)-secreting adenoma of the pituitary gland. Cushing syndrome due to an isolated adrenal adenoma is far less common than hypercortisolism due to a pituitary adenoma, but adrenalectomy is curative for primary adrenal tumors or for adrenal hyperplasia that persists despite efforts to resect a pituitary tumor. (See Schwartz 10th ed., p. 1580.)

23. All of the following imaging techniques are useful to localize a pheochromocytoma EXCEPT
    A. Computed tomography (CT) scan
    B. Magnetic resonance imaging (MRI) scan
    C. Metaiodobenzylguanidine (MIBG) scan
    D. Octreotide scan

Answer: D
Pheochromocytomas are solid tumors which appear on computed tomography (CT) scan as soft tissue masses. They are detected with 85 to 95% accuracy, but it is important to avoid intravenous-contrast enhancement when a pheochromocytoma is suspected; intravenous contrast can provoke a hypertensive crisis due to release of catecholamines. MR is useful to identify pheochromocytomas, both because they identify soft tissue masses, but also because this tumor tends to enhance on T2-weighted images. Radio-labeled metaiodobenzylguanidine (MIBG) is taken up avidly by the pheochromocytoma because its structure is similar to norepinephrine. Therefore the MIBG scan can localize an occult tumor. Octreotide scans are not used for pheochromocytoma as the tumor does not overexpress somatostatin receptors. (See Schwartz 10th ed., p. 1586.)

24. Pheochromocytomas can secrete excess amounts of all of the following EXCEPT
    A. Dopa (L-dihydroxyphenylalanine)
    B. Dopamine
    C. Norepinephrine
    D. Epinephrine

Answer: A
Extra-adrenal pheochromocytomas (also known as *paragangliomas*) secrete norepinephrine, because these sites lack the enzyme (phenylethanolamine *N*-methyltransferase) which converts norepinephrine to epinephrine. Adrenal pheochromocytomas secrete both epinephrine and norepinephrine as well as dopamine. Some pheochromocytomas secrete only dopamine, and patients with these tumors may be normotensive. (See Schwartz 10th ed., p. 1586.)

25. The preoperative preparation of a patient with pheochromocytoma should include all of the following EXCEPT
    A. An alpha-adrenergic blocker such as phentolamine.
    B. A beta-adrenergic blocker such as propranolol.
    C. Intravenous hydration to avoid volume depletion.
    D. Systemic steroids to avoid adrenal insufficiency.

Answer: D
The preoperative preparation of a patient with a catecholamine-secreting tumor includes alpha-hypertension, a beta-adrenergic blocker to prevent tachycardia, and volume replacement to avoid hypotension due to alpha- and beta-blockers. Steroids are not needed to prevent adrenal insufficiency. (See Schwartz 10th ed., p. 1586.)

26. A follow-up CT scan in a 60-year-old patient with previous nephrolithiasis reveals a 1.5-cm hypovascular round lesion with clear margins in the right adrenal gland. The patient is not hypertensive, hyperglycemic, or hypokalemic. Urinary catechol metabolites are within normal limits, and serum cortisol and ACTH levels are normal. Which course is advisable?
    A. Repeat CT scan and chemical tests annually.
    B. Percutaneous FNAB.
    C. Adrenal venous sampling for cortisol, renin, and angiotensin.
    D. Laparoscopic adrenalectomy.

Answer: A

The adrenal "incidentaloma" is an increasingly common finding with the ubiquitous use of CT scanning, with an incidence of 0.4 to 4.4%. A variety of benign and malignant lesions can account for these findings, and a distant history of malignancy elsewhere should raise the possibility of metastatic disease. Primary malignancy of the adrenal gland is rare, and the functioning tumors are excluded by screening tests for cortisol and catecholamine excess. In the absence of symptoms associated with adrenally disease, annual follow-up of these lesions with imaging and chemical tests seems prudent. (See Schwartz 10th ed., p. 1589.)

27. Advantages of laparoscopic adrenalectomy compared with open adrenalectomy include all of the following EXCEPT
    A. Decreased incidence of wound infection
    B. Decreased length of hospital stay
    C. Decreased operative time
    D. Decreased narcotic analgesic use

Answer: C

Laparoscopic (videoscopic) approaches to adrenalectomy have been shown to be advantageous for several outcomes including wound complications, analgesic use, and length of hospital stay. These advantages are in balance to adverse considerations including length of operative time and cost. (See Schwartz 10th ed., p. 1591.)

28. In patients who undergo bilateral adrenalectomy in treatment of Cushing disease after failed attempts at resection of an ACTH-secreting pituitary adenoma, the subsequent development of Nelson syndrome is associated with all of the following EXCEPT
    A. Hyperpigmentation
    B. Diminished visual fields
    C. Loss of hearing
    D. Headaches

Answer: C

Nelson syndrome describes symptoms due to the progressive enlargement of a persistent ACTH-secreting pituitary fossa tumor. These symptoms include hyperpigmentation, visual field loss, headaches, and extraocular muscle palsies. Interference with the olfactory nerve is not part of the syndrome. (See Schwartz 10th ed., p. 1594.)

CHAPTER 39

Pediatric Surgery

1. Operative management of a newborn with the chest X-ray shown in Fig. 39-1 should occur
   A. Immediately after birth
   B. Within 24 hours
   C. Within 72 hours
   D. None of the above

Answer: D
The diagnosis of congenital diaphragmatic hernia (CDH) is made by chest X-ray, with the vast majority of infants developing immediate respiratory distress and pulmonary hypertension. CDH care has improved considerably through effective use of improved methods of ventilation and timely cannulation for extracorporeal membrane oxygenation. In the past, correction of the hernia was believed to be a surgical emergency, and patients underwent surgery shortly after birth. It is now accepted that the presence of persistent pulmonary hypertension that results in right-to-left shunting across the patent foramen ovale or the ductus arteriosus and the degree of pulmonary hypoplasia are the leading causes of cardiorespiratory insufficiency. Current management therefore is directed toward managing the pulmonary hypertension, which is usually seen within 7 to 10 days, but in some infants, may take up to several weeks. (See Schwartz 10th ed., Figure 39-3, pp. 1604–1605.)

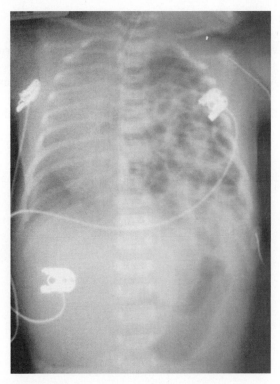

FIG. 39-1. Chest X-ray showing a left congenital diaphragmatic hernia.

2. Which of the following is most consistent with pyloric stenosis?
   A. Na 140 Cl 110 K 4.2 HCO$_3$ 26
   B. Na 142 Cl 90 K 5.2 HCO$_3$ 39
   C. Na 140 Cl 95 K 4.0 HCO$_3$ 18
   D. Na 139 Cl 85 K 3.2 HCO$_3$ 36

Answer: D

Infants with hypertrophic pyloric stenosis (HPS) develop a hypochloremic, hypokalemic metabolic alkalosis. The urine pH level is high initially, but eventually drops because hydrogen ions are preferentially exchanged for sodium ions in the distal tubule of the kidney as the hypochloremia becomes severe (paradoxical aciduria). The diagnosis of pyloric stenosis usually can be made on physical examination by palpation of the typical "olive" in the right upper quadrant and the presence of visible gastric waves on the abdomen. When the olive cannot be palpated, ultrasound (US) can diagnose the condition accurately in 95% of patients. Criteria for US diagnosis include a channel length of over 16 mm and pyloric thickness over 4 mm. (See Schwartz 10th ed., pp. 1613–1614.)

3. An infant presents to the emergency room with bilious emesis and irritability. Physical examination is notable for abdominal tenderness and erythema of the abdominal wall. Abdominal X-ray demonstrates dilated proximal bowel with air-fluid levels. What is the most appropriate next step in management, after resuscitation?
   A. Upper gastrointestinal series
   B. Barium enema
   C. Gastrostomy
   D. Laparotomy

Answer: D

The cardinal symptom of intestinal obstruction in the newborn is bilious emesis. Prompt recognition and treatment of neonatal intestinal obstruction can truly be lifesaving. Bilious vomiting is usually the first sign of volvulus, and all infants with bilious vomiting must be evaluated rapidly to ensure that they do not have intestinal malrotation with volvulus. The child with irritability and bilious emesis should raise particular suspicions for this diagnosis. If left untreated, vascular compromise of the midgut initially causes bloody stools, but eventually results in circulatory collapse. Additional clues to the presence of advanced ischemia of the intestine include erythema and edema of the abdominal wall, which progresses to shock and death. It must be re-emphasized that the index of suspicion for this condition must be high, since abdominal signs are minimal in the early stages. Abdominal films show a paucity of gas throughout the intestine with a few scattered air-fluid levels. When these findings are present, the patient should undergo immediate fluid resuscitation to ensure adequate perfusion and urine output followed by prompt exploratory laparotomy. (See Schwartz 10th ed., p. 1617.)

4. Which of the following statements regarding Hirschsprung disease is FALSE?
   A. Constipation and abdominal distention are classic symptoms.
   B. Approximately 20% of cases are diagnosed beyond the newborn period.
   C. The underlying pathology is characterized by an absence of ganglion cells in Auerbach plexus.
   D. Decompressive ostomy should involve distal, nondilated bowel.

Answer: D

Hirschsprung disease is characterized by the absence of ganglion cells in Auerbach plexus and hypertrophy of associated nerve trunks. It is thought to result from a defect in the migration of neural crest cells, which migrate from cephalad to caudad. In children who do not respond to nonoperative treatment, a decompressive stoma is required. It is important to ensure that this stoma is placed in ganglion-containing bowel, which must be confirmed by frozen section at the time of stoma creation. The hypertrophied, dilated portion of the intestine in Hirschsprung disease contains normal ganglion cells, and it is in the narrow segment of the colon distal to the dilated portion that ganglion cells are absent. (See Schwartz 10th ed., p. 1625.)

5. The most common form of esophageal atresia (EA) is
   A. Pure EA (no fistula)
   B. Pure TEF (no atresia)
   C. EA with distal tracheoesophageal fistula
   D. EA with proximal tracheoesophageal fistula

Answer: C
The five major varieties of esophageal atresia (EA) and tracheoesophageal fistula (TEF) are shown in Fig. 39-2. The most commonly seen variety is EA with distal TEF (type C), which occurs in approximately 85% of the cases in most series. The next most frequent type is pure EA (type A), occurring in 8 to 10% of patients, followed by TEF without EA (type E). This occurs in 8% of cases and is also referred to as an *H-type fistula,* based on the anatomic similarity to that letter (Fig. 39-3). EA with fistula between both proximal and distal ends of the esophagus and trachea (type D) is seen in approximately 2% of cases, and type B, EA with TEF between proximal esophagus and trachea, is seen in approximately 1% of all cases. (See Schwartz 10th ed., Figure 39-8 and 39-9, pp. 1608–1609.)

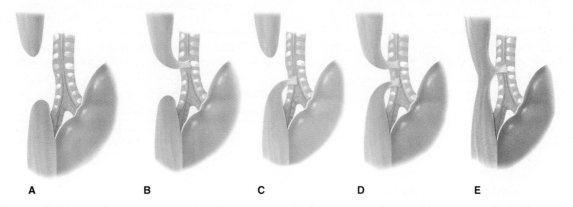

FIG. 39-2. The five varieties of esophageal atresia and tracheoesophageal fistula. **A.** Isolated esophageal atresia. **B.** Esophageal atresia with tracheoesophageal fistula between proximal segment of esophagus and trachea. **C.** Esophageal atresia with tracheoesophageal fistula between distal esophagus and trachea. **D.** Esophageal atresia with fistula between both proximal and distal ends of esophagus and trachea. **E.** Tracheoesophageal fistula without esophageal atresia (H-type fistula).

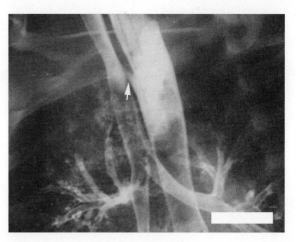

FIG. 39-3. Barium esophagram showing H-type tracheoesophageal fistula (arrow).

6. The predicted 4-year survival rate of a child with a Wilms tumor that is confined to one kidney and is grossly excised is
   A. 24%
   B. 38%
   C. 68%
   D. 97%

Answer: D
Following nephroureterectomy for Wilms tumor, the need for chemotherapy and/or radiation therapy is determined by the histology of the tumor and the clinical stage of the patient (Table 39-1). Essentially, patients who have disease confined to one kidney that is completely excised surgically receive a short course of chemotherapy and can expect a 97% 4-year survival, with tumor relapse rare after that time. Patients with

more advanced disease or with unfavorable histology receive more intensive chemotherapy and radiation. Even in stage IV, cure rates of 80% are achieved. The survival rates are worse in the small percentage of patients considered to have unfavorable histology. (See Schwartz 10th ed., Table 39-3, p. 1639.)

TABLE 39-1	Staging of Wilms tumor

Stage I: Tumor limited to the kidney and completely excised.

Stage II: Tumor that extends beyond the kidney but is completely excised. No residual tumor is apparent at or beyond the margins of excision. The tumor was biopsied, or there was local spillage of tumor confined to the flank.

Stage III: Residual tumor confined to the abdomen. Lymph nodes in the renal hilus, the periaortic chains, or beyond contain tumor. Diffuse peritoneal contamination by the tumor, such as by spillage of tumor beyond the flank before or during surgery or by tumor growth that has penetrated through the peritoneal surface. Implants are found on the peritoneal surfaces. Tumor extends beyond the surgical margins either microscopically or grossly. Tumor is not completely resectable because of local infiltration into vital structures.

Stage IV: Hematogenous metastases.

Stage V: Bilateral renal involvement.

Source: Reproduced with permission from D'Angio GJ, Breslow N, Beckwith JB, et al. Treatment of Wilms' tumor. Results of the Third National Wilms' Tumor Study. *Cancer.* 64(2):349-360;1989. Copyright © 1989 American Cancer Society.

7. A premature infant boy has been started on enteral feeds shortly after birth, but develops feeding intolerance 2 weeks postnatally. He displays abdominal tenderness, distention, and bloody stools. An abdominal radiograph is obtained and is shown in Fig. 39-4. What should be the next step in management?
   A. Nasogastric decompression, parenteral nutrition, broad-spectrum antibiotics.
   B. Laparotomy, excision of the affected bowel with ostomy formation.
   C. Laparotomy, reduction of the volvulus, division of adhesions, appendectomy.
   D. Water-soluble contrast enema.

Answer: A

The radiograph demonstrates pneumatosis intestinalis, in conjunction with the clinical scenario described, describes Bell stage II necrotizing enterocolitis (NEC). In all infants suspected of having NEC, feedings are discontinued, a nasogastric tube is placed, total parenteral nutrition (TPN) is started, and broad-spectrum parenteral antibiotics are given. The infant is resuscitated, and inotropes are administered to maintain perfusion as needed. Intubation and mechanical ventilation may be required to maintain oxygenation. Subsequent treatment may be influenced by the particular stage of NEC that is present. Patients with Bell stage II disease merit close observation. Serial physical examinations are performed looking for the development of diffuse peritonitis, a fixed mass, progressive abdominal wall cellulitis, or systemic sepsis. If infants fail to improve after several days of treatment or if abdominal radiographs show a fixed intestinal loop, consideration should be given to exploratory laparotomy. (See Schwartz 10th ed., Figure 39-19, pp. 1619–1620.)

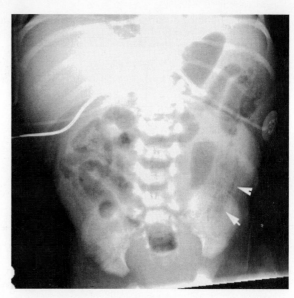

FIG. 39-4. Abdominal radiograph of infant with necrotizing enterocolitis. Arrows point to area of pneumatosis intestinalis.

8. An infant girl is found to have persistent jaundice after birth. A metabolic screen is normal, ultrasound demonstrates an absent gallbladder, and a technetium-99m iminodiacetic acid scan shows radionuclide that is concentrated in the liver but not excreted into the intestine. Which of the following is true?
   A. This condition is usually managed nonoperatively.
   B. Surgery should be performed within 60 days of life.
   C. Cystoenterostomy provides adequate biliary drainage.
   D. Most of these patients will not require transplantation.

Answer: B
This patient has biliary atresia, a rare disease characterized by fibroproliferative obliteration of the biliary tree, which progresses toward hepatic fibrosis, cirrhosis, and end-stage liver failure. Surgical treatment is the first-line therapy, consisting of creation of a hepatoportoenterostomy (Kasai procedure). Numerous studies suggest that the likelihood of surgical success is inversely related to the age at the time of portoenterostomy. Infants treated prior to 60 days of life are more likely to achieve successful and long-term biliary drainage than older infants. Although the outlook is less favorable for patients after the 12th week, it is reasonable to proceed with surgery even beyond this time point, as the alternative is certain liver failure. Approximately one-third of patients remain symptom-free after portoenterostomy; the remainder requires liver transplantation due to progressive liver failure. Independent risk factors that predict failure of the procedure include bridging liver fibrosis at the time of surgery and postoperative cholangitic episodes. (See Schwartz 10th ed., pp. 1628–1629.)

9. The leading cause of death for children older than 1 year of age is
   A. Malignancy
   B. Infection
   C. Injury
   D. Congenital anomalies

Answer: C
Injury is the leading cause of death among children older than 1 year. In fact, trauma accounts for almost half of all pediatric deaths, more than cancer, congenital anomalies, pneumonia, heart disease, homicide, and meningitis combined. Motor vehicle collisions are the leading cause of death in people age 1 to 19 years, followed by homicide or suicide (predominantly with firearms) and drowning. Unintentional injuries account for 65% of all injury-related deaths in children younger than 19 years. Each year, approximately 20,000 children and teenagers die as a result of injury in the United States. For every child who dies from an injury, it is calculated that 40 others are hospitalized and 1120 are treated in emergency departments. An estimated 50,000 children acquire permanent disabilities each year, most of which are the result of head injuries. Thus, the problem of pediatric trauma continues to be one of the major threats to the health and well-being of children. (See Schwartz 10th ed., p. 1642.)

10. A "double bubble" on an abdominal radiograph in an infant is characteristic of
    A. Duodenal atresia
    B. Jejunal atresia
    C. Meconium ileus
    D. Pyloric stenosis

Answer: A

Whenever the diagnosis of duodenal obstruction is entertained, malrotation and midgut volvulus must be excluded. Other causes of duodenal obstruction include duodenal atresia, duodenal web, stenosis, annular pancreas, or duodenal duplication cyst. The classic finding on abdominal radiography is the "double bubble" sign, which represents the dilated stomach and duodenum (Fig. 39-5). In association with the appropriate clinical picture, this finding is sufficient to confirm the diagnosis of duodenal obstruction. (See Schwartz 10th ed., Figure 39-13, p. 1615.)

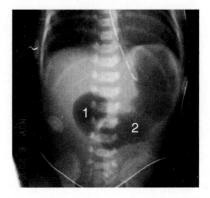

FIG. 39-5. Abdominal X-ray showing "double bubble" sign in a newborn infant with duodenal atresia. The two "bubbles" are numbered.

11. The defect in gastroschisis is
    A. To the left of the umbilicus
    B. To the right of the umbilicus
    C. Through the umbilicus
    D. Superior to the umbilicus

Answer: B

Gastroschisis represents a congenital anomaly characterized by a defect in the anterior abdominal wall through which the intestinal contents freely protrude. Unlike omphalocele, there is no overlying sac and the size of the defect is usually <4 cm. The abdominal wall defect is located at the junction of the umbilicus and normal skin and is almost always to the right of the umbilicus (Fig. 39-6), whereas for omphalocele the umbilical cord inserts into the sac. The umbilicus becomes partly detached, allowing free communication with the abdominal cavity. The appearance of the bowel provides some information with respect to the in utero timing of the defect. The intestine may be normal in appearance, suggesting that the rupture occurred relatively late during the pregnancy. More commonly, however, the intestine is thick, edematous, discolored, and covered with exudate, implying a more long-standing process. (See Schwartz 10th ed., Figure 39-31, p. 1633.)

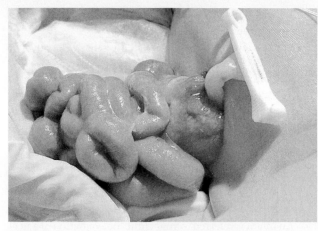

FIG. 39-6. Gastroschisis in a newborn. Note the location of the umbilical cord, and the edematous, thickened bowel.

12. The initial treatment for a pure EA (no fistula) is
    A. Repair of the EA.
    B. Repair of the EA with placement of a gastrostomy.
    C. Repair of the EA, Nissen fundoplication, and placement of a gastrostomy.
    D. Gastrostomy alone.

Answer: D

Primary EA (type A) represents a challenging problem, particularly if the upper and lower ends are too far apart for an anastomosis to be created. Under these circumstances, treatment strategies include placement of a gastrostomy tube and performing serial bougienage to increase the length of the upper pouch. This occasionally allows for primary anastomosis to be performed. Occasionally, when the two ends cannot be brought safely together, esophageal replacement is required, using either a gastric pull-up, reverse gastric tube, or colon interposition. (See Schwartz 10th ed., p. 1612.)

13. The most common branchial cleft fistula originates from the
    A. First branchial cleft
    B. Second branchial cleft
    C. Third branchial cleft
    D. Fourth branchial cleft

Answer: B

Paired branchial clefts and arches develop early in the fourth gestational week. The first cleft and the first, second, third, and fourth pouches give rise to adult organs. The embryologic communication between the pharynx and the external surface may persist as a fistula. A fistula is seen most commonly with the second branchial cleft, which normally disappears, and extends from the anterior border of the sternocleidomastoid muscle superiorly, inward through the bifurcation of the carotid artery, and enters the posterolateral pharynx just below the tonsillar fossa. In contrast, a third branchial cleft fistula passes posterior to the carotid bifurcation. The branchial cleft remnants may contain small pieces of cartilage and cysts, but internal fistulas are rare. A second branchial cleft sinus is suspected when clear fluid is noted draining from the external opening of the tract at the anterior border of the lower third of the sternomastoid muscle. Rarely, branchial cleft anomalies occur in association with biliary atresia and congenital cardiac anomalies, an association that is referred to as Goldenhar complex. (See Schwartz 10th ed., p. 1602.)

14. Which of the following is characteristic of congenital lobar emphysema?
    A. It results from dilatation of the airways associated with chronic suppurative disease.
    B. Its arterial blood supply characteristically comes directly from the aorta.
    C. It most commonly involves the upper lobes of the lungs.
    D. Resection is usually performed due to risk of malignant degeneration.

Answer: C
Congenital lobar emphysema is a condition manifested during the first few months of life as a progressive hyperexpansion of one or more lobes of the lung. It usually occurs in the upper lobes of the lung (left greater than right), and is caused by intrinsic bronchial obstruction from poor bronchial cartilage development or extrinsic compression. Treatment is resection of the affected lobe, which can be safely performed using either an open or thoracoscopic approach. The other choices describe bronchiectasis, pulmonary sequestration, and congenital pulmonary airway malformation, respectively. (See Schwartz 10th ed., pp. 1605–1607.)

15. An infant is referred to your clinic for evaluation of a neck mass. On physical examination, the patient has a left lateral neck mass with his head rotated to the opposite side. Which of the following is the most likely diagnosis?
    A. Thyroglossal duct cyst
    B. Torticollis
    C. Thymic cyst
    D. Lymphatic malformation

Answer: B
The management of neck masses in children is determined by their location and the length of time that they have been present. Neck lesions are found either in the midline or lateral compartments. Midline masses include thyroglossal duct remnants, thyroid masses, thymic cysts, or dermoid cysts. Lateral lesions include branchial cleft remnants, lymphatic malformations (previously known as *cystic hygroma*), vascular malformations, salivary gland tumors, torticollis, and lipoblastoma. The presence of a lateral neck mass in infancy in association with rotation of the head toward the opposite side of the mass indicates the presence of congenital torticollis. This lesion results from fibrosis of the sternocleidomastoid muscle, and is histologically characterized by the deposition of collagen and fibroblasts around atrophied muscle cells. In the vast majority of cases, physical therapy based on passive stretching of the affected muscle is of benefit. Rarely, surgical transection of the sternocleidomastoid may be indicated. (See Schwartz 10th ed., pp. 1601–1603.)

16. A 9-month-old boy presents with two episodes of vomiting as well as episodes of colicky pain. His abdominal examination is notable for upper abdominal tenderness, and his stools are guaiac-positive. US demonstrates a target sign, and he is then taken for an air-contrast enema. What is the likelihood that he will need operative intervention?
    A. 25%
    B. 50%
    C. 75%
    D. 90%

Answer: A
Patients with intussusception should be assessed for the presence of peritonitis and for the severity of systemic illness. In the absence of peritonitis, the child should undergo radiographic reduction. The air enema is diagnostic and may also be curative, and it is the preferred method of diagnosis and treatment of intussusception. Air is introduced with a manometer, and the pressure that is administered is carefully monitored. Under most instances, this should not exceed 120 mm Hg. Successful reduction is marked by free reflux of air into multiple loops of small bowel and symptomatic improvement as the infant suddenly becomes pain-free. Unless both of these signs are observed, it cannot be assumed that the intussusception is reduced. If reduction is unsuccessful and the infant remains stable, the infant should be brought back to the radiology suite for a repeat attempt at reduction after a few hours. This strategy has improved the success rate of nonoperative reduction in many centers. In addition, hydrostatic reduction with barium may be useful if pneumatic reduction is unsuccessful. The overall success rate of radiographic reduction varies based on the experience of the center and is typically between 60 and 90%. (See Schwartz 10th ed., p. 1622.)

17. A newborn is found to have a blind rectal pouch on examination. Which of the following are not associated with this condition?
    A. EA
    B. Cardiac defects
    C. Omphalocele
    D. Tethered spinal cord

Answer: C

The patient is described to have an imperforate anus, the embryologic basis of which involves failure of descent of the urorectal septum, resulting in a blind rectal pouch that often has a fistulous tract. Approximately 60% of patients have an associated malformation, the most common of which is a urinary tract defect (approximately 50% of patients). Skeletal defects are also seen, with the sacrum most commonly involved. Spinal cord anomalies, especially tethered cord, are common, particularly in children with high lesions. Gastrointestinal anomalies occur, most commonly EA. Cardiac anomalies may be noted, and occasionally patients present with a constellation of defects as part of the VACTERRL syndrome (*v*ertebral anomalies, *a*norectal anomalies, *c*ardiac defects, *t*racheoesophageal fistula, *r*enal anomalies, and *r*adial *l*imb hyperplasia). (See Schwartz 10th ed., p. 1627.)

18. Which type of choledochal cyst arises from the intraduodenal portion of the common bile duct?
    A. Type I
    B. Type II
    C. Type III
    D. Type IV

Answer: C

Choledochal cysts refer to a spectrum of congenital biliary tract disorders, with a cyst wall composed of fibrous tissue and devoid of mucosal lining. Type I cysts are characterized by fusiform dilatation of the bile duct, type II by isolated diverticula protruding from the wall of the common bile duct, and type III cysts arise from the intraduodenal portion of the common bile duct (also known as *choledochoceles*). Type IVA consists of multiple dilatations of the intrahepatic and extrahepatic bile ducts, whereas Type IVB involves only the extrahepatic bile ducts. Lastly, type V (Caroli disease) cysts are all intrahepatic, and usually consist of multiple dilatations. Cysts can lead to abdominal pain, cholangitis, pancreatitis, as well as a biliary tract malignancy. (See Schwartz 10th ed., p. 1630.)

19. Which of the following is not characteristic of prune-belly syndrome?
    A. Bilateral intra-abdominal testes
    B. Dilatation of the ureters
    C. Dilatation of the urinary bladder
    D. Malformed renal parenchyma

Answer: D

Prune-belly syndrome refers to a disorder that is characterized by extremely lax lower abdominal musculature, dilated urinary tract including the bladder, and bilateral undescended testes. The term prune-belly syndrome appropriately describes the wrinkled appearance of the anterior abdominal wall that characterizes these patients. The incidence is significantly higher in men, and patients manifest a variety of comorbidities, the most significant of which is pulmonary hypoplasia, which is not survivable in the most severe cases. Skeletal abnormalities include dislocation or dysplasia of the hip and pectus excavatum. Approximately 80% of these patients will have some degree of vesicoureteral reflux, which can predispose to urinary tract infection. Despite the marked dilatation of the urinary tract, most children with prune-belly syndrome have adequate renal parenchyma for growth and development. (See Schwartz 10th ed., p. 1634.)

20. Undescended testes are usually repaired by what age?
    A. 6 months
    B. 1 year of age
    C. 2 years of age
    D. 4 years of age

Answer: C

Men with bilateral undescended testicles are often infertile. When the testicle is not within the scrotum, it is subjected to a higher temperature, resulting in decreased spermatogenesis. Mengel and coworkers studied 515 undescended testicles by histology and demonstrated a decreasing presence of spermatogonia after 2 years of age. Despite orchidopexy, the incidence of infertility is approximately two times higher in men with unilateral orchidopexy compared with men with normal testicular descent. Consequently, it is now recommended that the undescended testicle be surgically repositioned by 1 year of age. (See Schwartz 10th ed., p. 1636.)

CHAPTER 40

Urology

1. Which of the following is INCORRECT concerning the anatomy of the penis?
   A. The paired corpora spongiosum functions as one compartment due to vascular interconnections.
   B. *Priapism* is defined as a persistent erection of more than 4 hours' duration.
   C. The corpora cavernosum are enclosed by the tunica albuginea.
   D. The corpora cavernosum and spongiosum are surrounded by Bucks fascia.

Answer: A
The corpora cavernosum are the paired, cylinder-like structures that are the main erectile bodies of the penis. The corpora cavernosum consist of a tough outer layer called the *tunica albuginea* and spongy, sinusoidal tissue inside that fills with blood to result in erection. The two corpora cavernosum have numerous vascular interconnections, so they function as one compartment. Surrounding all three bodies of the penis are the outer dartos fascia and the inner Buck fascia. (See Schwartz 10th ed., p. 1652.)

2. Which of the following is true about bladder cancer?
   A. For patients with bladder cancer invading into the bladder muscle (T2 lesion) immediate radiotherapy followed by surgery offers the best chance of cure.
   B. Patients with limited lymph node involvement may be cured by surgery alone.
   C. Continent neobladders have yet to be successfully utilized in patients undergoing cystectomy.
   D. Intravesical chemotherapy prior to surgery is routinely used for bladder cancers invading into the bladder muscle (T2 lesion).

Answer: B
For patients who have disease invading into bladder muscle (T2), immediate (within 3 months of diagnosis) cystectomy with extended lymph node dissection offers the best chance of survival. Patients with limited lymph node involvement may be cured with surgery alone. Patients have multiple reconstructive options, including continent and noncontinent urinary diversions. The orthotopic neobladder has emerged as a popular urinary diversion for patients without urethral involvement. This diversion type involves the detubularization of a segment of bowel, typically distal ileum, which is then refashioned into a pouch that is anastomosed to the proximal urethra (neobladder) or to the skin (continent cutaneous diversion). Patients with non–muscle-invasive bladder cancer (confined to the bladder mucosa or submucosa) can be managed with transurethral resection alone and adjuvant intravesical (instilled into the bladder) chemotherapy/immunotherapy. (See Schwartz 10th ed., pp. 1653–1654.)

3. Which of the following is true concerning testicular cancer?
   A. Most common malignancy in men between 15 and 35 years.
   B. Most commonly presents as a painful enlarging mass.
   C. Initial workup includes chest, abdominal, and brain imaging.
   D. Most common site of metastases is to the lungs.

Answer: A
Testicular cancer is the most common solid malignancy in men between 15 and 35 years. Chest and abdominal imaging must be performed to evaluate for evidence of metastasis. The most common site of spread is the retroperitoneal lymph nodes extending from the common iliac vessels to the renal vessels. (See Schwartz 10th ed., p. 1654.)

4. Which of the following statements about kidney cancer is FALSE?
   A. Lesions are usually solid but can be cystic.
   B. May be sporadic or hereditary.
   C. Surgical debulking can improve survival in patients who present with metastatic disease.
   D. Patients are not curable (and therefore should not be operated on) if tumor thrombus extends proximally into the vena cava.

Answer: D
Renal tumors are usually solid, but they also can be cystic. Most cases of renal cell carcinoma (RCC) are sporadic, but many hereditary forms have been described. Up to 20 to 30% of patients may present with metastatic disease, in which case, surgical debulking can improve survival, as shown in randomized controlled trials. Up to 10% of RCC invades the lumen of the renal vein or vena cava. The degree of venous extension directly impacts the surgical approach. Patients with thrombus below the level of the liver can be managed with cross-clamping above and below the thrombus and extraction from a cavotomy at the insertion of the renal vein. (See Schwartz 10th ed., pp. 1655–1656.)

5. Which of the following is FALSE concerning carcinoma of the prostate?
   A. Annual digital rectal examination and serum prostate-specific antigen (PSA) determinations are recommended beginning at age 55.
   B. Lung metastasis is less common than bone metastasis.
   C. Radical prostatectomy is associated with a 5% incidence of permanent urinary incontinence.
   D. Once prostate cancer has spread, it is no longer curable but can be contained by lowering serum testosterone and/ or by administration of androgen receptor blockers.

Answer: C
The American Urological Association has advised for screening for men 55 to 69 years of age. The most common site of spread of prostate cancer is the pelvic lymph nodes and bone. Radical prostatectomy is associated with early incontinence and erectile dysfunction (ED) (depending on nerve sparing). Incontinence improves significantly with time, with <1% of men in experienced hands suffering severe long-term problems with urinary control. (See Schwartz 10th ed., pp. 1657–1658.)

6. Concerning ureteric trauma, which of the following is true?
   A. Retrograde pyelogram is the most sensitive test to detect ureteral injury.
   B. Bladder mobilization is not integral to repair of ureteric injury.
   C. Kidney mobilization is not integral to repair of ureteric injury.
   D. Use of ureteric stents is not useful in predicting postrepair strictures.

Answer: A
A retrograde pyelogram is the most sensitive test for ureteral injury. Partial injuries can be primarily repaired, although all devitalized tissue must be debrided to avoid delayed tissue breakdown and urinoma formation. Ureteral stents should be placed in this situation to facilitate healing without stricture. Midurethral level injuries can be treated with a uretero-ureterostomy if a spatulated, tension-free repair can be achieved. For longer defects, the bladder can be mobilized and brought up to the psoas muscle (psoas hitch). For additional length, a tubularized flap of bladder (Boari flap) can be created and anastomosed to the remaining ureter. (See Schwartz 10th ed., pp. 1659–1660.)

7. Treatment of acute urinary retention may include all of the following EXCEPT
   A. Coude catheterization.
   B. Fluid replacement using 1:1 mL of D5W.
   C. Placement of a suprapubic drainage tube.
   D. Continuous bladder irrigation if hematuria is the cause of retention.

Answer: B
Treatment should include placement of a urethral catheter as quickly as possible. However, benign prostatic hyperplasia (BPH) or urethral strictures often make the placement of a catheter difficult. For men with BPH, a coude (French for curved) catheter is helpful in negotiating past the angulation in the prostatic urethra. Placement of a suprapubic tube approximately two fingerbreadths above the pubic symphysis may be needed. If hematuria is the cause of retention, continuous bladder irrigation often is necessary to prevent clot formation. Fluid replacement typically is 0.5 mL of 0.45 normal saline for every 1 mL of urine output above 200 mL in 1 hour, although sodium and potassium supplementation requirements depend on the electrolyte status of the patient. (See Schwartz 10th ed., pp.1661–1662.)

8. Regarding testicular torsion, which of the following is FALSE?
   A. Undescended testicle is a risk factor.
   B. Decreased blood flow relative to contralateral testicle demonstrable by ultrasound.
   C. Testicular salvage decreases to <5% if surgery is delayed >6 hours.
   D. Surgical exploration should include fixation of the contralateral testicle.

Answer: C
Risk factors for torsion include undescended testis, testicular tumor, and a "bell-clapper" deformity—poor gubernacular fixation of the testicles to the scrotal wall. The diagnosis is made by clinical history and examination, but can be supported by a Doppler ultrasound, which typically shows decreased intratesticular blood flow relative to the contralateral testis. Immediate surgical exploration can salvage an ischemic testis. More than 80% of testes can be salvaged if surgery is performed within 6 hours; this rate decreases to <20% as time lapses beyond 12 hours. At the time of surgery, the contralateral testes must also be explored and fixed to the dartos fascia due to the possibility that the same anatomic defect allowing torsion exists on the contralateral side. (See Schwartz 10th ed., pp. 1662–1663.)

9. All of the following are true concerning priapism EXCEPT
   A. *Priapism* is defined as a persistent erection for >4 hours unrelated to sexual stimulation.
   B. Etiologic factors include sickle cell disease, malignancy, total parenteral nutrition, penile shaft fractures.
   C. Low flow priapism can be confirmed with a penile blood gas determination.
   D. Treatment may require injection of phenylephrine.

Answer: B
Priapism is a persistent erection for more than 4 hours unrelated to sexual stimulation. Risk factors include sickle cell disease or trait, malignancy, medications, cocaine abuse, certain antidepressants, and total parenteral nutrition. Low-flow priapism can be confirmed with a penile blood gas of the cavernosal bodies demonstrating hypoxic, acidotic blood. Injection of phenylephrine (up to 200 mg in 20 mL normal saline) into the corporal bodies may be required. (See Schwartz 10th ed., p. 1663.)

10. Which of the following is true concerning BPH?
    A. Consequences of BPH include gross hematuria, chronic infection, bladder calculi, urinary retention, and paraphimosis.
    B. Medical treatment includes alpha blockers.
    C. Transurethral resection can lead to transurethral resection syndrome.
    D. Electrovaporization of the prostate should be avoided because of the danger of closed-space thermal injury.

Answer: A
Besides voiding symptoms, consequences of BPH include gross hematuria, infections due to incomplete emptying, bladder calculi, and urinary retention. Over time, incomplete emptying may lead to chronic bladder overdistention that can result in a de-functionalized bladder. Medical treatment of BPH is usually the first step. Alpha blockers act on α-receptors in the smooth muscle of the prostate and decrease its tone. Transurethral resection of the prostate is the mainstay of endoscopic surgical BPH treatment. It is extremely effective at improving flow and decreasing residual urine. Complications are rare but include incontinence and excessive fluid absorption of the hypotonic irrigating solution used during resection, resulting in the transurethral resection syndrome. It is due to hyponatremia and fluid overload, and although rare, can result in death. Mental status changes and pulmonary edema are managed by diuresis and sodium supplementation with hypertonic saline in severe cases. Because of these rare, but potentially dangerous side effects, laser or electrovaporization of the prostate has grown popular. It is associated with very limited fluid absorption, and saline can be used because there is no monopolar electrocautery. (See Schwartz 10th ed., p. 1665.)

11. Which of the following is true concerning urolithiasis?
    A. May affect up to 20% of the population over the course of a lifetime.
    B. Most common type is calcium oxalate lithiasis.
    C. Most patients will benefit from a chronic urinary acidification program.
    D. Study of choice for diagnosis is contrast computed tomography (CT) scanning.

Answer: B

Urolithiasis, or urinary calculus disease, may affect up to 10% of the population over the course of a lifetime. Calculi are crystalline aggregates of one or more components, most commonly calcium oxalate. Computed tomography (CT) scans will demonstrate all calculi except those composed of crystalline-excreted indinavir, an antiretroviral medication. For this reason, noncontrast CT scans have become the study of choice to evaluate for urolithiasis. Patients with recurrent stones will benefit from examination of stone composition and 24-hour urine metabolic workup to determine the underlying etiology. Better hydration is useful for all etiologies. Additionally, most patients will benefit from alkalization of the urine (eg, potassium citrate). (See Schwartz 10th ed., p. 1666.)

CHAPTER 41

Gynecology

1. Concerning human papillomavirus (HPV) vaccination, which of the following is FALSE?
   A. Two HPV vaccines have been developed and approved by the U.S. Food and Drug Administration (FDA).
   B. Both vaccines generate high concentrations of neutralizing antibodies to HPV L1 protein.
   C. Prospective randomized clinical trials have demonstrated that vaccination prevents nearly 100% of HPV subtype-specific precancerous cell changes.
   D. HPV immunizations prevents 90% of all cervical cancers.

Answer: D

Two human papillomavirus (HPV) vaccines have been developed and approved by the U.S. Food and Drug Administration (FDA). Vaccination generates high concentrations of neutralizing antibodies to HPV L1 protein, the antigen in both vaccines. Several randomized clinical trials involving approximately 35,000 young women have shown that both Gardasil and Cervarix prevent nearly 100% of the HPV subtype-specific precancerous cervical cell changes for up to 4 years after vaccination among women who were not infected at the time of vaccination. Cervical cancer screening continues to play an important role in detection and treatment of cervical intraepithelial neoplasia (CIN) II/III and prevention of cervical cancer in these high-risk patients. Cervical cancer screening continues to be of great importance since HPV immunization will not prevent approximately 25 to 30% of cervical cancers in HPV-naïve women and does not protect against the development of cancer in women already infected with carcinogenic HPV types. (See Schwartz 10th ed., pp. 1681–1682.)

2. Concerning uterine leiomyomas, all of the following are true EXCEPT
   A. Most common pelvic tumor.
   B. Has a racial predilection.
   C. Classified according to anatomic location.
   D. Rarely necessitates hysterectomy.

Answer: D

Leiomyomas, also known colloquially as *fibroids,* are the most common female pelvic tumor and occur in response to growth of the uterine smooth muscle cells (myometrium). They are common in the reproductive years, and by age 50, at least 60% of white and up to 80% of black women are (or have been) affected. Leiomyomas are described according to their anatomic location (Fig. 41-1) as intramural, subserosal, submucosal, pedunculated, cervical, and rarely ectopic. Most are asymptomatic; however, abnormal uterine bleeding caused by leiomyomas is the most common indication for hysterectomy in the United States. (See Schwartz 10th ed., Figure 41-9, pp. 1683–1684.)

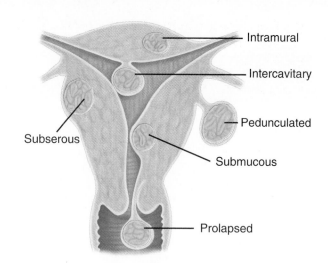

FIG. 41-1. Types of uterine myomas.

3. Which of the following concerning endometriosis is FALSE?
   A. More common in infertile women.
   B. Etiology is inflammation-induced.
   C. Can involve the thoracic cavity.
   D. Can cause increase in serum CA-125.

Answer: B

Endometriosis is especially prevalent in patients suffering from chronic pelvic pain (80%) and infertility (20–50%). The pathophysiology of endometriosis is poorly understood; etiologic theories explaining dissemination of endometrial glands include retrograde menstruation, lymphatic and vascular spread of endometrial glands, and coelomic metaplasia. Endometriosis commonly involves the ovaries, pelvic peritoneal surfaces, and uterosacral ligaments. Other possible sites include the rectovaginal septum, sigmoid colon, intraperitoneal organs, retroperitoneal space, ureters, incisional scars, umbilicus, and even the thoracic cavity. Endometriosis can also cause increases in serum cancer antigen 125 (CA-125). (See Schwartz 10th ed., pp. 1689–1690.)

4. Pregnancy-related surgical conditions include all of the following EXCEPT
   A. Trauma-related hypovolemia may be compounded by pregnancy-induced decreases in systemic vascular resistance.
   B. Gastric motility is decreased, leading to increased risk of aspiration.
   C. Increased likelihood of thromboembolic events due to increase in several coagulation factors induced by pregnancy.
   D. Fetal autoregulation of blood pressure during all three trimesters of pregnancy.

Answer: D

Trauma-related hypovolemia may be compounded by pregnancy-induced decreases in systemic vascular resistance. Gastric motility is decreased, increasing the risk of aspiration. Several coagulation factors are also increased in pregnancy, increasing the likelihood for thromboembolic events. It should also be recognized that the fetus will be impacted significantly by maternal hypotension, as blood may be shunted away from the uterus. Only the third-trimester fetus has any ability to autoregulate in the context of decreased uterine blood flow and oxygen delivery. (See Schwartz 10th ed., p. 1691.)

5. Typical indications for cesarean delivery include all of the following EXCEPT
   A. Questionable fetal status
   B. Breech presentation
   C. Cephalopelvic disproportion
   D. Maternal coagulopathy

Answer: D

Typical indications for cesarean delivery include nonreassuring fetal status, breech or other malpresentations, triplet and higher order gestations, cephalopelvic disproportion, failure to progress, placenta previa, and active genital herpes. (See Schwartz 10th ed., p. 1693.)

6. Pelvic floor dysfunction include all of the following EXCEPT
   A. Urinary incontinence
   B. Pelvic organ prolapse
   C. Fecal incontinence
   D. Dyspareunia

Answer: D

Pelvic floor disorders can be categorized, from an urogyne-cologic perspective, into three main topics: female urinary incontinence and voiding dysfunction, pelvic organ prolapse, and disorders of defecation. (See Schwartz 10th ed., p. 1694.)

7. All of the following are true concerning stress incontinence EXCEPT
   A. Can be due to lack of urethrovaginal support.
   B. Can be due to intrinsic sphincter deficiency.
   C. Goal of surgical repair is to create a partial urethral obstruction.
   D. Urethral reimplantation is sometimes necessary if other approaches fail.

Answer: D

Stress incontinence is believed to be caused by lack of ure-throvaginal support (urethral hypermobility) or intrinsic sphincter deficiency (ISD). ISD is a term applied to a subset of stress-incontinent patients who have particularly severe symptoms, including urine leakage with minimal exertion. This condition is often recognized clinically as the low pressure or "drainpipe" urethra. The urethral sphincter mechanism in these patients is severely damaged, limiting coaptation of the urethra. Standard surgical procedures used to correct stress incontinence share a common feature: partial urethral obstruction that achieves urethral closure under stress. (See Schwartz 10th ed., p. 1695.)

8. Concerning vulvar carcinoma, all of the following are true EXCEPT
   A. Etiology may be due to an HPV-dependent pathway of carcinogenesis.
   B. Approximately 50% are squamous lesions.
   C. Hematogenous dissemination is rare.
   D. Staging and primary surgical treatment are typically performed as a single procedure.

Answer: B

Evidence supports an HPV-dependent pathway of carcino-genesis with risks factors similar to vulvar intraepithelial neo-plasia (VIN) in the majority of cases. Vulvar carcinomas are squamous in 90% of cases. Spread of vulvar carcinoma is by direct local extension and via lymphatic microembolization. Hematogenous spread is uncommon. Staging and primary surgical treatment are typically preformed as a single procedure and tailored to the individual patient. (See Schwartz 10th ed., p. 1696.)

9. Which of the following is true concerning endometrial carcinoma?
   A. Third most common gynecological malignancy.
   B. Equally frequent in menopausal and postmenopausal women.
   C. Risk factors include obesity, smoking.
   D. Use of combination oral contraception pills has a protective effect.

Answer: C

Endometrial cancer is the most common gynecologic malignancy and fourth most common cancer in women. It is most common in menopausal women in the fifth decade of life; up to 15 to 25% of cases occur prior to menopause, and 1 to 5% occur before age 40. Risk factors for the most common type of endometrial cancer include increased exposure to estrogen without adequate opposition by progesterone, either endogenous (obesity, chronic anovulation) or exogenous (hormone replacement). Additional risk factors include diabetes, Lynch II syndrome (hereditary nonpolyposis colorectal cancer), and prolonged use of tamoxifen. Tamoxifen is a mixed agonist/antagonist ligand for the estrogen receptor. It is an agonistic in the uterus and an antagonistic to the breast and ovary. Protective factors for endometrial cancer include smoking and use of combination oral contraceptive pills. (See Schwartz 10th ed., pp. 1698–1699.)

10. Which of the following is FALSE concerning epithelial ovarian cancer (EOC) risk factors?
    A. Risk factors include early menarche.
    B. Risk factors include late menopause.
    C. Risk factors include previous hysterectomy.
    D. Risk factors include nulliparity.

Answer: C

Risk factors for development of epithelial ovarian cancer (EOC) include events that appear to increase the number of lifetime ovulations (eg, early menarche, late menopause, nulliparity), whereas events that decrease the number of ovulations decrease risk (eg, pregnancy, breastfeeding, oral contraceptives). Additionally, a history of tubal ligation or hysterectomy also decreases EOC risk. (See Schwartz 10th ed., p. 1701.)

11. The objectives of surgery in EOC include which of the following?
    A. Establishing histological diagnosis
    B. Surgical staging
    C. Surgical cytoreduction
    D. A, B, and C

Answer: D

The objectives of surgery in EOC are threefold. The first is to make the histologic diagnosis. The second is to assess the extent of disease through complete surgical staging. The third objective is (complete when feasible) surgical cytoreduction or debulking. (See Schwartz 10th ed., p. 1701.)

CHAPTER 42

Neurosurgery

1. Electromyography (EMG) and nerve conduction studies (NCS) are useful for assessing the function of
   A. Peripheral nerves
   B. Bilateral carotid arteries
   C. Intracranial liquids
   D. Spinal nerves

Answer: A

Electromyography and nerve conduction studies (EMG/NCS) are useful for assessing the function of peripheral nerves. EMG records muscle activity in response to a proximal stimulation of the motor nerve. NCS record the velocity and amplitude of the nerve action potential. EMG/NCS typically is performed approximately 3 to 4 weeks after an acute injury, as nerves distal to the injury continue to transmit electrical impulses normally until degeneration of the distal nerve progresses. (See Schwartz 10th ed., p. 1712.)

2. The lesion that can cause mass effect and rapidly kill the patient is
   A. Inferior fossa lesions
   B. Posterior fossa lesions
   C. Progressive obtundation
   D. Bradycardial lesions

Answer: B

The posterior fossa (brain stem and cerebellum) requires special consideration because the volume of the posterior fossa within the cranial vault is small. Posterior fossa lesions such as tumors, hemorrhage, or stroke can cause mass effect that can rapidly kill the patient in two ways. Occlusion of the fourth ventricle can lead to acute obstructive hydrocephalus, raised intracranial pressure (ICP), herniation, and eventually death. This mass effect can also lead directly to brain stem compression (Fig. 42-1). Symptoms of brain stem compression include hypertension, agitation, and progressive obtundation, followed rapidly by brain death. A patient exhibiting any of these symptoms needs an emergent neurosurgical evaluation for possible ventriculostomy or suboccipital craniectomy (removal of the bone covering the cerebellum). This situation is especially critical, as expeditious decompression can lead to significant functional recovery. (See Schwartz 10th ed., Figure 42-5, pp. 1714–1715.)

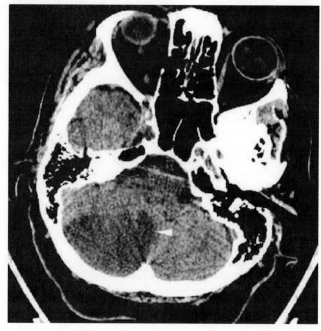

FIG. 42-1. Maturing cerebellar stroke seen as a hypodense area in the right cerebellar hemisphere (*arrowhead*) on head computed tomography (CT) in a patient with rapidly progressing obtundation 2 days after the initial onset of symptoms. Swelling of the infarcted tissue causes posterior fossa mass effect. The fourth ventricle is obliterated and not visible, and the brain stem is being compressed.

3. According to the Glasgow Coma Scale (GCS), a patient with a head injury score of 5 is classified as
   A. Mild
   B. Moderate
   C. Severe
   D. Seizure

Answer: D

Traumatic brain injury (TBI) can be classified as mild, moderate, or severe. For patients with a history of head trauma, classification is as follows: severe head injury if the GCS score is 3 to 8, moderate head injury if the Glasgow Coma Scale (GCS) score is 9 to 12, and mild head injury if the GCS score is 13 to 15. Many patients present to emergency rooms and trauma bays with a history of TBI. A triage system must be used to maximize resource utilization while minimizing the chance of missing occult or progressing injuries. (See Schwartz 10th ed., p. 1718.)

4. In regard to the halo test, a positive indicator for cerebrospinal fluid (CFS) when tinged with blood will show the following when dropped on an absorbent tissue
   A. A single ring with a darker center spot containing blood components surrounded by a light halo of CFS.
   B. A double ring with a darker center spot containing blood components surrounded by a light halo of CFS.
   C. A single ring with a lighter center spot containing CFS surrounded by a darker halo of blood components.
   D. A double ring with a lighter center spot containing CFS surrounded by a darker halo of blood components.

Answer: B

Copious clear drainage from the nose or ear makes the diagnosis of cerebrospinal fluid (CSF) leakage obvious. Often, however, the drainage may be discolored with blood or small in volume if some drains into the throat. The halo test can help differentiate. Allow a drop of the fluid to fall on an absorbent surface such as a facial tissue. If blood is mixed with CSF, the drop will form a double ring, with a darker center spot containing blood components surrounded by a light halo of CSF. If this test is indeterminate, the fluid can be sent for beta-2 transferrin testing, a carbohydrate-free isoform of transferrin exclusively found in the CSF. (See Schwartz 10th ed., pp. 1716–1717.)

5. Neurapraxia is defined as
   A. The disruption of axons and myelin.
   B. The disruption of axons and endoneurial tubes.
   C. The temporary failure of nerve function without physical axonal disruption.
   D. The temporary failure of nerve function with physical axonal disruption.

Answer: C
Neurapraxia is defined as the temporary failure of nerve function without physical axonal disruption. Axon degeneration does not occur. Return of normal axonal function occurs over hours to months, often in the 2- to 4-week range. (See Schwartz 10th ed., p. 1026.)

6. A patient who withdraws from pain, is mumbling inappropriate words, and opens his eyes to pain has a GCS score of
   A. 3
   B. 6
   C. 9
   D. 12

Answer: C
See Table 42-1. (See Schwartz 10th ed., Table 42-2, p. 1712.)

TABLE 42-1	The Glasgow Coma Scale score[a]					
Motor Response		**Verbal Response**		**Eye-Opening Response**	
Obeys commands	6	Oriented	5	Opens spontaneously	4
Localizes to pain	5	Confused	4	Opens to speech	3
Withdraws from pain	4	Inappropriate words	3	Opens to pain	2
Flexor posturing	3	Unintelligible sounds	2	No eye opening	1
Extensor posturing	2	No sounds	1		
No movement	1				

[a]Add the three scores to obtain the Glasgow Coma Scale (GCS) score, which can range from 3 to 15. Add "T" after the GCS if intubated and no verbal score is possible. For these patients, the GCS can range from 3T to 10T.

7. The most common malignant tumor of the brain is
   A. Ependymoma
   B. Astrocytoma
   C. Ganglioglioma
   D. Teratoma

Answer: B
Astrocytoma is the most common primary central nervous system (CNS) neoplasm. The term *glioma* often is used to refer to astrocytomas specifically, excluding other glial tumors. Astrocytomas are graded from I to IV. Grades I and II are referred to as *low-grade astrocytoma*, grade III as *anaplastic astrocytoma*, and grade IV as *glioblastoma multiforme* (GBM). Prognosis varies significantly between grades I/II, III, and IV, but not between I and II. Median survival is 8 years after diagnosis with a low-grade tumor, 2 to 3 years with an anaplastic astrocytoma, and roughly 1 year with a GBM. GBMs account for almost two-thirds of all astrocytomas, anaplastic astrocytomas account for two-thirds of the rest, and low-grade astrocytomas the remainder. Figure 42-2 demonstrates the typical appearance of a GBM. (See Schwartz 10th ed., Figure 42-20, pp. 1733–1734.)

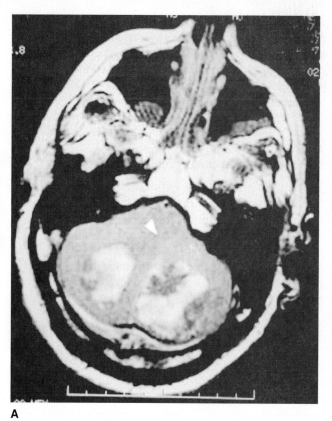
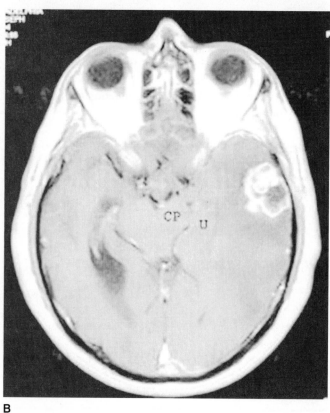

FIG. 42-2. A. Postcontrast T1-weighted axial magnetic resonance imaging (MRI) demonstrating a ring-enhancing lesion in the anteromedial right temporal lobe with central necrosis (*dark area*) consistent with glioblastoma multiforme. **B.** T2-weighted axial MRI with extensive bright signal signifying peritumoral edema seen with glioblastoma multiformes.

8. A 25-year-old man is seen in the emergency department after he struck his head against the windshield in an automobile accident. He opens his eyes and withdraws his arm during painful stimulation of his hand. He responds verbally to questions with inappropriate words. His GCS score is
   A. 6
   B. 9
   C. 12
   D. 15

Answer: B
The initial assessment of the trauma patient includes the primary survey, resuscitation, secondary survey, and definitive care. Neurosurgical evaluation begins during the primary survey with the determination of the GCS score (usually referred to simply as the *GCS*) for the patient. The GCS is determined by adding the scores of the best responses of the patient in each of three categories. The motor score ranges from 1 to 6, verbal from 1 to 5, and eyes from 1 to 4. The GCS therefore ranges from 3 to 15, as detailed in Table 42-1. Tracheal intubation or severe facial or eye swelling can impede verbal and eye responses. In these circumstances, the patient is given the score of 1 with a modifier, such as verbal "1T" where T = tube. (See Schwartz 10th ed., p. 1715.)

9. The most common level of cervical radiculopathy from cervical disc herniation is
   A. C4–C5
   B. C5–C6
   C. C6–C7
   D. C7–T1

Answer: C
The cervical nerve roots exit the central canal above the pedicle of the same-numbered vertebra and at the level of the higher adjacent intervertebral disc. For example, the C6 nerve root passes above the C6 pedicle at the level of the C5–C6 discs. The cervical nerve roots may be compressed acutely by disc herniation, or chronically by hypertrophic degenerative changes of the discs, facets, and ligaments. Table 42-2 summarizes the effects of various disc herniations. Most patients with acute disc herniations. Most patients with acute disc herniations will improve without surgery, nonsteroidal anti-inflammatory drugs (NSAIDs), or cervical traction may help alleviate symptoms. Patients whose symptoms do not resolve

or who have significant weakness should undergo decompressive surgery. The two main options for nerve root decompression are anterior cervical discectomy and fusion (ACDF) and posterior cervical foraminotomy (keyhole foraminotomy). ACDF allows more direct access to and removal of the pathology (anterior to the nerve root). However, the procedure requires fusion because discectomy causes a collapse of the interbody space and instability will likely occur. Fig. 42-3 demonstrates a C6–C7 ACDF with the typical interposed graft and plating system. Keyhole foraminotomy allows for decompression without requiring fusion, but it is less effective for removing centrally located canal pathology. (See Schwartz 10th ed., Table 42-6 and Figure 42-27, pp. 1740–1741.)

TABLE 42-2	Cervical disc herniations and symptoms by level				
Level	**Frequency (%)**	**Root Injured**	**Reflex**	**Weakness**	**Numbness**
C4–C5	2	C5	—	Deltoid	Shoulder
C5–C6	19	C6	Biceps	Biceps brachii	Thumb
C6–C7	69	C7	Triceps	Wrist extensors (wrist drop)	Second and third digits
C7–T1	10	C8	—	Hand intrinsics	Fourth and fifth digits

Source: Adapted with permission from Greenberg MS. *Handbook of Neurosurgery,* 7th ed. New York: Thieme; 2010, Table 18-18, p. 461.

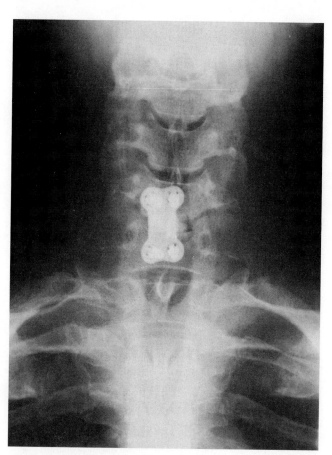
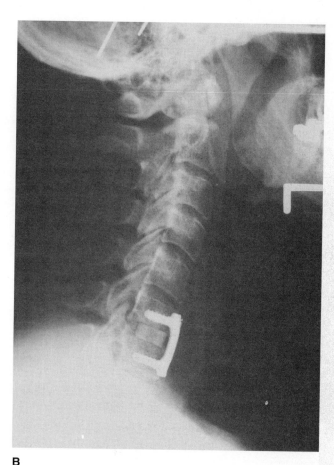

A   **B**

FIG. 42-3. A. Anteroposterior cervical spine X-ray showing the position of an anterior cervical plate used for stabilization after C6–C7 discectomy. Patient presented with right triceps weakness and dysesthesias in the right fifth digit. Magnetic resonance imaging (MRI) revealed a right paracentral C6–C7 herniated disc compressing the exiting C7 nerve root. **B.** Lateral cervical spine X-ray of the same patient clearly demonstrates the position of the plate and screws. The allograft bone spacer placed in the drilled-out disc space is also apparent.

10. A 35-year-old mother of two children, 5 and 6 years, has had amenorrhea and galactorrhea for the past 12 months. Her serum prolactin level is elevated, and radiographs of her skull show an "empty sella." The most likely diagnosis is
   A. Menopause
   B. Pregnancy
   C. Pituitary tumor
   D. Sheehan syndrome

Answer: C

Pituitary adenomas arise from the anterior pituitary gland (adenohypophysis). Tumors <1 cm diameter are considered microadenomas; larger tumors are macroadenomas. Pituitary tumors may be functional (ie, secrete endocrinologically active compounds at pathologic levels) or nonfunctional (ie, secrete nothing or inactive compounds). Functional tumors are often diagnosed when quite small, due to endocrine dysfunction. The most common endocrine syndromes are Cushing disease, due to adrenocorticotropic hormone secretion, Forbes-Albright syndrome, due to prolactin secretion, and acromegaly, due to growth hormone secretion. Nonfunctional tumors are typically diagnosed as larger lesions causing mass effects such as visual field deficits due to compression of the optic chiasm or panhypopituitarism due to compression of the gland. Figure 42-4 demonstrates a large pituitary adenoma. Hemorrhage into a pituitary tumor causes abrupt symptoms of headache, visual disturbance, decreased mental status, and endocrine dysfunction. This is known as *pituitary apoplexy.* (See Schwartz 10th ed., Figure 42-23, pp. 1735–1736.)

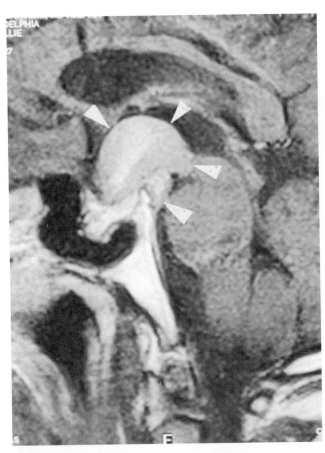

FIG. 42-4. Postcontrast T1-weighted sagittal magnetic resonance imaging (MRI) demonstrating a large sellar/suprasellar lesion (*arrowheads*) involving the third ventricle superiorly and abutting the midbrain and pons posteriorly. The patient presented with progressive visual field and acuity loss. Pathology and laboratory work revealed a nonfunctioning pituitary adenoma.

11. The most common intradural extramedullary tumors in children are
    A. Ependymomas
    B. Astrocytomas
    C. Dermoids
    D. Teratomas

Answer: B

Astrocytomas are the most common intramedullary tumors in children, although they also occur in adults. They may occur at all levels, although more often in the cervical cord. The tumor may interfere with the CSF-containing central canal of the spinal cord, leading to a dilated central canal, referred to as *syringomyelia* (syrinx). Spinal astrocytomas are usually low grade, but complete excision is rarely possible due to the nonencapsulated, infiltrative nature of the tumor. As a result, patients with astrocytomas fare worse overall than patients with ependymomas. (See Schwartz 10th ed., pp. 1738–1739.)

12. Diabetics, intravenous (IV) drug abusers, and dialysis patients have an increased risk of contracting the CNS infection
    A. Pyogenic vertebral osteomyelitis
    B. Subdural empyema
    C. Discitis
    D. Epidural abscess

Answer: A

Pyogenic vertebral osteomyelitis is a destructive bacterial infection of the vertebrae, usually of the vertebral body. Vertebral osteomyelitis frequently results from hematogenous spread of distant disease, but may occur as an extension of adjacent disease, such as psoas abscess or perinephric abscess. *Staphylococcus aureus* and *Enterobacter* spp. are the most frequent etiologic organisms. Patients usually present with fever and back pain. Diabetics, IV drug abusers, and dialysis patients have increased incidence of vertebral osteomyelitis. Epidural extension may lead to compression of the spinal cord or nerve roots with resultant neurologic deficit. Osteomyelitis presents a lytic picture on imaging and must be distinguished from neoplastic disease. Adjacent intervertebral disc involvement occurs frequently with pyogenic osteomyelitis, but rarely with neoplasia. Plain films and computed tomography (CT) help assess the extent of bony destruction or deformity such as kyphosis. Magnetic resonance imaging (MRI) shows adjacent soft tissue or epidural disease. Most cases can be treated successfully with antibiotics alone, although the organism must be isolated to steer antibiotic choice. Blood cultures may be positive. Surgical intervention may be required for debridement when antibiotics alone fail, or for stabilization and fusion in the setting of instability and deformity. (See Schwartz 10th ed., p. 1745.)

CHAPTER 43

Orthopedic Surgery

1. Long bone fractures can be described as fitting any of the following recognized types EXCEPT
   A. Convoluted
   B. Transverse
   C. Oblique
   D. Spiral

Answer: A
Musculoskeletal injuries resulting from trauma include fractures of bones, damage to joints, and injuries to soft tissues. Long bone fractures can be described as *transverse, oblique, spiral, segmental,* or *comminuted.* (See Schwartz 10th ed., p. 1756.)

2. Goals of fracture reduction include all of the following EXCEPT
   A. Restore length
   B. Restore marrow integrity
   C. Restore rotation
   D. Restore angulation

Answer: B
Reduction is performed with axial traction and reversal of the mechanism of injury in order to restore length, rotation, and angulation. (See Schwartz 10th ed., p. 1757.)

3. Which of the following is true concerning compartment syndrome?
   A. Due to decreased intracompartmental pressure
   B. Typified by hyperesthesia
   C. Can be assessed by needles placed into affected compartment
   D. Pain relieved by passive muscle stretching

Answer: C
Compartment syndrome is an orthopedic emergency caused by significant swelling within a compartment of an injured extremity that jeopardizes blood flow to the limb. Increased pressure within the compartment compromises perfusion to muscles and can cause ischemia or necrosis. Patients complain of pain and numbness, and passive stretch of muscles within the compartment causes severe pain. While the diagnosis is based on clinical examination, pressures can be measured with needles placed into the compartment, which is necessary in unconscious patients who will not show these examination findings. (See Schwartz 10th ed., p. 1757.)

4. Shoulder dislocations are frequently associated with all of the following EXCEPT
   A. Injuries to labrum
   B. Humeral head fractures
   C. Seizures
   D. Axillary vasculature disruptions

Answer: D
The shoulder is one of the most commonly dislocated joints and most dislocations are anterior. They are often associated with injuries to the labrum (Bankart lesion), impression fractures of the humeral head (Hill-Sachs lesion), and rotator cuff tears. Posterior dislocations are associated with seizures or electric shock. Adequate radiographs are required to diagnose a shoulder dislocation, with the axillary view being the most critical. (See Schwartz 10th ed., p. 1759.)

5. Which of the following is NOT a component of the elbow dislocation "Terrible Triad"?
   A. Elbow dislocation
   B. Radial head fracture
   C. Coronoid fracture
   D. Radial nerve damage

Answer: D

A severe injury, known as the *Terrible Triad,* includes an elbow dislocation, a radial head fracture, and a coronoid fracture. These are unstable injuries and require repair of the torn lateral collateral ligament (LCL), fixation or replacement of the radial head, and possible fixation of the coronoid depending on the size of the fracture fragment. (See Schwartz 10th ed., p. 1759.)

6. Each of the following is associated with pelvic fracture EXCEPT
   A. Prompt operative intervention for pubic rami fractures.
   B. Life-threatening hemorrhage.
   C. Associated genitourinary (GU) injury.
   D. Displacement associated with two or more fractures in the pelvic ring.

Answer: A

Pelvic fractures are indicative of high energy trauma and are associated with head, chest, abdominal, and urogenital injuries. Hemorrhage from pelvic trauma can be life-threatening and patients can present with hemodynamic instability, requiring significant fluid resuscitation, and blood transfusions. The bleeding that occurs is often due to injury to the venous plexus in the posterior pelvis, though it can also be due to a large vessel injury such as a gluteal artery. Other associated injuries are bladder and urethral injuries that manifest with bleeding from the urethral meatus or blood in the catheter and need to be assessed with a retrograde urethrogram. The pelvis is a ring structure made up of the sacrum and the two innominate bones that are held together by strong ligaments. Because it is a ring, displacement can only occur if the ring is disrupted in two places. Displaced sacral fractures and iliac wing fractures are treated with screws or plates, while pubic rami fractures can usually be managed nonoperatively. (See Schwartz 10th ed., p. 1760.)

7. Which of the following is associated with hip fracture?
   A. More common in men than women.
   B. Mortality rate in first year after hip fracture is 25%.
   C. Usually managed nonoperatively.
   D. Traction with bed rest rather than early mobilization is the chief therapeutic goal.

Answer: B

Hip fractures are an extremely common injury seen in orthopedics and are associated with significant morbidity and mortality. They most often occur in elderly patients after ground level falls, are much more common in women than men, and occur more commonly in patients with osteoporosis. Patients who suffer hip fractures are at increased risk for many complications, including deep vein thrombosis, pulmonary embolism, pneumonia, deconditioning, pressure sores, and even death, as the mortality rate in the first year following a hip fracture is around 25%. One of the most important reasons for performing surgery is to prevent these complications, and getting patients out of bed and walking as soon as possible diminishes their risk. Therefore, surgery is almost always the treatment of choice for hip fractures. (See Schwartz 10th ed., pp. 1760–1761.)

8. Chronic unremitting back pain suggests all of the following possibilities EXCEPT
   A. Infection
   B. Malignancy (primary)
   C. Spinal cord infarction
   D. Metastatic disease

Answer: C

Back pain occurs in the majority of adults but is usually self-limited resolving in 1 to 2 weeks. Chronic unremitting back pain suggests the possibility of infection, malignancy, or metastatic disease. (See Schwartz 10th ed., p. 1771.)

9. Scoliosis curves are classified as any of the following possibilities EXCEPT
   A. Congenital
   B. Covascular
   C. Neurological
   D. Myogenic

Answer: B

Scoliotic curves are classified as congenital, degenerative, metabolic (mucopolysaccharidoses), neurogenic (cerebral palsy), and myogenic curves (muscular dystrophy). Idiopathic scoliosis is the most common form, and represents a spectrum of genetic disease. (See Schwartz 10th ed., p. 1771.)

10. Surgical management of arthritis includes all of the following EXCEPT
    A. Arthroplasty
    B. Osteotomy
    C. Arthrodesis
    D. Arthrolysis

Answer: D

A full description of surgical options can be found in section "Surgical Management of Arthritis." (See Schwartz 10th ed., pp. 1772–1773.)

Surgery of the Hand and Wrist

1. For vascular injuries to the hand requiring tourniquet, the maximum time the tourniquet should be applied to prevent tissue necrosis is
   A. 1 hour
   B. 2 hours
   C. 3 hours
   D. 4 hours

Answer: B

Initial treatment for an actively bleeding wound should be direct local pressure for not less than 10 continuous minutes. If this is unsuccessful, an upper extremity tourniquet inflated to 100 mm Hg above the systolic pressure should be used. One should keep this tourniquet time to less than 2 hours to avoid tissue necrosis. Once bleeding is controlled well enough to evaluate the wound, it may be cautiously explored to evaluate for bleeding points. One must be very cautious if attempting to ligate these to ensure that adjacent structures, such as nerves, are not included in the ligature. (See Schwartz 10th ed., p. 1799.)

2. Anesthetic agents with epinephrine should NOT be used in
   A. The fingertip
   B. The hand
   C. The wrist
   D. The forearm

Answer: A

A commonly held axiom is that epinephrine is unacceptable to be used in the hand. Several recent large series have dispelled this myth. Epinephrine should not be used in the fingertip and not in concentrations higher than 1:100,000 (ie, what is present in commercially available local anesthetic with epinephrine). Beyond that, its use is acceptable and may be useful in an emergency room (ER) where tourniquet control may not be available. Also, because most ER procedures are done under pure local anesthesia, many patients will not tolerate the discomfort of the tourniquet beyond 30 minutes. Epinephrine will provide hemostasis and also prolong the effect of the local anesthetic. (See Schwartz 10th ed., p. 1796.)

3. Most nondisplaced fractures do NOT require surgical treatment EXCEPT
   A. Those of the lunate bone of the wrist.
   B. Those of the capitate bone of the wrist.
   C. Those of the scaphoid bone of the wrist.
   D. All nondisplaced fractures require surgical treatment.

Answer: C

Most nondisplaced fractures do not require surgical treatment. The scaphoid bone of the wrist is a notable exception to this rule. Due to peculiarities in its vascular supply, particularly vulnerable at its proximal end, nondisplaced scaphoid fractures can fail to unite in up to 20% of patients even with appropriate immobilization. Recent developments in hardware and surgical technique have allowed stabilization of the fracture with minimal surgical exposure. One prospective randomized series of scaphoid wrist fractures demonstrated shortening of time to union by up to 6 weeks in the surgically treated group, but no difference in rate of union. Surgery may be useful in the younger, more active patient who would benefit from an earlier return to full activity. (See Schwartz 10th ed., pp. 1795–1796.)

4. A patient shown to have wasting at the interdigital web spaces, experiences numbness of the ring finger and exhibits Wartenberg sign on physical examination most likely is suffering from
   A. Cubital tunnel syndrome
   B. Carpal tunnel syndrome
   C. Pronator syndrome
   D. Anterior interosseous nerve syndrome

Answer: A

The ulnar nerve also innervates the dorsal surface of the small finger and ulnar side of the ring finger, so numbness in these areas can be explained by cubital tunnel syndrome. The patient may also report weakness in grip due to effects on the flexor digitorum profundus (FDP) tendons to the ring and small fingers and the intrinsic hand muscles. Patients with advanced disease may complain of inability to fully extend the ring and small finger interphalangeal (IP) joints.

Physical examination for cubital tunnel syndrome begins with inspection. Look for wasting in the hypothenar eminence and the interdigital web spaces. When the hand rests flat on the table, the small finger may rest in abduction with respect to the other fingers; this is called Wartenberg sign. Tinel sign is often present at the cubital tunnel. Elbow flexion test will often be positive. Grip strength and finger abduction strength should be compared to the unaffected side. Froment sign can be tested by placing a sheet of paper between the thumb and index finger and instructing the patient to hold on to the paper while the examiner pulls it away without flexing the finger or thumb (this tests the strength of the adductor pollicis and first dorsal interosseous muscles). If the patient must flex the index finger and/or thumb (FDP-index and flexor pollicis longus [FPL], both median nerve supplied) to maintain traction on the paper, this is a positive response. (See Schwartz 10th ed., p. 1806.)

5. The most common primary malignant tumor of the hand is
   A. Melanoma
   B. Basal cell carcinoma
   C. Squamous cell carcinoma (SCC)
   D. Epithelioid sarcoma

Answer: C

Squamous cell carcinoma (SCC) is the most common primary malignant tumor of the hand, accounting for 75 to 90% of all malignancies of the hand. Eleven percent of all cutaneous SCC occurs in the hand. It is the most common malignancy of the nail bed. Risk factors include sun exposure, radiation exposure, chronic ulcers, immunosuppression, xeroderma pigmentosa, and actinic keratosis. (See Schwartz 10th ed., p. 1817.)

6. Necrotizing infections
   A. Often present with pain out of proportion to findings.
   B. Often have discharge present.
   C. Debridement should begin following confirmation by way of radiograph findings.
   D. Oral antibiotics should begin immediately.

Answer: A

Bacteria spread along the fascial layer, resulting in the death of soft tissues, which is in part due to the extensive blood vessel thrombosis that occurs. An inciting event is not always identified. Immunocompromised patients and those who abuse drugs or alcohol are at greater risk, with intravenous drug users having the highest increased risk. The infection can by mono- or polymicrobial, with group A β-hemolytic *Streptococcus* being the most common pathogen, followed by α-hemolytic *Streptococcus*, *Staphylococcus* aureus, and anaerobes. Prompt clinical diagnosis and treatment are the most important factors for salvaging limbs and saving life. Patients will present with pain out of proportion with findings. Appearance of skin may range from normal to erythematous or maroon with edema, induration, and blistering. Crepitus may occur if a gas-forming organism is involved. "Dirty dishwater fluid" may be encountered as a scant grayish fluid, but often there is little to no discharge. There may be no appreciable leukocytosis. The infection can progress rapidly and can lead to septic shock and disseminated intravascular coagulation. Radiographs may reveal gas formation, but they must not delay emergent debridement once the diagnosis is suspected. Intravenous antibiotics should be started immediately to cover gram-positive, gram-negative, and anaerobic bacteria. Patients will require multiple debridements, and the spread of infection is normally wider than expected based on initial assessment. Necrotizing myositis, or myonecrosis, is usually caused by *Clostridium perfringens* due to heavily contaminated wounds. Unlike necrotizing fasciitis, muscle is universally involved and found to be necrotic. Treatment includes emergent debridement of all necrotic tissue along with empirical intravenous antibiotics. (See Schwartz 10th ed., p. 1811.)

7. The majority of acute cases of infections flexor tenosynovitis (FTS) are due to
   A. Systemic lupus erythematosus
   B. Chronic inflammation as a result of diabetes
   C. Rheumatoid arthritis (RA)
   D. Purulent infection

Answer: D

Flexor tenosynovitis (FTS) is a severe pathophysiologic state causing disruption of normal flexor tendon function in the hand. A variety of etiologies are responsible for this process. Most acute cases of FTS are due to purulent infection. FTS also can occur secondary to chronic inflammation as a result of diabetes, rheumatoid arthritis, crystalline deposition, overuse syndromes, amyloidosis, psoriatic arthritis, systemic lupus erythematosus, and sarcoidosis. (See Schwartz 10th ed., pp. 1811–1812.)

8. The most common soft tissue tumor of the wrist is
   A. Mucous cyst
   B. Ganglion cyst
   C. Lipoma
   D. Schwannoma

Answer: B

Ganglion cyst is the most common soft tissue tumor of the hand and wrist, comprising 50 to 70% of all soft tissue tumors in this region. They can occur at any age but are most common in the second to fourth decades with a slight predilection toward females. (See Schwartz 10th ed., p. 1815.)

9. All hand infections EXCEPT the following require surgical management
   A. Paronychia
   B. Felon
   C. Cellulitis
   D. Osteomyelitis

Answer: C

All hand infections other than cellulitis will require surgical management. Clinical examination, particularly noting the area of greatest tenderness and/or inflammation, is the single most useful diagnostic tool to localize any purulence requiring drainage. Specific recommendations for differentiating among the possible locations of hand infection are included in the diagnostic algorithm shown in Fig. 44-1. (See Schwartz 10th ed., Figure 44-23, p. 1814.)

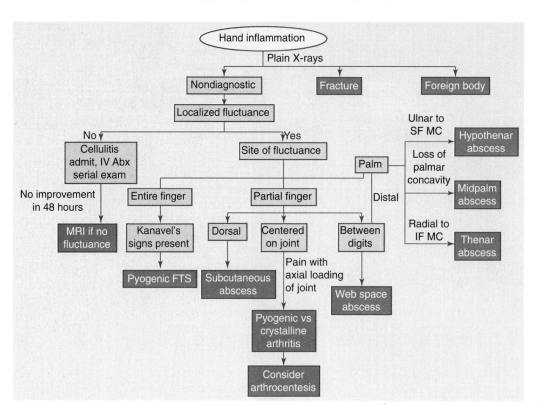

FIG. 44-1. Diagnostic algorithm. Diagnostic workup for a patient with hand inflammation to evaluate for infection. See text for details about particular infectious diagnoses. Abx = antibiotics; exam = examination; FTS = flexor tenosynovitis; IF MC = index finger metacarpal; IV = intravenous; MRI = magnetic resonance imaging; SF MC = small finger metacarpal.

10. Which of the following patient groups has a 1000-fold increased risk of developing squamous cell carcinoma (SCC)?
    A. Transplant patients on immunosuppression
    B. Patients with xeroderma pigmentosa
    C. Patients with actinic keratosis
    D. Patients exposed to inorganic arsenic

Answer: B

SCC is the most common primary malignant tumor of the hand, accounting for 75 to 90% of all malignancies of the hand. Eleven percent of all cutaneous SCC occurs in the hand. It is the most common malignancy of the nail bed. Risk factors include sun exposure, radiation exposure, chronic ulcers, immunosuppression, xeroderma pigmentosa, and actinic keratosis. Marjolin's ulcers represent malignant degeneration of old burn or traumatic wounds into an SCC and are a more aggressive type. Transplant patients on immunosuppression have a fourfold increased risk and patients with xeroderma pigmentosa have a 1000-fold increased risk of developing an SCC. They often develop as small, firm nodules or plaques with indistinct margins and surface irregularities ranging from smooth to verruciform or ulcerated (Fig. 44-2). They are locally invasive, with 2 to 5% lymph node involvement. Metastasis rates of up to 20% have been reported in radiation or burn wounds. Standard treatment is excision with 0.5- to 1.0-cm margins. Other treatment options include curettage and electrodessication, cryotherapy, and radiotherapy. (See Schwartz 10th ed., Figure 44-27, p. 1817.)

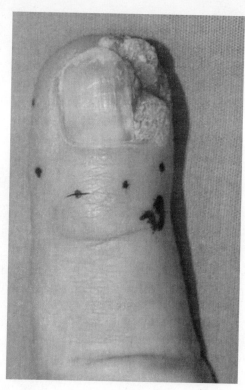

FIG. 44-2. Squamous cell carcinoma involving the nail fold and nail bed. Note the wart-like and ulcerated appearance.

11. Which of the following about enchondromas is true?
    A. Have never been reported in the trapezoid.
    B. Discovery is often prompted by patients presenting with hand pain.
    C. Are the most common malignant primary bone tumors.
    D. The most common location is the middle phalanges.

Answer: A

This is the most common primary benign bone tumor of the hand and wrist and is of cartilage origin. Up to 90% of all bone tumors in the hand and wrist are enchondromas, with 35 to 54% of all enchondromas occurring in the hand and wrist. They are often found incidentally on X-rays taken for other reasons (eg, hand trauma). They are usually solitary and favor the diaphysis of small tubular bones and are most common in the second and third decades of life. The most common location is in the proximal phalanges, followed by the metacarpals and then middle phalanges. Enchondroma has never been reported in the trapezoid. Presentation is usually asymptomatic, but pain may occur if there is a pathologic fracture or impending fracture. The etiology is believed to be from a fragment of cartilage from the central physis. Histology shows well-differentiated hyaline cartilage with lamellar bone and calcification. Two variants of enchondroma include Ollier disease (multiple enchondromatosis) and Maffucci syndrome (multiple enchondromatosis associated with multiple soft tissue hemangiomas). Malignant transformation is very rare in the solitary form, but there is a 25% incidence by age 40 in Ollier patients and a 100% life-time incidence in Maffucci patients. When malignant transformation does occur, it is almost uniformly a chondrosarcoma with pain and rapid growth. Diagnosis is usually made based on history, physical examination, and X-rays. There is a well-defined, multilobulated central lucency in the metaphysis or diaphysis that can expand causing cortical thinning or sometimes, thickening (Fig. 44-3). Further imaging is seldom needed, but a CT would be the study of choice. (See Schwartz 10th ed., Figure 44-29B, p. 1819.)

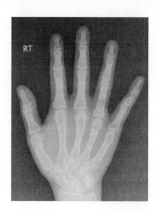

FIG. 44-3. Enchondroma. X-ray of the phalanx demonstrates a well-defined central lucency. Surrounding cortex may thin or thicken. Thinning of the cortex contributes to risk of pathologic fracture.

12. Proper handling of a traumatically amputated digit or limb includes which of the following?
    A. Place dry in a waterproof bag.
    B. Immerse in an antiseptic solution.
    C. Prep and wrapped in moistened gauze.
    D. Place on dry ice.

Answer: C

In preparation for replantation, the amputated part and proximal stump should be appropriately treated. The amputated part should be wrapped in moistened gauze and placed in a sealed plastic bag. This bag should then be placed in an ice water bath. Do not use dry ice, and do not allow the part to contact ice directly; frostbite can occur in the amputated part, which will decrease its chance of survival after replantation. Bleeding should be controlled in the proximal stump by as minimal a means necessary, and the stump should be dressed with a nonadherent gauze and bulky dressing. (See Schwartz 10th ed., p. 1800.)

Plastic and Reconstructive Surgery

CHAPTER 45

1. All of the following are true about split-thickness skin grafts EXCEPT
   A. Degree of contraction is dependent on amount of dermis in graft.
   B. High reliability of take.
   C. Healing with abnormal pigmentation more common in thin than thick grafts.
   D. Meshing grafts improve their ultimate cosmetic appearance.

Answer: D
Many of the characteristics of a split-thickness graft are determined by the amount of dermis present. Less dermis translates into less primary contraction (the degree to which a graft shrinks in surface area after harvesting and before grafting), more secondary contraction (the degree to which a graft shrinks during healing), and better chance of graft survival. Thin split grafts have low primary contraction, high secondary contraction, and high reliability of graft take, often even in imperfect recipient beds. Thin grafts, however, tend to heal with abnormal pigmentation and poor durability compared with thick split grafts and full-thickness grafts. Split grafts may be meshed to expand the surface area that can be covered. (See Schwartz 10th ed., p. 1832.)

2. Which of the following definitions is INCORRECT?
   A. Flap composition: Description of the tissue components within the flap.
   B. Flap contiguity: The position of a flap relative to its recipient bed.
   C. Pedicle: Bridge of tissue that remains between a flap and its source; blood vessels that nourish a flap.
   D. Free flap: Flaps that are completely detached from the body prior to their reimplantation with microvascular anastomoses.

Answer: B
The composition of a flap describes its tissue components. The contiguity of a flap describes its position related to its source. Distant flaps are transferred from a different anatomic region to the defect. They may remain attached to the source anatomic region (pedicled flaps) or may be transferred as free flaps by microsurgery. These are completely detached from the body, and their blood supply is reinstated by microvascular anastomoses to recipient vessels close to the defect. The term *pedicle* was originally used to describe a bridge of tissue that remains between a flap and its source, similar to how a peninsula remains attached to its mainland. However, as knowledge of flap blood supply and (micro)vascular anatomy has improved over the years, the term pedicle has increasingly become reserved for describing the blood vessels that nourish the flap. (See Schwartz 10th ed., p. 1833.)

3. Factors influencing the development of cleft lip/palate include all the following EXCEPT
   A. Increased parental age.
   B. Vitamin A deficiency during pregnancy.
   C. Infections during pregnancy.
   D. Smoking during pregnancy.

Answer: B
The cause of orofacial clefting is felt to be multifactorial. Factors that likely increase the incidence of clefting include increased parental age, drug use and infections during pregnancy, and smoking during pregnancy. (See Schwartz 10th ed., pp. 1840–1841.)

4. Principles of reconstructive surgery include all of the following EXCEPT
   A. Adequate restoration of lost anatomic components without residual deficits.
   B. Uncomplicated and timely wound healing.
   C. Individualization of specific reconstructive technique to specific patient deficit.
   D. Compromise of extent of tumor resection if needed for specific reconstructive surgical outcome.

Answer: D

The reconstructive surgeon aims to restore lost anatomic components adequately. Residual deficits, seemingly inconsequential, may progress to psychological morbidity, societal malacceptance, and social withdrawal. Uncomplicated and timely wound healing is important to allow adjuvant therapies when indicated and smooth discharge to home and occupation. Each defect can be addressed by a number of methods, but the technique must be decided for each individual patient. Although a more complex reconstruction might offer improved outcomes, it may bring an increased risk of complications. Some patients may therefore benefit from use of a simpler method with more acceptable anesthetic and operative risk rather than a gold-standard reconstruction. (See Schwartz 10th ed., p. 1862.)

CHAPTER 46

Anesthesia for the Surgical Patient

1. Malignant hyperthermia (MH) can develop after receiving general anesthesia. Triggering agents include, but are NOT limited to
   A. Halothane, isoflurane
   B. Desflurane
   C. Electroflurane
   D. Hypoflurane, osteoflurane

Answer: A

Malignant hyperthermia (MH) is a hereditary, life-threatening, hypermetabolic acute disorder, developing during or after receiving general anesthesia. The clinical incidence of MH is about 1:12,000 in children and 1:40,000 in adults. A genetic predisposition and one or more triggering agents are necessary to evoke MH. Triggering agents include all volatile anesthetics (eg, halothane, enflurane, isoflurane, sevoflurane, and desflurane) and the depolarizing muscle relaxant succinylcholine. Volatile anesthetics and/or succinylcholine cause a rise in the myoplasmic calcium concentration in susceptible patients, resulting in persistent muscle contraction. (See Schwartz 10th ed., p. 1918.)

2. Postoperative nausea and vomiting (PONV) typically occurs in what percentage of surgical cases?
   A. 10–15%
   B. 90%
   C. 20–30%
   D. None

Answer: C

Postoperative nausea and vomiting (PONV) typically occurs in 20 to 30% of surgical cases, with considerable variation in frequency reported between studies (range, 8–92%). PONV is generally considered a transient, unpleasant event carrying little long-term morbidity; however, aspiration of emesis, gastric bleeding, and wound hematomas may occur with protracted or vigorous retching or vomiting. Troublesome PONV can prolong recovery room stay and hospitalization and is one of the most common causes of hospital admission following ambulatory surgery. (See Schwartz 10th ed., p. 1915.)

3. The intentional dilution of blood volume often is referred to as
   A. Acute normovolemic hemodilution (ANH) anemia
   B. Acute hypovolemic normodilution (AHN) anemia
   C. Hypercoagulable hemodilution (HH) anemia
   D. None of the above

Answer: A

The intentional dilution of blood volume often is referred to as *acute normovolemic hemodilution* (ANH) anemia. ANH is a technique in which whole blood is removed from a patient, while the circulating blood volume is maintained with acellular fluid. Blood is collected via central lines with simultaneous infusion of crystalloid or colloid solutions. Collected blood is reinfused after major blood loss has ceased, or sooner, if indicated. Blood units are reinfused in the reverse order of collection. Under conditions of ANH, the increased plasma compartment becomes an important source of O_2, which is delivered to the tissues. (See Schwartz 10th ed., p. 1914.)

4. Hydroxyethyl starch (HES), gelatin, and albumin are several types of
   A. Crystalloids
   B. Coagulates
   C. Antigens
   D. Colloids

Answer: D

Several types of colloids are available, but three are most commonly used—hydroxyethyl starch (HES), gelatin, and albumin. The HES preparations differ from one another according to their concentration, molecular weight, and extent of hydroxy- ethylation or substitution, with resultant varying physiochemical properties. HES solutions most often are described according to their weight-averaged mean molecular weight in kilodaltons (kDa): high molecular weight (450 kDa), middle molecular weight (200 kDa, 270 kDa), and low molecular weight (130 kDa, 70 kDa). HES 450 kDa solutions are available in a normal saline solution (HES 450/NS) and in a lactated, balanced salt solution (HES 450/BS). Although all of these colloids are used in Europe, gelatins are not available in the United States, and the only HES preparations approved by the U.S. Food and Drug Administration are the 6% high molecular weight (450 kDa) formulations. (See Schwartz 10th ed., p. 1911.)

5. Of the options below, which is a stage of a patient undergoing inhalation induction?
   A. Confusion
   B. Aggression
   C. Excitement
   D. None of the above

Answer: C

Patients undergoing *inhalation induction* progress through three stages: (a) awake, (b) excitement, and (c) surgical level of anesthesia. Adult patients are not good candidates for this type of induction, as the smell of the inhalation agent is unpleasant and the excitement stage can last for several minutes, which may cause hypertension, tachycardia, laryngospasm, vomiting, and aspiration. Children, however, progress through stage 2 quickly and are highly motivated for inhalation induction as an alternative to the intravenous (IV) route. The benefit of postinduction IV cannulation is the avoidance of many presurgical anxieties, and inhalation induction is the most common technique for pediatric surgery. (See Schwartz 10th ed., p. 1909.)

6. Regional anesthesia may be useful in patients with
   A. Advanced liver disease
   B. Renal disease
   C. Diabetes mellitus
   D. Colorectal cancer

Answer: A

Regional anesthesia may be useful in patients with advanced liver disease, assuming coagulation status is acceptable. When general anesthesia is selected, administration of modest doses of volatile anesthetics with or without nitrous oxide or fentanyl often is recommended. Selection of nondepolarizing muscle relaxants should consider clearance mechanisms for these drugs. For example, patients with hepatic cirrhosis may be hypersensitive to mivacurium because of the lowered plasma cholinesterase activity. Perfusion to the liver is maintained by administering fluids (guided by filling pressures) and maintaining adequate systemic pressure and cardiac output. (See Schwartz 10th ed., p. 1907.)

7. P3 of the American Society of Anesthesiologists physical status classification system is which of the follow
   A. A normal healthy patient.
   B. A moribund patient who is not expected to survive without operation.
   C. A patient with severe systemic disease that is a constant threat to life.
   D. A patient with severe systemic disease.

Answer: D

American Society of Anesthesiologists physical status classification system

P1: A normal healthy patient.
P2: A patient with mild systemic disease.
P3: A patient with severe systemic disease.
P4: A patient with severe systemic disease that is a constant threat to life.

P5: A moribund patient who is not expected to survive without the operation.

P6: A declared brain-dead patient whose organs are being removed for donor purposes. (See Schwartz 10th ed., p. 1905.)

Answer: D

The physical examination is targeted primarily at the central nervous system (CNS), cardiovascular system, lungs, and upper airway. Specific areas to investigate are given in Table 46-1. (See Schwartz 10th ed., Table 46-5, p. 1904.)

8. During a preoperative physical examination, specific areas to investigate for the respiratory system include
   A. Consciousness; neurocognition; peripheral sensory
   B. Cervical spine mobility; visualize uvula; artificial teeth; thyromental distance
   C. Blood pressure; standing and sitting, bilateral; peripheral pulses; heart auscultation; heart rate; murmur; rhythm
   D. Auscultation of lungs; wheezes; rales

TABLE 46-1	Preoperative physical examination		
Central Nervous System	**Cardiovascular System**	**Respiratory System**	**Oral Airway**
Consciousness; neurocognition; peripheral sensory	Blood pressure; standing and sitting, bilateral; peripheral pulses; heart auscultation; heart rate; murmur; rhythm	Auscultation of lungs; wheezes; rales	Cervical spine mobility; visualize uvula; artificial teeth; thyromental distance

CHAPTER 47

Surgical Considerations in the Elderly

1. Physiologic aging, or "senescence," is defined as decreased functional reserve of critical organ systems. It is generally believed to occur at what age?
   A. 55 years
   B. 70 years
   C. 90 years
   D. No defined age

Answer: B
The cut off for the definition of *senescence* has increased from 55 years in the late 1960s to 70 years currently. This is a general definition as each patient should be assessed for their own capacity to respond to the stress of surgery. (See Schwartz 10th ed., p. 1923.)

2. Frailty is a major risk factor for postoperative complications. Which of the following measures does NOT contribute to frailty?
   A. Impaired cognition
   B. One or more falls in past 6 months
   C. Osteoporosis
   D. Hematocrit <35%

Answer: C
Frailty, disability (inability to perform more than one activity of daily living), and comorbidities such as anemia and hypoalbuminemia are the primary conditions which impact on the outcome of surgical procedures in the elderly. Each condition should be assessed preoperatively. (See Schwartz 10th ed., p. 1926.)

3. What is the most common indication for surgical intervention in the elderly?
   A. Coronary disease
   B. Appendiceal disease
   C. Long bone fracture
   D. Biliary tract disease

Answer: D
Biliary tract disease due to pigmented or cholesterol stone formation and acute cholecystitis are common problems in the elderly and most likely to lead to surgical intervention. The mortality risk of emergency cholecystectomy is four times that of elective cholecystectomy in the elderly. (See Schwartz 10th ed., p. 1924.)

4. What is the leading cause of postoperative morbidity and mortality in the elderly?
   A. Congestive heart failure
   B. Cerebrovascular accident
   C. Pneumonia
   D. Renal failure

Answer: A
Impaired cardiac reserve means that elderly patients cannot increase their ejection fraction as demand increases, but are dependent on ventricular filling and increased stroke volume to meet the need for increased output. Intravascular volume is therefore critically important, but fluid overload is poorly tolerated and can result in congestive heart failure. (See Schwartz 10th ed., pp. 1926–1927.)

5. Elderly patients with acute peritonitis may NOT present with typical symptoms of acute abdominal pain, fever, or leukocytosis due to an impaired immune response. A high index of suspicion is needed as the initial clinical diagnosis in elderly patients with acute appendicitis is correct in what percent of cases?
   A. Less than 50%
   B. 70–80%
   C. 90–95%
   D. 100%

Answer: A
In elderly patients with acute appendicitis or acute cholecystitis, one-third lack symptoms of abdominal pain, one-third are afebrile, and one-third have a normal white blood cell count. Therefore an "unimpressive" abdominal examination is irrelevant in the evaluation of the elderly patient whose tolerance for food has suddenly changed. (See Schwartz 10th ed., p. 1926.)

6. Determination of an elderly patient's nutritional status and reversal of malnutrition is important to prevent all of the following complications EXCEPT
    A. Poor wound healing
    B. Increased nosocomial infections
    C. Delayed functional recovery
    D. Adverse drug reactions

Answer: D
Poor nutritional status in elderly patients is common. It is estimated that 9 to 15% of patients older than 65 years are malnourished in the outpatient setting, and this increases to 12 to 50% in the acute hospital setting, and 25 to 60% in the chronically institutionalized. A formal nutritional assessment and preoperative nutritional repletion, if needed, can significantly reduce the incidence of postoperative complications. The incidence of postoperative complications is increased in patients with an albumin level <3.5 g/L. (See Schwartz 10th ed., p. 1929.)

7. In elderly patients undergoing heart valve replacement, bioprosthetic valves are preferred over synthetic valves because
    A. There is less need for anticoagulation which is hazardous in the elderly.
    B. The operative time is shorter which reduces the risk of pulmonary complications.
    C. Synthetic valves have a higher incidence of manufacturing defects.
    D. The extent of hemolysis is less with bioprosthetic valves.

Answer: A
Prolonged anticoagulation is more hazardous in the elderly where the risk of falls is increased. Even a fall from the standing position can result in a fatal intracranial bleed in an anticoagulated patient. (See Schwartz 10th ed., p. 1031.)

8. Cancer treatment in elderly patients is
    A. Always less successful.
    B. Complicated by the fact that clinical trials usually do not include elderly subjects.
    C. Recommended equally as in younger patients.
    D. Does not change overall life expectancy.

Answer: B
The frequency of referrals for surgical treatment of equivalent stage cancer is decreased in the elderly for virtually all tumors. Despite this, survival after surgery is nearly equivalent for same stage malignancy as in younger patients. The data derived from clinical trials of adjuvant and neoadjuvant therapy are less helpful for decision making in elderly patients because elderly subjects are usually not included in clinical studies. (See Schwartz 10th ed., p. 1931.)

9. Avoidance of surgical resection of breast cancer in an elderly patient is unacceptable because
    A. Mortality rates of breast surgery are very low in the elderly.
    B. Medical therapy (eg, tamoxifen) instead of surgery is equivalent to surgical outcomes.
    C. Of decreased life expectancy.
    D. Screening mammography is less useful in the elderly.

Answer: A
Elderly patients have a higher incidence of breast cancer than younger patients, and their mortality risk from breast surgery is less than 1%. Medical therapy is less effective than surgical removal of the primary tumor, and screening mammography reduces cancer-related mortality in patients up to age 75. (See Schwartz 10th ed., p. 1932.)

10. What is the likelihood that an asymptomatic, 2 cm, solitary pulmonary nodule seen on chest X-ray in a 70-year-old smoker is a malignancy?
    A. 25%
    B. 50%
    C. 70%
    D. 90%

Answer: C
Lung cancer is the leading cause of cancer-related death in patients older than 70 years. The peak incidence is between 75 and 79 years. Non–small-cell lung cancer accounts for roughly 80% of all cases. In cases of resectable primary lung cancer, resection remains the treatment of choice, with an expected survival of almost 3 years. (See Schwartz 10th ed., pp. 1933–1934.)

11. In elderly trauma patients, injuries from falls accounts for about 20% of etiologies. The management of these patients is complicated by all of the following factors EXCEPT
    A. Concurrent medication use including anticoagulants and beta blockers.
    B. Coexisting dementia and cerebrovascular disease.
    C. Underlying cardiac arrhythmias.
    D. Lack of advanced directives to guide clinical-care decisions.

Answer: D

Elderly trauma victims are more likely to have underlying organ-specific limitations and medication use which complicates resuscitation and hemostasis. They are also more likely to be undertriaged and treated at non-level 1 trauma centers. (See Schwartz 10th ed., p. 1935.)

12. Minimally invasive approaches to surgical treatment have been shown to be associated with reduced morbidity and mortality in elderly patients for all of the following EXCEPT
    A. Repair of abdominal aortic aneurysm.
    B. Removal of the gallbladder.
    C. Colon resection.
    D. Parathyroidectomy.

Answer: D

Minimally invasive approaches to surgical treatment have dramatically decreased mortality and morbidity rates in elderly subjects for aortic aneurysm repair, cholecystectomy, and colorectal surgery. Laparoscopic techniques or endovascular methods have enabled the surgical correction of multiple abdominal conditions with far less morbidity in the elderly than open surgical techniques. Neck surgery is usually well tolerated by elderly patients. (See Schwartz 10th ed., p. 1936.)

13. The goals of palliative surgery include all of the following EXCEPT
    A. Relief of symptoms.
    B. Preservation of quality of life.
    C. Eradication (cure) of the disease.
    D. Prevention of complications of disease.

Answer: C

Palliative surgery is directed at preserving quality of life, avoiding devastating complications of disease, and relief of symptoms. It is not intended to alter the course of a disease process but is considered when surgical treatment can extend a meaningful existence for the patient. (See Schwartz 10th ed., p. 1938.)

14. The goals of ethical decision making in the elderly patient include all of the following EXCEPT
    A. Acknowledgement of medical futility.
    B. Clarify and follow patients' wishes regarding like-sustaining therapies.
    C. Respect patient's autonomy to decide the course of therapy.
    D. Abide by the wishes of the family if they conflict with those of the patient.

Answer: D

The primacy of the patient and his/her decisions regarding their own care is of greatest importance in the ethical care of the elderly surgical patient. A surrogate decision maker may be appointed by the patient, but that individual should decide medical decisions based on what they believe would be the choice of the patient. (See Schwartz 10th ed., p. 1930.)

15. The combined recommendations of the American College of Surgeons National Surgical Quality Improvement Program (ACS-NSQIP) and the American Geriatrics Society (AGS) have provide best practice guidelines for the preoperative evaluation of elderly surgical patients. These recommendations are required standards for training programs in which of the following specialties?
    A. General surgery residency training
    B. Cardiothoracic surgical residency training
    C. Vascular surgical residency training
    D. All of the above

Answer: D

The combined recommendations of American College of Surgeons National Surgical Quality Improvement Program (ACS-NSQIP) and the American Geriatrics Society (AGS) have been endorsed by all training programs under the aegis of the American College of Surgeons (ACS). (See Schwartz 10th ed., p. 1929.)

CHAPTER 48

Ethics, Palliative Care, and Care at the End of Life

1. Biomedical ethics is a system of analysis and deliberation which is intended to direct physicians and surgeons to moral "goodness" in patient care. It includes consideration of all of the following EXCEPT
   A. Autonomy: The patient's right to decide for himself/herself what care will be provided.
   B. Beneficence: The concept that proposed treatments will benefit the patient.
   C. Nonmaleficence: The avoidance of treatments which may harm the patient.
   D. Equipoise: The lack of a preference for one treatment over another.

Answer: D
The patient and the doctor decide together what treatment is in the best interest of the patient, and share the benefits and the burdens of this joint decision making. The physician's role is to clarify the indications, risks, and benefits of the possible treatment courses; the patient's role is to decide what course to take. (See Schwartz 10th ed., p. 1941.)

2. Living wills are documents which are meant to guide decision making when
   A. The patient's family cannot be contacted.
   B. The patient is rendered incompetent or unresponsive by an illness judged to be terminal.
   C. Multiple attempts at resuscitation have failed.
   D. The patient's family disagrees with the course of treatment.

Answer: B
Living wills are intended to guide decisions by physicians, family members, and/or surrogate decision makers when the patient himself/herself is unable to render an opinion and the condition or disease is judged to be terminal or "hopeless." (See Schwartz 10th ed., p. 1942.)

3. "Informed consent" implies all of the following EXCEPT
   A. The patient has been provided with the pertinent details of his/her diagnosis, prognosis, and the options for and risks of treatment.
   B. The information has been provided according to what a reasonable person would be expected to understand.
   C. The discussion of the options, risks, and possible hazards has been documented.
   D. There are witnesses to the discussion who also understand the discussion.

Answer: D
The "reasonable person" standard for informed consent has precedent in a 1972 court case which rejected the notion that "simple consent" for treatment was sufficient. The court decided that the facts of diagnosis, treatment options, and risks that a "reasonable person" would want to know should be included in the discussion to obtain consent for treatment. There is no requirement for witness documentation when the patient is believed to be competent to handle their own affairs. (See Schwartz 10th ed., p. 1942.)

4. When discussing possible surgical options with a patient, it is appropriate to do all of the following EXCEPT
   A. Document that the patient is capable of rendering informed consent.
   B. Ask the patient to identify a surrogate health care decision maker in the event he/she is incapable of deciding treatment choices.
   C. Avoid discussing the "pain and suffering" aspects of a treatment plan.
   D. Provide an opportunity for the patient to ask questions or to deliberate with others if the condition permits.

Answer: C

The obligation of the surgeon is to ensure that the patient is competent and understands the discussion of treatment options. If the condition is not an emergency, the patient should be allowed to consult with others or to ask for time to consider their response. All aspects of the expected course and treatment options, including symptoms, side-effects and complications, should be discussed. (See Schwartz 10th ed., p. 1944.)

CHAPTER 49

Global Surgery

1. Patients in rural and developing locales often have difficulty accessing health care and undergoing surgical interventions. Interest in global surgery has grown significantly in recent years due in part to all of the following EXCEPT
   A. Trained surgeons migrating to areas of need.
   B. Improved control of acute infectious diseases previously the cause of significant morbidity.
   C. Technology allowing improved access to health care information and training.
   D. Recognition of the cost-effectiveness of surgery as a public health intervention.

Answer: A

Although much of the world remains with limited access to surgery, this is changing. Patients who have been denied surgical care previously due to concerns about cost and access are no longer being ignored. Over time, it has become apparent that the patients in need of surgical care are those who have the greatest socioeconomic impact on society (ie, young, otherwise healthy and productive members of society). Offering a potential cure via surgery allows the patient to return to normal function and contribute to society in a meaningful way; improving the infrastructure of the country. Many trained physicians, especially surgeons, who planned to return to areas of need find that the lack of resources and infrastructure hamper their opportunity for development. Therefore, fully trained surgeons tend to remain in larger, more developed areas. While this is seen across the globe, migration of practitioners to economically and culturally favorable locales impacts Low and Middle Income Countries (LMICs) more, as they have a higher burden of diseased patients with fewer health care workers and a steeper gradient from developed to developing areas of their country. (See Schwartz 10th ed., pp. 1960–1962 and 1970–1976.)

2. A 24-year-old man in Tanzania is traveling without helmet on the back of a motorbike sideswipes a large truck. He is brought in to the hospital and found to have rib fractures, a femur fracture, and a traumatic brain injury. If one wanted to calculate the impact of this injury on his life, one could calculate a Disability Adjusted Life Year (DALY) score. What components make up this score?
   A. Years of life lived.
   B. Severity of illness and years of life lived with that disability.
   C. Patient quality of life and years of life lived with impaired quality of life.
   D. Years of life lost, compared to country average, and a weighted calculation of life years lived with disability.

Answer: D

The Disability Adjusted Life Year (DALY) score is a measure of overall disease burden expressed as the number of years lost due to ill-health, disability, or early death. The DALY has become commonly used in public health in dealing with the Health Impact Assessment. DALYs deal with potential life years lost due to premature death or disability. This combines morbidity and mortality into a single metric. Health liabilities are typically measured in Years of Life Lost (YLL). However, YLL does not take into account disability, often expressed as Years Lived with Disability (YLD). DALYs are calculated by taking the sum of these two components. A valuation of the "severity" of the disability must be made to accurately account for the degree of patient disability.

$$DALY = YLL + YLD$$

The DALY reflects chronic illness and amount of time a person remains affected. One DALY is equal to 1 year of healthy life lost. DALY can be applied to a multitude of conditions including physical, psychiatric, and neurologic conditions. (See Schwartz 10th ed., pp. 1973–1974.)

3. After you establish an advanced surgical department in a foreign country, a 55-year-old woman presents with right upper quadrant pain of 3 months occurring after every meal. An ultrasound shows a thickened gallbladder wall and pericholecystic fluid and a diagnosis of cholecystitis is made. The patient undergoes a laparoscopic cholecystectomy. The World Health Organization's (WHO) 10 basic and essential objectives for safe surgical practice focus on all of the following EXCEPT

   A. Preparing for life-threatening loss of airway or respiratory function.
   B. Minimizing surgical-site infection.
   C. Minimizing cost and length of hospital stay for the patient.
   D. Communicating critical patient information.

Answer: C

Surgeons strive to constantly improve morbidity and mortality of their patients. In resource-limited areas access to certain pre and postop interventions or monitoring may be limited and in order to minimize complications, the World Health Organization (WHO) enacted the Safe Surgery Saves Lives Initiative. This campaign targeted preventable injuries and was found to have a 50% decrease in mortality. The 10 objectives for safe surgery include: identifying the correct patient and site, prevention of harm and pain, preparing for life-threatening airway compromise, preparing for high-risk blood loss, avoiding allergic reactions or reactions to drugs, minimizing surgical-site infections, preventing retained sponges, identifying all surgical specimens, effective hand-offs of patient information, and routine patient surveillance (Table 49-1). (See Schwartz 10th ed., Table 49-2, p. 1968.)

TABLE 49-1	Ten basic and essential objectives for safe surgery (WHO[a])
1.	Operate on the correct patient at the correct site
2.	Use method known to prevent harm from anesthetic administration, while protecting the patient from pain
3.	Recognize and effectively prepare for life-threatening loss of airway or respiratory function
4.	Recognize and effectively prepare for risk of high blood loss
5.	Avoid inducing any allergic or adverse drug reaction known to be a significant risk for the patient
6.	Consistently use method known to minimize risk of surgical site infection
7.	Prevent inadvertent retention of instruments or sponges in surgical wounds
8.	Secure and accurately identify all surgical specimens
9.	Effectively communicate and exchange critical patient information for the safe conduct of the operation
10.	Establish routine surveillance of surgical capacity, volume, and results

[a]Data from WHO Guidelines for Safe Surgery 2009. http://whqlibdoc.who.int/publications/2009/9789241598552_eng.pdf.

4. A 50-year-old man presents to a clinic in Cameroon with abdominal pain. On further questioning, you learn that he lives 60 miles from the nearest hospital and has not seen a physician in years. The patient is counseled regarding screening colonoscopy, which he undergoes and multiple polyps are noted. The patient is referred to for surgery. Factors which must be considered that impact surgical services include

   A. Socioeconomic status of the patient and cultural background.
   B. Accessibility of facilities to the patient.
   C. Availability and training level of supporting specialties (anesthesia, nursing, etc).
   D. All of the above.

Answer: D

Three factors, among many others, that must be considered when planning surgical care in low-resource settings are listed above. It is important for surgeons to understand and acknowledge their patients circumstances and customs while considering the physical and human resources of their environment. Safe and effective surgical care in low-resource setting requires careful attention to several fields traditionally outside of surgical training—such as logistics, business, public policy, engineering, and public health. (See Schwartz 10th ed., pp. 1974–1975.)

5. A 55-year-old East African woman presents with a palpable mass in her right breast that has been present for several years. You are concerned for cancer and know her case fatality rate is significantly higher than a similar patient in North America. Why?
   A. Later presentation to care.
   B. Limited access to screening.
   C. Lack of access to surgical care.
   D. All of the above.

Answer: D

Patients in LMICs bear a substantial proportion of the global burden of cancer morbidity and mortality. In the year 2030, the proportion of new cancer cases from LMICs is expected to be at least 70% with nearly two-thirds of global cancer deaths in LMICs. Cancer mortality is inversely associated with the strength of a country's health system, which is reflected in patient access to screening and treatment as well as the ease with which patient can access medical care. (See Schwartz 10th ed., p. 1958.)

6. When considering surgical care in LMICs, "task shifting" is often talked about as a way to provide surgical care while additional surgeons are trained and recruited. What does this term refer to?
   A. Shifting care from rural areas to established centers.
   B. Training nonsurgeon physicians and midlevel practitioners to provide basic surgical care.
   C. Establishing a system that allows selected surgical disease to be treated medically.
   D. Shifting the tasks of surgical care from western medical staff to local staff.

Answer: B

Task shifting involves training nonsurgeon physicians, nurses, midwives, and advanced care practitioners to provide basic surgical or anesthetic care. This may be an inevitable fact of life in LMICs and the surgeon shortage is prodigious. Task shifting in this way may allow services that were only available under fully trained surgeons to be more accessible and mitigate the significant surgeon's shortage in many LMICs. Concerns about quality of care, supervision, and the impact on surgeon's professional development remain areas of debate. (See Schwartz 10th ed., pp. 1960–1962.)

7. You are planning to work abroad but a colleague mentions that "surgery is too expensive" in LMICs and you should focus on providing mosquito netting instead. You disagree, which of the following answers could help you support your case.
   A. Surgical treatment is often primary prevention for additional disease (eg, Cesarean sections help prevent obstetrical fistulae).
   B. A number of studies demonstrate that surgical care is below the $100/DALY threshold set by the World Bank for cost-effective care.
   C. District hospital level surgical service can be provide for $11-33/DALY averted.
   D. All of the above.

Answer: D

A common question raised to proponents of surgical care in LMICs is one of cost. A number of independent studies as well as work by the World Bank and WHO show that, while nothing is free, the burden of surgical disease is so huge in LMICs and the surgical need so high that even relatively cost-effective interventions can cost-effectively reduce the burden of human disease. Compared to other public health initiates, developing basic and emergency surgical care at a district hospital level is as cost-effective, or even more so, than typical health programs such as HIV-AIDS treatment or measles immunization! Surgeons truly are the front line of global public health. (See Schwartz 10th ed., pp. 1972–1974.)

Note: Page numbers followed by *t* indicate tables; those followed by *f* indicate figures.